DISEASE MANAGEMENT
SOURCEBOOK
THIRD EDITION

Health Reference Series

DISEASE MANAGEMENT
SOURCEBOOK

THIRD EDITION

Basic Consumer Health Information about Coping with Chronic and Serious Illnesses,
Navigating the Healthcare System, Communicating with Healthcare Providers,
Assessing Healthcare Quality, and Making Informed Healthcare Decisions, Including
Facts about Second Opinions, Hospitalization, Surgery, and Medications

Along with a Section about Children with Chronic Conditions, Information about
Legal, Financial, and Insurance Issues, a Glossary of Related Terms, and Directories
of Additional Resources

OMNIGRAPHICS

615 Griswold St., Ste. 520, Detroit, MI 48226

Bibliographic Note

Because this page cannot legibly accommodate all the copyright notices, the Bibliographic Note portion of the Preface constitutes an extension of the copyright notice.

* * *

OMNIGRAPHICS
Angela L. Williams, Managing Editor

* * *

ISBN 978-0-7808-1776-0
E-ISBN 978-0-7808-1777-7

Library of Congress Cataloging-in-Publication Data

Names: Williams, Angela, 1963- editor.

Title: Disease management sourcebook / edited by Angela L. Williams.

Description: Third edition. | Detroit, MI: Omnigraphics, 2020. | Series: Health reference series | Includes bibliographical references and index. | Summary: "Provides basic consumer health information about managing serious and chronic illness, navigating the healthcare system and finding and evaluating health information, patient rights and responsibilities, assistive technologies, and tips for dealing with legal, financial, and health insurance matters. Includes index, online access, glossary of related terms, and other resources."-- Provided by publisher.

Identifiers: LCCN 2019046079 (print) | LCCN 2019046080 (ebook) | ISBN 9780780817760 (library binding) | ISBN 9780780817777 (ebook)

Subjects: LCSH: Chronic diseases--Treatment. | Consumer education.

Classification: LCC RC108.D58 2020 (print) | LCC RC108 (ebook) | DDC 616/.044--dc23

LC record available at https://lccn.loc.gov/2019046079

LC ebook record available at https://lccn.loc.gov/2019046080

This book is printed on acid-free paper meeting the ANSI Z39.48 Standard. The infinity symbol that appears above indicates that the paper in this book meets that standard.

Printed in the United States

Table of Contents

Part 2. Working with Healthcare Providers and the Healthcare System

Part 5. Managing Chronic Disease

Part 6. Children and Chronic Disease

Part 7. Legal, Financial, and Insurance Issues That Impact Disease Management

Part 8. Additional Help and Information

Preface

ABOUT THIS BOOK

Making informed healthcare decisions is vital to everyone. It is particularly important to those who are living with chronic illnesses, such as cardiovascular disease, diabetes, and cancer. According to the Centers for Disease Control and Prevention (CDC), about 6 in 10 people in the United States have chronic diseases and 4 in 10 have multiple chronic diseases. Researchers estimate that only 12 percent of U.S. adults have proficient health literacy. In other words, nearly 9 out of 10 adults may lack the skills needed to manage their health and prevent disease. Low health literacy has been linked to poor health outcomes such as higher rates of hospitalization and less frequent use of preventive services. Both these outcomes are associated with higher healthcare costs.

Disease Management Sourcebook, Third Edition addresses these concerns by providing facts about navigating the healthcare system, communicating with healthcare providers, and finding and evaluating health information. It covers patient rights and responsibilities, privacy, medical errors, and healthcare fraud. It explains assistive technologies available to help people who have chronic illnesses and provides tips for dealing with legal, financial, and health-insurance matters. Facts about medications—including prescription, generic, over-the-counter, and counterfeit drugs—are included. The concluding chapter features a glossary and directories of resources for patients and their families and caregivers.

HOW TO USE THIS BOOK

This book is divided into parts and chapters. Parts focus on broad areas of interest. Chapters are devoted to single topics within a part.

Part 1: Facts about Serious and Chronic Illnesses presents an overview of disease management in the United States. It includes information about risk factors for chronic disease and symptoms that may indicate serious health conditions or medical emergencies. It describes common screening and diagnostic tests and offers tips for finding support after receiving a diagnosis.

Part 2: Working with Healthcare Providers and the Healthcare System provides information about effective communication in a doctor's office or hospital setting. Topics include making decisions in consultation with the doctor, second opinions, understanding medical specialties and alternative medicine, clinical trials, and laboratory services. Basic information is also provided about choosing a hospital and undergoing surgery, and issues related to healthcare quality are addressed.

Part 3: Health Literacy and Making Informed Health Decisions discusses the skills that are essential for making knowledgeable healthcare choices. Developments in health information technology are discussed. Insight into eHealth literacy is provided, and patients' rights and responsibilities are also discussed. Patient privacy rights, informed consent, medical errors, and healthcare fraud are also covered.

Part 4: Prescription and Over-the-Counter Medications provides information about what medications do and how to use them safely. It discusses purchasing and using prescription, generic, and over-the-counter drugs. Details on common drug interactions, adverse drug reactions, purchasing prescription drugs online, counterfeit and misused drugs, and imported drugs and safety concerns are also provided.

Part 5: Managing Chronic Disease offers guidelines for self-management practices, including tips for dealing with pain, stress, and depression. Infection prevention, assistive technology, and transitional and palliative-care options are explained. The part concludes with tips for caregivers of individuals with chronic diseases.

Part 6: Children and Chronic Disease presents authoritative information about serious illness in children for parents and caregivers. It provides information on pediatric palliative care and the pediatric intensive-care unit. It offers guidelines to help schools provide medical support for students with asthma, diabetes, and other chronic conditions, and provides information about finding camps for children with special health needs.

Part 7: Legal, Financial, and Insurance Issues That Impact Disease Management includes information about healthcare benefit laws, the Americans with Disabilities Act, and the Family and Medical Leave Act. It describes advance directives and explains how to access free or reduced-cost healthcare. It also includes information on health insurance and provides guidelines for purchasing health insurance. In addition, it discusses topics such as health savings accounts, medical discount plans, and the insurance claim process.

Part 8: Additional Help and Information includes a glossary of related terms and directories of resources for information about disease management, health insurance, and financial assistance for medical treatments.

BIBLIOGRAPHIC NOTE

This volume contains documents and excerpts from publications issued by the following U.S. government agencies: Administration for Community Living (ACL); Agency for Healthcare Research and Quality (AHRQ); Centers for Disease Control and Prevention (CDC); Centers for Medicare & Medicaid Services (CMS); *Eunice Kennedy Shriver* National Institute of Child Health and Human Development (NICHD); Federal Communications Commission (FCC); Federal Trade Commission (FTC); Genetics Home Reference (GHR); Health Resources and Services Administration (HRSA); National Cancer Institute (NCI); National Center for Complementary and Integrative Health (NCCIH); National Institute of Biomedical Imaging and Bioengineering (NIBIB); National Institute of Diabetes and Digestive and Kidney Diseases (NIDDK); National Institute of General Medical Sciences (NIGMS); National Institute of Mental Health (NIMH); National Institute of Nursing Research (NINR); National Institute on Aging (NIA); National Institutes of Health (NIH); *NIH News in Health*; Office of Disease Prevention and Health Promotion (ODPHP); Office of the National Coordinator for Health Information Technology (ONC); Substance Abuse and Mental Health Services Administration (SAMHSA); U.S. Department of Education (ED); U.S. Department of Health and Human Services (HHS); U.S. Department of Justice (DOJ); U.S. Department of Labor (DOL); U.S. Food and Drug Administration (FDA); and USA.gov.

It may also contain original material produced by Omnigraphics and reviewed by medical consultants.

ABOUT THE *HEALTH REFERENCE SERIES*

The *Health Reference Series* is designed to provide basic medical information for patients, families, caregivers, and the general public. Each volume takes a particular topic and provides comprehensive coverage. This is especially important for people who may be dealing with a newly diagnosed disease or a chronic disorder in themselves or in a family member. People looking for preventive guidance, information about disease warning signs, medical statistics, and risk factors for health problems will also find answers to their questions in the *Health Reference Series*. The *Series*, however, is not intended to serve as a tool for diagnosing illness, in prescribing treatments, or as a substitute for the physician–patient relationship. All people concerned about medical symptoms or the possibility of disease are encouraged to seek professional care from an appropriate healthcare provider.

A NOTE ABOUT SPELLING AND STYLE

Health Reference Series editors use *Stedman's Medical Dictionary* as an authority for questions related to the spelling of medical terms and *The Chicago Manual of*

Style for questions related to grammatical structures, punctuation, and other editorial concerns. Consistent adherence is not always possible, however, because the individual volumes within the *Series* include many documents from a wide variety of different producers, and the editor's primary goal is to present material from each source as accurately as is possible. This sometimes means that information in different chapters or sections may follow other guidelines and alternate spelling authorities. For example, occasionally a copyright holder may require that eponymous terms be shown in possessive forms (Crohn's disease vs. Crohn disease) or that British spelling norms be retained (leukaemia vs. leukemia).

MEDICAL REVIEW

Omnigraphics contracts with a team of qualified, senior medical professionals who serve as medical consultants for the *Health Reference Series*. As necessary, medical consultants review reprinted and originally written material for currency and accuracy. Citations including the phrase "Reviewed (month, year)" indicate material reviewed by this team. Medical consultation services are provided to the *Health Reference Series* editors by:

Dr. Vijayalakshmi, MBBS, DGO, MD
Dr. Senthil Selvan, MBBS, DCH, MD
Dr. K. Sivanandham, MBBS, DCH, MS (Research), PhD

OUR ADVISORY BOARD

We would like to thank the following board members for providing initial guidance on the development of this series:

- Dr. Lynda Baker, Associate Professor of Library and Information Science, Wayne State University, Detroit, MI
- Nancy Bulgarelli, William Beaumont Hospital Library, Royal Oak, MI
- Karen Imarisio, Bloomfield Township Public Library, Bloomfield Township, MI
- Karen Morgan, Mardigian Library, University of Michigan-Dearborn, Dearborn, MI
- Rosemary Orlando, St. Clair Shores Public Library, St. Clair Shores, MI

HEALTH REFERENCE SERIES UPDATE POLICY

The inaugural book in the *Health Reference Series* was the first edition of *Cancer Sourcebook* published in 1989. Since then, the *Series* has been enthusiastically received by librarians and in the medical community. In order to maintain the standard of providing high-quality health information for the layperson the editorial staff at Omnigraphics felt it was necessary to implement a policy of updating volumes when warranted.

Medical researchers have been making tremendous strides, and it is the purpose of the *Health Reference Series* to stay current with the most recent advances. Each decision to update a volume is made on an individual basis. Some of the considerations include how much new information is available and the feedback we receive from people who use the books. If there is a topic you would like to see added to the update list, or an area of medical concern you feel has not been adequately addressed, please write to:

Managing Editor
Health Reference Series
Omnigraphics
615 Griswold St., Ste. 520
Detroit, MI 48226

Part 1 | **Facts about Serious and Chronic Illnesses**

Chapter 1 | Chronic Diseases in the United States

Chronic diseases are defined broadly as "conditions that last one year or more and require ongoing medical attention or limit activities of daily living or both." Chronic diseases, such as heart disease, cancer, and diabetes are the leading causes of death and disability in the United States.

Many chronic diseases are caused by a shortlist of risk behaviors:

- Tobacco use and exposure to secondhand smoke
- Poor nutrition, including diets low in fruits and vegetables and high in sodium and saturated fats
- Lack of physical activity
- Excessive alcohol use

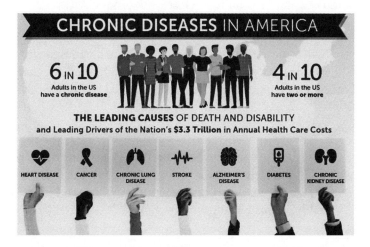

Figure 1.1. Statistics on Chronic Diseases in the United States *(Source: "Chronic Diseases in America," Centers for Disease Control and Prevention (CDC))*

This chapter includes text excerpted from "About Chronic Diseases," Centers for Disease Control and Prevention (CDC), October 23, 2019.

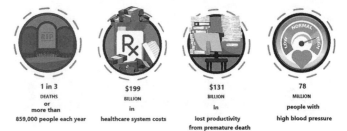

1 in 3	$199	$131	78
DEATHS	BILLION	BILLION	MILLION
or	in	in	people with
more than	healthcare system costs	lost productivity	high blood pressure
859,000 people each year		from premature death	

Figure 1.2. Statistics on Heart Disease and Stroke in the United States (*Source: "Division for Heart Disease and Stroke Prevention at a Glance," Centers for Disease Control and Prevention (CDC)*)

HEALTH AND ECONOMIC COSTS OF CHRONIC DISEASES

About 90 percent of the nation's $3.3 trillion in annual healthcare expenditures are for people with chronic and mental-health conditions.

Chronic diseases have significant health and economic costs in the United States. Preventing chronic diseases, or managing symptoms when prevention is not possible, can reduce these costs.

Heart Disease and Stroke

Nothing kills more Americans than heart disease and stroke. More than 859,000 Americans die of heart disease or stroke every year—that is one-third of all deaths. These diseases take an economic toll as well, costing the U.S. healthcare system $199 billion per year and causing $131 billion in lost work productivity.

Cancer

Each year in the United States, more than 1.6 million people are diagnosed with cancer, and almost 600,000 die from it, making cancer the second leading cause of death. The cost of cancer care continues to rise and is expected to reach almost $174 billion by 2020.

Diabetes

More than 30 million Americans have diabetes, and another 84 million adults in the United States have a condition called "prediabetes," which puts them at risk for type 2 diabetes. Diabetes can cause heart disease, kidney failure, and blindness, and costs the U.S. healthcare system and employers $237 billion every year.

Obesity

Obesity affects almost 1 in 5 children and 1 in 3 adults, putting people at risk for chronic diseases such as diabetes, heart disease, and some cancers. Over a quarter of all Americans 17 to 24 years of age are too heavy to join the military. Obesity costs the U.S. healthcare system $147 billion a year.

Chronic Diseases in the United States

Arthritis

Arthritis affects 54.4 million adults in the United States, which is about 1 in 4 adults. It is a leading cause of work disability in the United States, one of the most common chronic conditions, and a common cause of chronic pain. The total costs attributable to arthritis and related conditions were about $304 billion in 2013. Of this amount, nearly $140 billion was for medical costs and $164 billion was for indirect costs associated with lost earnings.

Alzheimer Disease

Alzheimer disease (AD), a type of dementia, is an irreversible, progressive brain disease that affects about 5.7 million Americans. It is the sixth leading cause of death among all adults and the fifth leading cause for those ages 65 or older. In 2010, the costs of treating AD were estimated to fall between $159 billion to $215 billion. By 2040, these costs are projected to jump to between $379 billion to $500 billion annually.

Epilepsy

In the United States, about 3 million adults and 470,000 children and teens younger than 18 have active epilepsy—meaning that they have been diagnosed by a doctor, had a recent seizure, or both. Adults with epilepsy report worse mental health, more cognitive impairment, and barriers in social participation compared to adults without epilepsy. Average direct healthcare costs for a person with epilepsy range from $10,200 to $47,900 per year.

Tooth Decay

Cavities (also called "tooth decay") are one of the most common chronic diseases in the United States. One in 5 children aged 6 to 11 years and 1 in 4 adults have untreated cavities. Untreated cavities can cause pain and infections that may lead to problems eating, speaking, and learning. On average, over 34 million school hours are lost and over $45 billion is lost in productivity each year due to unplanned (emergency) dental care.

Chapter 2 | Family History Is Important to Your Health

Chapter Contents

Section 2.1 | **What Is Family Health History?**

This section includes text excerpted from "Family Health History: The Basics," Centers for Disease Control and Prevention (CDC), October 3, 2019.

A family health history is a record of the diseases and health conditions in your family. You and your family members share genes.* You may also have behaviors in common, such as exercise habits and what you like to eat. You may live in the same area and come into contact with similar things in the environment. Family history includes all of these factors, any of which can affect your health.

A gene is a part of deoxyribonucleic acid (DNA) that carries the information needed to make a protein. People inherit one copy of each gene from their mother and one copy from their father. The genes that a person inherits from her or his parents can determine many things. For example, genes affect what a person will look like and whether the person might have certain diseases.

HOW CAN YOU COLLECT YOUR FAMILY HEALTH HISTORY?

You may know a lot about your family health history or only a little. To get the complete picture, use family gatherings as a time to talk about health history. If possible, look at death certificates and family medical records. Collect information about your parents, sisters, brothers, half-sisters, half-brothers, children,

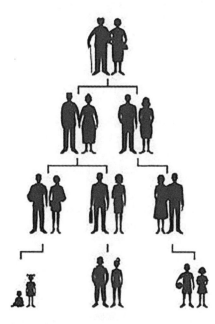

Figure 2.1. Family Tree

9

grandparents, aunts, uncles, nieces, and nephews. Include information on major medical conditions, causes of death, age at disease diagnosis, age at death, and ethnic background. Be sure to update the information regularly and share what you have learned with your family and doctor. You can use the Surgeon General's web-based tool "My Family Health Portrait" (phgkb.cdc.gov/FHH/html/index. html) to keep track of the information.

WHY IS FAMILY HEALTH HISTORY IMPORTANT FOR YOUR HEALTH?

Most people have a family health history of at least one chronic disease, such as cancer, heart disease, or diabetes. If you have a close family member with a chronic disease, you may be more likely to develop that disease yourself, especially if more than one close relative has (or had) the disease or a family member got the disease at a younger age than usual.

Collect your family health history information before visiting the doctor, and take it with you. Even if you do not know all of your family health history information, share what you do know. Family health history information, even if incomplete, can help your doctor decide which screening tests you need and when those tests should start.

HOW CAN YOU USE YOUR FAMILY HEALTH HISTORY TO IMPROVE YOUR HEALTH?

You cannot change your genes, but you can change unhealthy behaviors, such as smoking, not exercising or being active, and poor eating habits. If you have a family health history of disease, you may have the most to gain from lifestyle changes and screening tests. In many cases, healthy living habits can reduce your risk for diseases that run in your family. Screening tests, such as blood sugar testing, mammograms, and colorectal cancer screening, help find early signs of disease. Finding disease early can often mean better health in the long run.

Knowing Is Not Enough—Act on Your Family Health History!

- **Has your mother or sister had breast cancer?** Talk with your doctor about whether having a mammogram earlier is right for you.
- **Does your mom, dad, sister, or brother have diabetes?** Ask your doctor how early you should be screened for diabetes.
- **Did your mom, dad, brother, or sister get colorectal (colon) cancer before age 50?** Talk with your doctor about whether you should start getting colonoscopies earlier or have them done more often.

Section 2.2 | **Family Health History and Chronic Disease**

This section includes text excerpted from "Family Health History and Chronic Disease," Centers for Disease Control and Prevention (CDC), October 3, 2019.

If you have a family health history of a chronic disease such as cancer, heart disease, diabetes, or osteoporosis, you are more likely to get that disease yourself. Share your family health history with your doctor, who can help you take steps to prevent disease and catch it early if it develops.

BREAST AND OVARIAN CANCER AND FAMILY HEALTH HISTORY

If you are a woman with a family health history of breast cancer or ovarian cancer, you may be more likely to get these cancers yourself. Collecting your family health history of breast, ovarian, and other cancers and sharing this information with your doctor can help you find out if you are at higher risk. If you have had breast, ovarian, or other cancers, make sure that your family members know about your diagnosis.

Your doctor might consider your family health history in deciding when you should start mammography screening for breast cancer. If you are a woman with a parent, sibling, or child with breast cancer, you are at higher risk for breast cancer. Based on current recommendations, you should consider talking to your doctor about starting mammography screening in your forties. In some cases, your doctor might recommend genetic counseling, and a genetic counselor might recommend genetic testing based on your family health history. Breast, ovarian, and other cancers are sometimes caused by inherited mutations in *BRCA1, BRCA2,* and other genes. A genetic counselor can help determine which genetic mutations you should be tested for based on your personal and family health history of cancer, ancestry, and other factors.

When collecting your family health history:
- Include your parents, sisters, brothers, children, grandparents, aunts, uncles, nieces, and nephews
- List any cancers that each relative had and at what age she or he was diagnosed. For relatives who have died, list age and cause of death.
- Remember that breast and ovarian cancer risk does not just come from your mother's side of the family—your father's relatives with breast, ovarian, and other cancers matter, too!
- Update your family health history on a regular basis and let your doctor know about any new cases of breast, ovarian, or other cancers.
- If you are concerned about your personal or family health history of breast, ovarian, or other cancer, talk with your doctor. Whether or not you have a family health history of breast or ovarian cancer, you can take steps to help lower your risk of breast cancer and ovarian cancer.

DIABETES AND FAMILY HEALTH HISTORY

If you have a mother, father, sister, or brother with diabetes, you are more likely to get diabetes yourself. You are also more likely to have prediabetes. Talk to your doctor about your family health history of diabetes. Your doctor can help you take steps to prevent or delay diabetes, and reverse prediabetes if you have it.

Over 30 million people have diabetes. People with diabetes have levels of blood sugar that are too high. The different types of diabetes include type 1 diabetes, type 2 diabetes, and gestational diabetes. Diabetes can cause serious health problems, including heart disease, kidney problems, stroke, blindness, and the need for lower-leg amputations.

Even if you have a family health history of diabetes, you can prevent or delay type 2 diabetes by eating healthier, being physically active, and maintaining or reaching a healthy weight. This is especially important if you have prediabetes, and taking these steps can reverse prediabetes.

HEART DISEASE AND FAMILY HEALTH HISTORY

If you have a family health history of heart disease, collect information about your relatives with heart disease, including the age at which they were diagnosed. This is especially important if you have a parent, brother, or sister with heart disease. Share this information with your doctor so you can work together on steps to lower your chances of getting heart disease.

These steps can include:

- Eating a healthy diet
- Being physically active
- Maintaining a healthy weight
- Not smoking
- Limiting your alcohol use
- Checking your cholesterol
- Controlling your blood pressure
- Managing your diabetes, if you have it
- Having doctor-recommended screening tests done
- Taking medication if needed to treat high cholesterol, high blood pressure, or diabetes

HEREDITARY HEMOCHROMATOSIS

Hereditary hemochromatosis is a disorder in which the body can build up too much iron in the skin, heart, liver, pancreas, pituitary gland, and joints. It is a genetic disorder that can cause severe liver disease and other health problems. Early diagnosis and treatment are critical to prevent complications from the disorder. If you have a family health history of hemochromatosis, talk to your doctor about testing for hereditary hemochromatosis.

Family History Is Important to Your Health

Hereditary hemochromatosis is most commonly caused by certain variants in the *HFE* gene. If you inherit two of these variants, one from each parent, you have hereditary hemochromatosis and are at risk for developing high iron levels. If you have a family member, especially a sibling, who is known to have hereditary hemochromatosis, talk to your doctor about genetic testing for hereditary hemochromatosis.

OSTEOPOROSIS AND FAMILY HEALTH HISTORY

If one of your parents has had a broken bone, especially a broken hip, you may need to be screened earlier for osteoporosis. This is a medical condition in which bones become weak and are more likely to break. Share your family health history with your doctor. Your doctor can help you take steps to strengthen weak bones and prevent broken bones.

As of now, screening for osteoporosis is recommended for women who are 65 years old or older and for women who are 50 to 64 and have certain risk factors, including having a parent who has broken a hip. This screening uses several factors to determine how likely you are to have osteoporosis. Talk to your doctor if you have concerns about osteoporosis.

Chapter 3 | Risk Factors for Preventable Chronic Diseases

There are four main risk factors for preventable chronic diseases, including:
- Excessive alcohol use
- Poor nutrition
- Lack of physical activity
- Tobacco use

EXCESSIVE ALCOHOL USE

Excessive alcohol use is responsible for about 88,000 deaths a year in the United States, including 1 in 10 total deaths among working-age adults who are 20 to 64 years of age. In 2010, excessive alcohol use cost the U.S. economy $249 billion, or $2.05 a drink. About 40 percent of these costs were paid by federal, state, and local governments.

Excessive alcohol use includes binge drinking, heavy drinking, and any alcohol use by pregnant women or anyone younger than 21. Binge drinking is defined as "consuming 4 or more drinks on an occasion for a woman" or "5 or more drinks on an occasion for a man." Heavy drinking is defined as "consuming 8 or more drinks per week for a woman" or "15 or more drinks per week for a man."

Binge drinking is responsible for over half the deaths and three-quarters of the costs due to excessive alcohol use. The Centers for Disease Control and Prevention (CDC) estimates that 37 million U.S. adults—or 1 in 6—binge drink about once a week, consuming an average of 7 drinks per binge. As a result, U.S. adults consume about 17 billion binge drinks annually, or about 470 binge drinks per binge drinker. Further, 9 in 10 adults who binge drink do not have an alcohol-use disorder (AUD).

This chapter includes text excerpted from "About Chronic Diseases," Centers for Disease Control and Prevention (CDC), October 23, 2019.

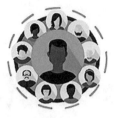
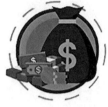

1 in 10 total deaths
among
working-age adults

$249 Billion
in
economic costs each year

Figure 3.1. How Excessive Alcohol Use Impacts the United States

The Health Effects of Excessive Alcohol Use
Chronic Health Effects

Over time, excessive alcohol use can lead to the development of chronic diseases and other serious problems, including AUD and problems with learning, memory, and mental health. Chronic health conditions that have been linked to excessive alcohol use include the following:

- **High blood pressure, heart disease, and stroke.** Binge drinking and heavy drinking can cause heart disease, including cardiomyopathy (disease of the heart muscle), as well as irregular heartbeat, high blood pressure, and stroke.
- **Liver disease.** Excessive alcohol use takes a toll on the liver and can lead to fatty liver disease (steatosis), hepatitis, fibrosis, and cirrhosis.
- **Cancer.** Excessive alcohol use can contribute to cancers of the mouth and throat, larynx (voice box), esophagus, colon and rectum, liver, and breast (in women). The less alcohol a person drinks, the lower the risk of cancer.

Immediate Health Effects

Excessive alcohol use has immediate effects that increase the risk of many harmful health conditions, including the following:

- **Injuries, violence, and poisonings.** Drinking too much alcohol increases the risk of injuries, including motor vehicle crashes, falls, drowning, and burns. It also increases the risk of violence, including homicide, suicide, sexual assault, and intimate partner violence (IPV). Alcohol also contributes to poisonings and overdoses from opioids and other substances.
- **Unintended pregnancy and sexually transmitted infections (STIs).** People who binge drink are more likely to have unprotected sex and

multiple sex partners. These activities increase the risk of unintended pregnancy and STI, including human immunodeficiency virus (HIV).

- **Poor pregnancy outcomes.** There is no known safe amount of alcohol use during pregnancy. Alcohol use during pregnancy can cause fetal alcohol spectrum disorders (FASDs) in infants. It may also increase the risk of miscarriage, premature birth, stillbirth, and sudden infant death syndrome (SIDS).

POOR NUTRITION

Good nutrition is essential for keeping Americans healthy across their lifespan. A healthy diet helps children grow and develop properly and reduces their risk of chronic diseases, including obesity. Adults who eat a healthy diet live longer and have a lower risk of obesity, heart disease, type 2 diabetes, and certain cancers. Healthy eating can help people with chronic diseases manage these conditions and prevent complications.

Most Americans, however, do not eat a healthy diet. Although breastfeeding is the ideal source of nutrition for infants, only 1 in 4 is exclusively breastfed through 6 months of age as recommended. Fewer than 1 in 10 adults and adolescents eat enough fruits and vegetables, and 9 in 10 Americans ages 2 years or older consume more than the recommended amount of sodium.

In addition, 6 in 10 young people ages 2 to 19 years and 5 in 10 adults consume a sugary drink daily. Processed foods and sugary drinks add unneeded sodium, saturated fats, and sugar to diets, increasing the risk of chronic diseases.

The Harmful Effects of Poor Nutrition
Overweight and Obesity

Eating a healthy diet, along with getting enough physical activity and sleep, can help children grow up healthy and prevent overweight and obesity. In the United States, 19 percent of young people ages 2 to 19 years and 40 percent of adults have obesity, which can put them at risk for heart disease, type 2 diabetes, and some cancers. In addition, obesity costs the U.S. healthcare system $147 billion a year.

Heart Disease and Stroke

Two of the leading causes of heart disease and stroke are high blood pressure and high blood cholesterol. Getting too much sodium can lead to high blood pressure. *Dietary Guidelines for Americans 2015–2020* recommends getting less than 2,300 mg a day, but Americans consume more than 3,400 mg a day on average. Over 70 percent of the sodium that Americans eat comes from packaged, processed, store-bought, and restaurant foods. Eating foods low in saturated fats and high in fiber, along with regular physical activity, can help prevent high blood cholesterol.

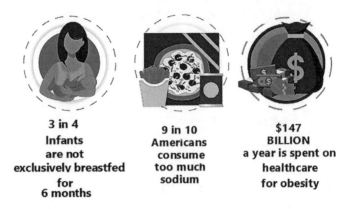

3 in 4
Infants
are not
exclusively breastfed
for
6 months

9 in 10
Americans
consume
too much
sodium

$147
BILLION
a year is spent on
healthcare
for obesity

Figure 3.2. How Poor Nutrition Impacts the United States

Type 2 Diabetes

People who are overweight or have obesity are at increased risk of type 2 diabetes compared to those at a normal weight because, over time, their bodies become less able to use the insulin they make. More than 84 million U.S. adults—or 1 in 3 people—have prediabetes, and 90 percent of them do not know they have it. In the last 20 years, the number of adults diagnosed with diabetes has more than doubled as the U.S. population has aged and become heavier.

Cancer

An unhealthy diet can increase the risk of some cancers. Overweight and obesity are associated with at least 13 types of cancer, including endometrial (uterine) cancer, breast cancer in postmenopausal women, and colorectal cancer. These cancers make up 40 percent of all cancers diagnosed.

Deficits in Brain Function

The brain develops most quickly from the start of pregnancy to a child's second birthday. Having low levels of iron during pregnancy and early childhood is associated with mental and behavioral delays in children. Ensuring that iodine levels are high enough during pregnancy also helps a growing fetus have the best brain development possible.

LACK OF PHYSICAL ACTIVITY

Many Americans live in communities that are not designed for physical activity. Only 1 in 4 U.S. adults and 1 in 5 high-school students get the recommended levels of physical activity. Not getting enough physical activity comes with high health and financial costs. It can contribute to heart disease, type 2 diabetes, several cancers, and obesity. In addition, low levels of physical activity are associated with $117 billion in healthcare costs every year.

Risk Factors for Preventable Chronic Diseases

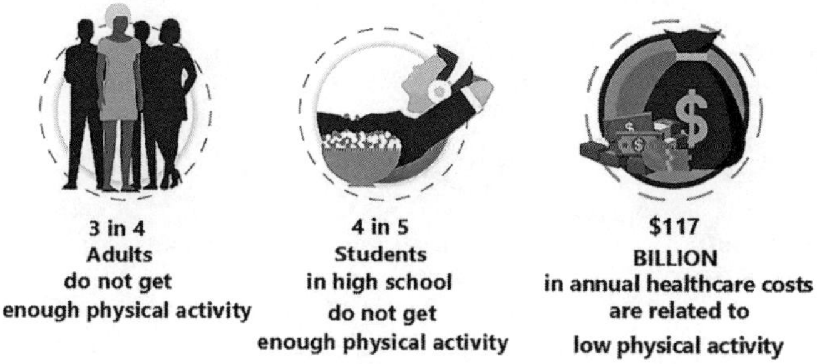

3 in 4
Adults
do not get
enough physical activity

4 in 5
Students
in high school
do not get
enough physical activity

$117
BILLION
in annual healthcare costs
are related to
low physical activity

Figure 3.3. Facts about Physical Activity

People of all ages and conditions can benefit from more physical activity, including aerobic and muscle-strengthening exercises, according to the new *Physical Activity Guidelines for Americans*, Second Edition. Physical activity contributes to normal growth and development, reduces the risk of several chronic diseases, and helps people function better throughout the day and sleep better at night. Even short bouts of physical activity can improve health and wellness.

The Harmful Effects of Not Getting Enough Physical Activity
Heart Disease
Not getting enough physical activity can lead to heart disease—even for people who have no other risk factors. It can also increase the likelihood of developing other heart disease risk factors, including obesity, high blood pressure, high blood cholesterol, and type 2 diabetes.

Type 2 Diabetes
Not getting enough physical activity can raise a person's risk of developing type 2 diabetes. Physical activity helps control blood sugar (glucose), weight, and blood pressure and helps raise "good" cholesterol and lower "bad" cholesterol. Adequate physical activity can also help reduce the risk of heart disease and nerve damage, which are often problems for people with diabetes.

Cancer
Getting the recommended amount of physical activity can lower the risk of many cancers, including cancers of the bladder, breast, colon, uterus, esophagus, kidney, lung, and stomach. These effects apply regardless of weight status.

The Health Benefits of Physical Activity
The *Physical Activity Guidelines for Americans*, Second Edition presents findings on the benefits of regular physical activity, which include:
- Improved sleep
- Increased ability to perform everyday activities

| 480,000 People die each year because of cigarette smoking | 58 MILLION nonsmokers are exposed to secondhand smoke | $170 BILLION is spent each year to treat smoking-related diseases |

Figure 3.4. Impact of Smoking

- Improved cognitive ability and a reduced risk of dementia
- Improved bone and musculoskeletal health

In addition, getting enough physical activity, along with eating a healthy diet, is the best way to maintain a healthy weight. People who want to lose weight may need to get more physical activity and reduce calorie intake.

TOBACCO USE

Tobacco use is the leading cause of preventable disease, disability, and death in the United States. As of 2017, about 34 million U.S. adults smoke cigarettes. Every day, about 2,000 young people under 18 smoke their first cigarette, and more than 300 become daily cigarette smokers. Cigarette smoking causes more than 480,000 deaths annually, including 41,000 deaths from secondhand smoke. For every American who dies because of smoking, at least 30 are living with a serious smoking-related illness.

Smoking-related illness costs society over $300 billion each year, including $170 billion in direct medical costs. These costs could be reduced if young people do not smoke and smokers are helped to quit.

The Harmful Effects of Tobacco Use

Cigarette smoking leads to disease and disability and harms nearly every organ of the body. Smoking causes cancer, heart disease, stroke, lung diseases, type 2 diabetes, and other chronic health conditions. The impact also extends beyond the smoker. For example, smoking during pregnancy increases the risk of premature birth (being born too early) and SIDS.

Secondhand smoke, which affects 58 million nonsmoking Americans, also causes stroke, lung cancer, and coronary heart disease (CHD) in adults. Children who are exposed to secondhand smoke are at increased risk of SIDS, impaired lung function, acute respiratory infections (ARIs), middle-ear disease, and more frequent and severe asthma attacks.

Risk Factors for Preventable Chronic Diseases

Cancer

Cigarette smoking causes several forms of cancer, including about 90 percent of lung cancer deaths. Nonsmokers who are exposed to secondhand smoke at home or work have a 20 percent to 30 percent higher risk of getting lung cancer. Smoking also causes cancers of the voice box (larynx), mouth and throat, esophagus, bladder, kidney, liver, pancreas, cervix, colon, rectum, and stomach, as well as a type of blood cancer called "acute myeloid leukemia" (AML). In addition, smoking can interfere with cancer treatment, increasing the risk of recurrence, more serious complications, and death.

Heart Disease and Stroke

Cigarette smoking is a major cause of heart disease and stroke and causes 1 in every 4 deaths from heart disease and stroke. Nonsmokers who breathe secondhand smoke at home or work have a 25 percent to 30 percent higher risk of heart disease and a 20 percent to 30 percent higher risk of stroke. Smoking can damage the body by:

- Raising triglycerides (a type of fat in the blood) and lowering high-density lipoprotein (HDL) or "good" cholesterol
- Making blood sticky and more likely to clot, which can block blood flow to the heart and brain
- Damaging cells that line blood vessels, increasing the buildup of plaque (fat, cholesterol, calcium, and other substances) in blood vessels, and causing blood vessels to thicken and narrow

Lung Disease

Cigarette smoking can cause lung disease by damaging the airways and the small air sacs (alveoli) found in the lungs. It can cause chronic obstructive pulmonary disease (COPD), which includes emphysema and chronic bronchitis. Smoking accounts for as many as 8 in 10 COPD-related deaths. If you have asthma, tobacco smoke can trigger an asthma attack or make an attack worse.

Diabetes

The risk of developing type 2 diabetes is 30 percent to 40 percent higher for current smokers than nonsmokers. The more cigarettes a person smokes, the higher their risk of type 2 diabetes. People with diabetes who smoke are more likely than nonsmokers to have trouble controlling their blood sugar and to have serious complications, including:

- Heart disease and kidney disease
- Poor blood flow in the legs and feet that can lead to infections, ulcers, and amputation (surgery to remove a body part, such as toes or feet)
- Retinopathy (an eye disease that can cause blindness)
- Peripheral neuropathy (nerve damage in the arms and legs that causes numbness, pain, weakness, and poor coordination)

Chapter 4 | How You Can Prevent Chronic Diseases

Many chronic diseases are caused by key risky behaviors. By making healthy choices, you can reduce your likelihood of getting a chronic disease and improve your quality of life.

QUIT SMOKING

Stopping smoking (or never starting) lowers your risk of serious health problems, such as heart disease, cancer, type 2 diabetes, and lung disease, as well as premature death—even for longtime smokers. Take the first step and call 800-784-8669 for FREE support.

EAT HEALTHY

Eating healthy helps prevent, delay, and manage heart disease, type 2 diabetes, and other chronic diseases. A balanced diet of fruits, veggies, whole grains, lean meats, and low-fat dairy products is important at any age. If you are overweight, losing even five to seven percent of your body weight can help prevent or delay type 2 diabetes.

GET REGULAR PHYSICAL ACTIVITY

Regular physical activity can help you prevent, delay, or manage chronic diseases. Aim for moderate physical activity (such as brisk walking or gardening) for at least 150 minutes a week.

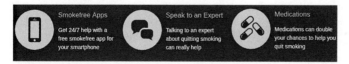

Figure 4.1. Tools for Smokers Who Want to Quit *(Source: "Quit Now," BeTobaccoFree.gov, U.S. Department of Health and Human Services (HHS))*

This chapter includes text excerpted from "How You Can Prevent Chronic Diseases," Centers for Disease Control and Prevention (CDC), July 30, 2019.

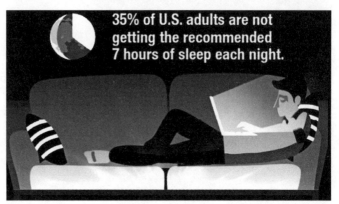

35% of U.S. adults are not getting the recommended 7 hours of sleep each night.

Figure 4.2. Statistics on Sleep Deprivation among the U.S. Adults *(Source: "Did You Get Enough Sleep Last Night?" Centers for Disease Control and Prevention (CDC))*

AVOID DRINKING TOO MUCH ALCOHOL

Over time, excessive drinking can lead to high blood pressure, various cancers, heart disease, stroke, and liver disease. By not drinking too much, you can reduce these health risks.

GET SCREENED

To prevent chronic diseases or catch them early, visit your doctor regularly for preventive services.

GET ENOUGH SLEEP

Insufficient sleep has been linked to the development and poor management of diabetes, heart disease, obesity, and depression. Adults should get at least seven hours of sleep daily.

KNOW YOUR FAMILY HISTORY

If you have a family history of a chronic disease, such as cancer, heart disease, diabetes, or osteoporosis, you may be more likely to develop that disease yourself. Share your family health history with your doctor, who can help you take steps to prevent these conditions or catch them early.

MAKE HEALTHY CHOICES IN SCHOOL, AT WORK, AND IN THE COMMUNITY

By making healthy behaviors part of your daily life, you can prevent conditions such as high blood pressure or obesity, which raises your risk of developing the most common and serious chronic diseases.

Chapter 5 | **Choosing Your Doctor**

Finding a main doctor (often called your "primary doctor" or "primary-care doctor") with whom you feel comfortable talking is the first step in good medical communication. It is also a way to ensure your good health. This doctor gets to know you and what your health is usually like. She or he can help you make medical decisions that suit your values and daily habits and can keep in touch with other medical specialists and healthcare providers you may need.

If you do not have a primary doctor or are not at ease with the one you currently see, now may be the time to find a new doctor. Whether you have just moved to a new city, changed insurance providers, or had a bad experience with your doctor or medical staff, it is worthwhile to spend time finding a doctor you can trust.

People sometimes hesitate to change doctors because they worry about hurting their doctor's feelings. But doctors understand that different people have different needs. They know it is important for everyone to have a doctor with whom they are comfortable.

Primary-care physicians frequently are family practitioners, internists, or geriatricians. Here are some suggestions that can help you find a doctor who meets your needs.

DECIDE WHAT YOU ARE LOOKING FOR IN A DOCTOR

A good first step is to make a list of qualities that matter to you. Do you care if your doctor is a woman or a man? Is it important that your doctor has evening office hours, is associated with a specific hospital or medical center, or speaks your language? Do you prefer a doctor who has an individual practice or one who is part of a group so that you can see one of your doctor's partners if your doctor is not available? After you have made your list, go back over it and decide which qualities are most important and which are nice, but not essential.

This chapter includes text excerpted from "How to Choose a Doctor You Can Talk To," National Institute on Aging (NIA), National Institutes of Health (NIH), May 17, 2017.

IDENTIFY SEVERAL POSSIBLE DOCTORS

Once you have a general sense of what you are looking for, ask friends and relatives, medical specialists, and other health professionals for the names of doctors with whom they have had good experiences. Rather than just getting a name, ask about the person's experiences. For example, say: "What do you like about Dr. Smith?" and "Does this doctor take time to answer questions?" A doctor whose name comes up often may be a strong possibility.

If you belong to a managed-care plan—a health-maintenance organization (HMO) or preferred provider organization (PPO)—you may be required to choose a doctor in the plan or else you may have to pay extra to see a doctor outside the network. Most managed-care plans will provide information on their doctors' backgrounds and credentials. Some plans have websites with lists of participating doctors from which you can choose.

It may be helpful to develop a list of a few names you can choose from. As you find out more about the doctors on this list, you may rule out some of them. In some cases, a doctor may not be accepting new patients and you may have to make another choice.

What Are Health-Maintenance and Preferred-Provider Organizations?

Members of a health-maintenance organization pay a set monthly fee no matter how many (or few) times they see a doctor. Usually, there are no deductibles or claims forms, but you will have a copayment for doctor visits and prescriptions. Each member chooses a primary-care doctor from within the HMO network. The primary-care doctor coordinates all care and, if necessary, refers members to specialists.

A preferred-provider organization is a network of doctors and other health-care providers. The doctors in this network agree to provide medical services to health-plan members of the preferred-provider organization at discounted costs. Members can choose to see any doctor at any time, but choosing to see an out-of-network doctor will cost more than seeing a member of the preferred-provider organization network.

CONSULT REFERENCE SOURCES

The American Medical Association's (AMA) Doctor Finder website (doctorfinder.ama-assn.org/doctorfinder/html/patient.jsp) and the American Board of Medical Specialties' (ABMS) Certification Matters™ database (www.abms. org/verify-certification/certification-matters-service-for-patients-and-families/) can help you find doctors in your area. These websites do not recommend individual doctors, but they do provide a list of doctors you may want to consider. MedlinePlus, a website from the U.S. National Library of Medicine (NLM) at the National Institutes of Health (NIH), has a comprehensive list of directories, which may also be helpful. For a list of doctors who participate in Medicare, visit www.medicare.gov/physiciancompare.

Do not forget to call your local or state medical society to check if complaints have been filed against any of the doctors you are considering.

What Does "Board Certified" Mean?

Doctors who are board certified received extra training after regular medical school. They also passed an exam certifying their expertise in specialty areas. Examples of specialty areas are general internal medicine, family medicine, geriatrics, gynecology, and orthopedics. The ABMS has a database of all board-certified physicians that is updated daily. You can also call toll-free to verify a doctor's certification at 866-275-2267. Board certification is one way to learn about a doctor's medical expertise, but it does not tell you about the doctor's communication skills.

LEARN ABOUT THE DOCTORS YOU ARE CONSIDERING

Once you have narrowed your list to two or three doctors, call their offices. The office staff is a good source of information about the doctor's education and qualifications, office policies, and payment procedures. Pay attention to the office staff—you will have to communicate with them often!

You may want to set up an appointment to meet and talk with a doctor you are considering. She or he is likely to charge you for such a visit. After the appointment, ask yourself if this doctor is a person with whom you can work well. If you are not satisfied, schedule a visit with one of your other candidates.

When learning about a doctor, consider asking questions such as:
- Do you have many older patients?
- How do you feel about involving my family in care decisions?
- Can I call or e-mail you or your staff when I have questions? Do you charge for the telephone or e-mail time?
- What are your thoughts about complementary or alternative treatments?

MAKE A CHOICE

When making a decision about which doctor to choose, you might want to ask yourself questions such as:
- Did the doctor give me a chance to ask questions?
- Was the doctor really listening to me?
- Could I understand what the doctor was saying? Was I comfortable asking her or him to say it again?

Once you have chosen a doctor, make your first actual care appointment. This visit may include a medical history and a physical exam. Be sure to bring your medical records, or have them sent from your former doctor. Bring a list of your current medicines or put the medicines in a bag and take them with you. If you have not already met the doctor, ask for extra time during this visit to ask any questions you have about the doctor or the practice.

Chapter 6 | Is It a Medical Emergency?

Patients with chronic medical conditions often become so accustomed to managing their own treatment, from pills and injections to pain control, that they often wait too long to call their doctor when their condition worsens. As a result, studies show that the majority of frequent visitors to emergency rooms (ERs) are patients with chronic illnesses. And since emergency care can cost two-to-three times as much as an office visit, clearly it is better to make an appointment with the regular doctor than wait until an ER trip becomes necessary. But how can a patient and her or his family tell when the situation worsens to the point at which there is no alternative?

WHEN TO GO TO THE EMERGENCY ROOM

In some instances, such as with injuries that result in copious bleeding, it is obvious when emergency treatment is necessary. But when people deal with the symptoms of chronic illnesses on a daily basis, it can be more difficult to determine the point at which home care is no longer an option. The best way for the patient and caregivers to gain this knowledge is to have a conversation with the doctor and ask for a detailed description of the types of signs associated with the particular condition that could indicate an emergency. By becoming intimately familiar with the day-to-day symptoms and management of the condition, patients and their families will be better prepared to determine steps to take if the illness worsens.

In general, some signs that a visit to an ER or call to 911 may be necessary include:

- Stopped breathing, or extreme difficulty breathing
- Loss of consciousness
- Uncontrollable bleeding
- Pain that is significantly beyond that normally experienced as a result of the condition

"Is It a Medical Emergency?" © 2017 Omnigraphics. Reviewed December 2019.

- Severe pain in the chest or jaw
- Changes in vision
- High fever, especially with a stiff neck
- Sudden headache
- Seizures
- Uncontrollable vomiting
- Changes in mental state, such as confusion
- Sudden paralysis, weakness, or dizziness
- Unusual abdominal pain
- Severe allergic reaction, such as in response to a new medication
- Coughing or vomiting blood
- The patient's sense that something about the condition has changed

Note that when the patient is a child who is too young to describe symptoms or changes in a medical condition, it falls to the parent or guardian to be vigilant for signs that might constitute an emergency. All of the above indicators are applicable to infants and toddlers as well, but other signs can include:

- Turning blue
- Continuing loose stools
- Hard to wake up
- Fast heartbeat for an extended period of time
- Dry mouth
- Dry diapers for more than 18 hours
- A body part that is cold or pale

WHAT TO DO IN AN EMERGENCY SITUATION

The advice given most often about emergencies is to remain calm. And as trite as that might sound, a panic-stricken relative or caregiver will not be able to respond appropriately or describe the situation to a first responder or medical professional in such a way as to ensure the fastest and best treatment for the patient. And if the patient is alone when the emergency occurs, her or his physical response to panic (rapid heartbeat, increased breathing rate, sweating, or dizziness) can exacerbate the condition itself. In addition to maintaining composure, other steps to be taken include the following:

- **Call 911 if necessary.** Certain situations leave no room for doubt that an immediate trained response is required. For example, if the patient has stopped breathing, is bleeding profusely, or has lost consciousness, she or he needs qualified emergency medical technicians (EMTs) and an ambulance.
- **Assess the need for first aid.** In extreme, life-threatening cases, such as when breathing has stopped or there is no pulse, cardiopulmonary

resuscitation (CPR) or other first aid needs to be administered immediately. Caregivers for patients with some chronic conditions should undergo training in order to learn proper first-aid techniques.

- **Resist the urge to transport the patient.** Although it may seem faster than waiting for an ambulance, transporting a patient in extreme distress, such as lost consciousness or stopped breathing, can delay treatment and make matters worse. It is better to call 911 and follow the operator's instructions.

- **Prepare for the ER visit.** If it is determined that the patient may be transported safely, advanced preparation can save time at the hospital. Bring a list of the patient's medications, allergies, and immunizations, as well as the name and contact information of her or his regular doctor.

- **If unsure what to do, call a professional.** If the situation is not immediately life-threatening, and you are not sure if an ER visit is necessary, call the patient's doctor or another medical professional familiar with her or his condition. In addition, many health systems and insurance companies offer 24-hour consultation lines, which can help make an assessment.

URGENT-CARE FACILITIES

Urgent-care facilities are available for patients whose doctors are unavailable or when illness occurs outside of the physician's normal office hours, and they can serve as a viable alternative to the emergency room in certain cases. Although many of their services are designed to treat such medical situations as flu, sprains and fractures, fever, and minor lacerations, they are well-equipped to handle many of the problems associated with chronic illnesses. For example, if the condition results in dehydration, an urgent-care center can provide IV fluids while monitoring the patient's vital signs, or if pain intensifies beyond the control of the patient's normal medication, the clinic can respond with appropriate treatment.

BEING PREPARED

Obviously, it is not possible to prevent all medical emergencies, especially in the case of patients with chronic conditions. But advanced preparation can lessen the severity and allay some anxiety if an emergency does occur. Some ways to prepare for an emergency include:

- Keep contact information handy for doctors, hospitals, urgent-care clinics, professional caregivers, and emergency advice lines.
- Have a list of medications (including dosages), allergies, and immunizations ready in advance.

- Ask the doctor for a written medical history for the patient and keep it ready for EMTs or emergency-room personnel.
- Keep an appropriately equipped first-aid kit on hand.
- Be sure the patient is seeing her or his doctor for regularly scheduled appointments and is following the doctor's instructions carefully.
- Learn first-aid basics, including CPR.

Depending on the particular condition, there may be other, more specific ways to prepare for a crisis situation. The best thing to do is to discuss this with the physician supervising the case and ask about additional steps you can take to be prepared.

References

1. Kaneshiro, Neil K., MD, MHA. "When to Use the Emergency Room—Child," MedlinePlus, National Institutes of Health (NIH), November 20, 2014.
2. Martin, Laura J., MD, MPH, ABIM. "When to Use the Emergency Room—Adult," MedlinePlus, National Institutes of Health (NIH), October 27, 2014.
3. "Medical Emergency," Tufts University Office of Emergency Management, n.d.
4. English, Taunya. "Chronic Conditions: When Do You Call the Doctor?" Center for Advancing Health (CFAH), n.d.
5. "What to Do in an Emergency," American College of Emergency Physicians (ACEP), n.d.
6. "When Should I Go to the Emergency Department?" Progressive Emergency Physicians, n.d.

Chapter 7 | Common Screening and Diagnostic Tests

Chapter Contents

Section 7.1 | Screening Tests: What You Need to Know

This section contains text excerpted from the following sources: Text under the heading "What Are the Screening Tests?" is excerpted from "Health Screening," MedlinePlus, National Institutes of Health (NIH), January 3, 2017; Text under the heading "Benefits and Harms of Screening Tests" is excerpted from "To Screen or Not to Screen?" *NIH News in Health*, National Institutes of Health (NIH), March 2017.

WHAT ARE SCREENING TESTS?

Screenings are tests that look for diseases before you have symptoms. Screening tests can find diseases early, when they are easier to treat. You can get some screenings in your doctor's office. Others need special equipment, so you may need to go to a different office or clinic.

Some conditions that doctors commonly screen for include:
- Breast cancer and cervical cancer in women
- Cancers
- Colorectal cancer
- Depression
- Diabetes
- Heart disease
- High blood pressure
- High cholesterol
- Obesity
- Osteoporosis
- Overweight and obesity
- Pregnancy issues
- Prostate cancer in men
- Sexually transmitted infections (STIs)

Which tests you need depends on your age, sex, family history, and whether you have risk factors for certain diseases. After a screening test, ask when you will get the results and whom to talk to about them.

BENEFITS AND HARMS OF SCREENING TESTS

Catching chronic health conditions early—even before you have symptoms—seems like a great idea. That is what screening tests are designed to do. Some screenings can reduce your risk of dying from the disease. But sometimes, experts say, a test may cause more harm than good. Before you get a test, talk with your doctor about the possible benefits and harms to help you decide what is best for your health.

Screening tests are given to people who seem healthy to try to find unnoticed problems. They are done before you have any signs or symptoms of the disease. They come in many forms. Your doctor might take your health history and perform a physical exam to look for signs of health or disease. They can also include lab tests of blood, tissue, or urine samples or imaging procedures that look inside your body.

"I wouldn't say that all people should just simply get screening tests," says Dr. Barnett S. Kramer, a cancer prevention expert at the National Institutes of Health (NIH). "Patients should be aware of both the potential benefits and the harms when they're choosing what screening tests to have and how often."

Teams of experts regularly look at all the evidence about the balance of benefits and harms of different screening tests. They develop guidelines for who should be screened and how often.

Every screening test comes with its own risks. Some procedures can cause problems such as bleeding or infection. A positive screening test can lead to further tests that come with their own risks.

"Most people who feel healthy are healthy," says Kramer. "So a negative test to confirm that you're healthy doesn't add much new information." But mistakenly being told that you do or do not have a disease can be harmful. This is called a "misdiagnosis."

A "false negative" means that you are told you do not have the disease, but you do. This can cause problems if you do not pay attention to symptoms that appear later because you think you do not have the disease. A "false positive" means that you are told you may have the disease, but you do not. This can lead to unnecessary worry and potentially harmful tests and treatments that you do not need.

Even correctly finding a disease may not improve your health or help you live longer. You may learn you have an untreatable disease long before you would have. Or find out about a disease that never would have caused a problem. This is called "over-diagnosis." Some cancers, for example, never cause symptoms or become life-threatening. But if found by a screening test, they are likely to be treated. Cancer treatments can have harsh and long-lasting side effects. Currently, there is no way to know if the treatment will help you live longer.

An effective screening test may decrease your chances of dying of the condition. Most have not been shown to lengthen your overall life expectancy, Kramer explains. Their usefulness varies and may depend on your risk factors, age, or treatment options.

If you are at risk for certain health conditions—because of a family history or lifestyle exposures, such as smoking—you may choose to have screenings more regularly. If you are considering a screening, talk with your healthcare provider.

Ask Your Doctor about Screening Tests

- What is my chance of dying of the condition if I do or do not have the screening?

Common Screening and Diagnostic Tests

- What are the harms of the test? How often do they occur?
- How likely are false positive or false negative results?
- What are possible harms of the diagnostic tests if I get a positive screening result?
- What is the chance of finding a disease that would not have caused a problem?
- How effective are the treatment options?
- Am I healthy enough to take the therapy if you discover a disease?
- What are other ways to decrease my risk of dying of this condition? How effective are they?

Section 7.2 | Screening Tests for Women

This section includes text excerpted from "Women: Stay Healthy at Any Age," Agency for Healthcare Research and Quality (AHRQ), U.S. Department of Health and Human Services (HHS), May 2014. Reviewed December 2019.

Screenings are tests that look for diseases before you have symptoms. Blood-pressure checks and mammograms are examples of screenings. You can get some screenings, such as blood-pressure readings, at your doctor's office. Others, such as mammograms, need special equipment, so you may need to go to a different office. After a screening test, ask when you will see the results and who to talk to about them.

DISEASES AND CONDITIONS FOR WHICH WOMEN NEED TO GET SCREENED

Breast cancer. Talk with your healthcare team about whether you need a mammogram.

BRCA 1 and *BRCA 2* genes. If you have a family member with breast, ovarian, or peritoneal cancer, talk with your doctor or nurse about your family history. Women with a strong family history of certain cancers may benefit from genetic counseling and *BRCA* genetic testing.

Cervical cancer. Starting at age 21, get a Pap smear every 3 years until you are 65 years old. Women 30 years of age or older may choose to switch to a combination Pap smear and human papillomavirus (HPV) test every 5 years until the age of 65. If you are older than 65 or have had a hysterectomy, talk with your doctor or nurse about whether you still need to be screened.

Colon cancer. Between the ages of 50 and 75, get a screening test for colorectal cancer. Several tests—for example, a stool test or a colonoscopy—can detect this cancer. Your healthcare team can help you decide which is best for you. If you are between the ages of 76 and 85, talk with your doctor or nurse about whether you should continue to be screened.

Depression. Your emotional health is as important as your physical health. Talk to your healthcare team about being screened for depression, especially if during the last two weeks:

- You have felt down, sad, or hopeless
- You have felt little interest or pleasure in doing things

Diabetes. Get screened for diabetes (high blood sugar) if you have high blood pressure or if you take medication for high blood pressure. Diabetes can cause problems with your heart, brain, eyes, feet, kidneys, nerves, and other body parts.

Hepatitis C virus (HCV). Get screened one time for HCV infection if:

- You were born between 1945 and 1965
- You have ever injected drugs
- You received a blood transfusion before 1992

If you currently are an injection-drug user, you should be screened regularly.

High blood cholesterol. Have your blood cholesterol checked regularly with a blood test if:

- You use tobacco
- You are overweight or obese
- You have a personal history of heart disease or blocked arteries
- A male relative in your family had a heart attack before age 50 or a female relative before age 60

High blood pressure. Have your blood pressure checked at least every two years. High blood pressure can cause strokes, heart attacks, kidney and eye problems, and heart failure.

Human immunodeficiency virus (HIV). If you are 65 or younger, get screened for HIV. If you are older than 65, talk to your doctor or nurse about whether you should be screened.

Lung cancer. Talk to your doctor or nurse about getting screened for lung cancer if you are between the ages of 55 and 80, have a 30 pack-year smoking history, and smoke now or have quit within the past 15 years. (Your pack-year history is the number of packs of cigarettes smoked per day times the number of years you have smoked.) Know that quitting smoking is the best thing you can do for your health.

Overweight and obesity. The best way to learn if you are overweight or obese is to determine your body mass index (BMI). You can determine your BMI by entering your height and weight into a BMI calculator. A BMI between 18.5 and 25 indicates a normal weight. Persons with a BMI of 30 or higher may be obese. If you are obese, talk to your doctor or nurse about getting intensive behavioral counseling and help to lose weight. Overweight and obesity can lead to diabetes and cardiovascular disease (CVD).

Osteoporosis (bone thinning). Have a screening test at age 65 to make sure your bones are strong. The most common test is a dual-energy x-ray absorptiometry (DEXA) scan—a low-dose x-ray of the spine and hip. If you are younger than 65 and at high risk for bone fractures, you should also be screened. Talk with your healthcare team about your risk for bone fractures.

Sexually transmitted infections (STIs). STIs can make it hard to get pregnant, may affect your baby, and can cause other health problems. Get screened for chlamydia and gonorrhea infections if you are 24 years or younger and sexually active. If you are older than 24 years, talk to your doctor or nurse about whether you should be screened. Ask your doctor or nurse whether you should be screened for other STIs.

Section 7.3 | Screening Tests for Men

This section includes text excerpted from "Men: Stay Healthy at Any Age," Agency for Healthcare Research and Quality (AHRQ), U.S. Department of Health and Human Services (HHS), March 2014. Reviewed December 2019.

Screenings are tests that look for diseases before you have symptoms. Blood-pressure checks and tests for high blood cholesterol are examples of screenings. You can get some screenings, such as blood-pressure readings, in your doctor's office. Others, such as a colonoscopy, a test for colon cancer, need special equipment, so you may need to go to a different office.

After a screening test, ask when you will see the results and who you should talk to about them.

DISEASES AND CONDITIONS FOR WHICH MEN NEED TO GET SCREENED

Abdominal aortic aneurysm (AAA). If you are between the ages of 65 and 75 and have ever been a smoker (smoked 100 or more cigarettes in your lifetime), get screened once for abdominal aortic aneurysm. AAA is a bulging in your abdominal aorta, your largest artery. An AAA may burst, which can cause dangerous bleeding and death. An ultrasound, a painless procedure in which you lie on a table while a technician slides a medical device over your abdomen, will show whether an aneurysm is present.

Colon cancer. If you are between the ages of 50 and 75, get a screening test for colorectal cancer. Several different tests—for example, a stool test or a colonoscopy—can detect this cancer. Your healthcare team can help you decide which is best for you. If you are between the ages of 76 and 85, talk with your doctor or nurse about whether you should continue to be screened.

Depression. Your emotional health is as important as your physical health. Talk to your doctor or nurse about being screened for depression, especially if during the last two weeks:

- You have felt down, sad, or hopeless
- You have felt little interest or pleasure in doing things

Diabetes. Get screened for diabetes (high blood sugar) if you have high blood pressure or if you take medication for high blood pressure. Diabetes can cause problems with your heart, brain, eyes, feet, kidneys, nerves, and other body parts.

Hepatitis C virus (HCV). Get screened one time for HCV infection if:

- You were born between 1945 and 1965
- You have ever injected drugs
- You received a blood transfusion before 1992

If you currently are an injection-drug user, you should be screened regularly.

High blood cholesterol. If you are 35 or older, have your blood cholesterol checked regularly with a blood test. High cholesterol increases your chance of heart disease, stroke, and poor circulation. Talk to your doctor or nurse about having your cholesterol checked starting at age 20 if:

- You use tobacco
- You are overweight or obese
- You have diabetes or high blood pressure
- You have a history of heart disease or blocked arteries
- A man in your family had a heart attack before age 50 or a woman before age 60

High blood pressure. Have your blood pressure checked at least every two years. High blood pressure can cause strokes, heart attacks, kidney and eye problems, and heart failure.

Human immunodeficiency virus (HIV). If you are 65 or younger, get screened for HIV. If you are older than 65, ask your doctor or nurse whether you should be screened.

Lung cancer. Talk to your doctor or nurse about getting screened for lung cancer if you are between the ages of 55 and 80, have a 30 pack-year smoking history, and smoke now or have quit within the past 15 years. (Your pack-year history is the number of packs of cigarettes smoked per day times the number of years you have smoked.) Know that quitting smoking is the best thing you can do for your health.

Overweight and Obesity. The best way to learn if you are overweight or obese is to determine your body mass index (BMI). You can determine your BMI by entering your height and weight into a BMI calculator.

A BMI between 18.5 and 25 indicates a normal weight. Persons with a BMI of 30 or higher may be obese. If you are obese, talk to your doctor or nurse about getting intensive behavioral counseling and help to lose weight. Overweight and obesity can lead to diabetes and cardiovascular disease (CVD).

Section 7.4 | Laboratory-Developed Tests

This section includes text excerpted from "Laboratory Developed Tests," U.S. Food and Drug Administration (FDA), September 27, 2018.

A laboratory developed test (LDT) is a type of in vitro diagnostic (IVD) test that is designed, manufactured, and used within a single laboratory.

Laboratory developed tests can be used to measure or detect a wide variety of analytes (substances, such as proteins, chemical compounds, such as glucose or cholesterol, or deoxyribonucleic acid (DNA)), in a sample taken from a human body. Some LDTs are relatively simple tests that measure single analytes, such as a test that measures the level of sodium. Other LDTs are complex and may measure or detect one or more analytes. For example, some tests can detect many DNA variations from a single blood sample, which, such as levels of cholesterol or sodium, can be used to help diagnose a genetic disease. Various levels of chemicals, such as levels of cholesterol or sodium, can be measured to help diagnose a patient's state of health.

While the uses of an LDT are often the same as the uses of the U.S. Food and Drug Administration (FDA)-cleared or approved IVD tests, some labs may choose to offer their own test. For example, a hospital lab may run its own vitamin D assay, even though there is an FDA-cleared test for vitamin D on the market.

The FDA does not consider diagnostic devices to be LDTs if they are designed or manufactured completely, or partly, outside of the laboratory that offers and uses them.

Laboratory developed test are important to the continued development of personalized medicine, so it is important that IVDs are accurate so that patients and healthcare providers do not seek unnecessary treatments, delay needed treatments, or become exposed to inappropriate therapies.

Due to advances in technology and business models, LDTs have evolved and proliferated significantly since the FDA first obtained comprehensive authority to regulate all IVDs as devices in 1976. Some LDTs are now much more complex, have a nationwide reach, and present higher risks, such as detection of risk for breast cancer and Alzheimer disease (AD), which are similar to those of other IVDs that have undergone premarket review.

The FDA has identified problems with several high-risk LDTs, including:

- Claims that are not adequately supported with evidence
- Lack of appropriate controls yielding erroneous results
- Falsification of data

The FDA is concerned that people could initiate unnecessary treatment or delay or forego treatment altogether for a health condition, which could result in illness or death.

The FDA is aware of faulty LDTs that could have led to:

- Patients being over- or under-treated for heart disease
- Cancer patients being exposed to inappropriate therapies or not getting effective therapies
- Incorrect diagnosis of autism
- Unnecessary antibiotic treatments
- Exposure to unnecessary, harmful treatments for certain diseases such as Lyme disease

In 2010, the FDA announced its intent to reconsider its policy of enforcement discretion for LDTs and held a workshop to obtain input from stakeholders on such policy. The FDA used this feedback to develop an initial draft approach for LDT oversight and published draft guidance in 2014. The FDA solicited feedback on the draft LDT framework and notification guidances as well as held a public workshop.

Section 7.5 | **Home-Use Tests**

This section contains text excerpted from the following sources: Text in this section begins with excerpts from "Home Use Tests," U.S. Food and Drug Administration (FDA), April 4, 2019; Text under the heading "How You Can Get the Best Results with Home Use Tests" is excerpted from "How You Can Get the Best Results with Home Use Tests," U.S. Food and Drug Administration (FDA), December 28, 2017.

Home-use tests allow you to test for some diseases or conditions at home. These tests are cost-effective, quick, and confidential. Home-use tests can help:

Common Screening and Diagnostic Tests

- Detect possible health conditions when you have no symptoms, so that you can get early treatment and lower your chance of developing later complications (i.e., cholesterol testing, hepatitis testing)
- Detect specific conditions when there are no signs so that you can take immediate action (i.e., pregnancy testing)
- Monitor conditions to allow frequent changes in treatment (i.e., glucose testing to monitor blood sugar levels in diabetes)

Despite the benefits of home testing, you should take precautions when using home-use tests.

- See your healthcare provider regularly. Home-use tests are intended to help you with your healthcare, but they should not replace periodic visits to your doctor.
- Most tests are best evaluated together with your medical history, a physical exam, and other testing.
- Always see your doctor if you are feeling sick, are worried about a possible medical condition, or if the test instructions recommend you do so.
- Always use new test strips that are authorized for sale in the United States. The U.S. Food and Drug Administration (FDA) has issued a safety communication warning about the risks of using previously owned test strips or test strips that are not authorized for sale in the United States.

HOW YOU CAN GET THE BEST RESULTS WITH HOME-USE TESTS

Follow the tips listed here to use home-use tests as safely and effectively as possible.

- **Read the label and instructions carefully.** Review all instructions and pictures carefully to make sure you understand how to perform the test. Be sure you know:
    - What the test is for and what it is not for
    - How to store the test before you use it
    - How to collect and store the sample
    - When and how to run the test, including timing instructions
    - How to interpret the test
    - What might interfere with the test
    - The manufacturer's phone number (in case you have questions)
- **Use only tests regulated by the FDA.** There are several ways to find out if the FDA regulates a home-use test. You can ask your pharmacist or the vendor selling the test. If the FDA does not regulate the test, the U.S. government has not determined that the test is reasonably safe or effective, or substantially equivalent to another legally marketed device.

- **Follow all instructions.** You must follow all test instructions to get an accurate result. Most home tests require specific timing, materials, and sample amounts. You should also check the expiration dates and storage conditions before performing a test to make sure the components still work correctly.
- **Keep good records of your testing.**
- **Call the "800" telephone number listed on your home-use test if you have any questions.**
- **When in doubt, contact your doctor.** All tests can give false results. You should see your doctor if you believe your test results are wrong.
- **Do not change medications or dosages based on a home-use test without talking to your doctor.**

Section 7.6 | Direct-to-Consumer Genetic Testing

This section includes text excerpted from "Direct-to-Consumer Genetic Testing," Genetics Home Reference (GHR), National Institutes of Health (NIH), May 2018.

WHAT IS DIRECT-TO-CONSUMER GENETIC TESTING?

Most of the time, genetic testing is done through healthcare providers such as physicians, nurse practitioners, and genetic counselors. Healthcare providers determine which test is needed, order the test from a laboratory, collect and send the deoxyribonucleic acid (DNA) sample, interpret the test results, and share the results with the patient. Often, a health-insurance company covers part or all of the cost of testing.

Direct-to-consumer genetic testing is different: these genetic tests are marketed directly to customers via television, print advertisements, or the Internet, and the tests can be bought online or in stores. Customers send the company a DNA sample and receive their results directly from a secure website or in a written report. Direct-to-consumer genetic testing provides people access to their genetic information without necessarily involving a healthcare provider or health-insurance company in the process.

Dozens of companies currently offer direct-to-consumer genetic tests for a variety of purposes. The most popular tests use genetic variations to make predictions about health, provide information about common traits, and offer clues about a person's ancestry. The number of companies providing direct-to-consumer genetic testing is growing, along with the range of health conditions and traits covered by these tests. Because there is currently little regulation of direct-to-consumer genetic testing services, it is important to assess the quality of available services before pursuing any testing.

Other names for direct-to-consumer genetic testing include "DTC genetic testing," "direct-access genetic testing," "at-home genetic testing," and "home DNA testing." Ancestry testing (also called "genealogy testing") is also considered a form of direct-to-consumer genetic testing.

WHAT KINDS OF DIRECT-TO-CONSUMER GENETIC TESTS ARE AVAILABLE?

With so many companies offering direct-to-consumer genetic testing, it can be challenging to determine which tests will be most informative and helpful to you. When considering testing, think about what you hope to get out of the test. Some direct-to-consumer genetic tests are very specific (such as paternity tests), while other services provide a broad range of health, ancestry, and lifestyle information.

Some of the major types of direct-to-consumer genetic tests are discussed below.

Disease Risk and Health

The results of these tests estimate your genetic risk of developing several common diseases, such as celiac disease, Parkinson disease (PD), and Alzheimer disease (AD). Some companies also include a person's carrier status for less common conditions, including cystic fibrosis (CF) and sickle cell disease. A carrier is someone who has one copy of a gene mutation that, when present in two copies, causes a genetic disorder. The tests may also look for genetic variations related to other health-related traits, such as weight and metabolism (how a person's body converts nutrients from food into energy).

Ancestry or Genealogy

The results of these tests provide clues about where a person's ancestors might have come from, their ethnicity, and genetic connections between families.

Kinship

The results of these tests can indicate whether tested individuals are biologically related to one another. For example, kinship testing can establish whether one person is the biological father of another (paternity testing). The results of direct-to-consumer kinship tests, including paternity tests, are usually not admissible in a court of law.

Lifestyle

The results of these tests claim to provide information about lifestyle factors, such as nutrition, fitness, weight loss, skincare, sleep, and even your wine preferences, based on variations in your DNA. Many of the companies that offer this kind of testing also sell services, products, or programs that they customize on the basis of your test results.

Before choosing a direct-to-consumer genetic test, find out what kinds of health, ancestry, or other information will be reported to you. Think about whether there is any information you would rather not know. In some cases, you can decline to find out specific information if you tell the company before it delivers your results.

WHAT ARE THE BENEFITS AND RISKS OF DIRECT-TO-CONSUMER GENETIC TESTING?

Direct-to-consumer genetic testing has both benefits and limitations, although they are somewhat different than those of genetic testing ordered by a healthcare provider.

Benefits

- Direct-to-consumer genetic testing promotes awareness of genetic diseases.
- It provides personalized information about your health, disease risk, and other traits.
- It may help you be more proactive about your health.
- It does not require approval from a healthcare provider or health insurance company.
- It is often less expensive than genetic testing obtained through a healthcare provider.
- DNA sample collection is usually simple and noninvasive, and results are available quickly.
- Your data is added to a large database that can be used to further medical research. Depending on the company, the database may represent up to several million participants.

Risks and Limitations

- Tests may not be available for the health conditions or traits that interest you.
- This type of testing cannot tell definitively whether you will or will not get a particular disease.
- Unexpected information that you receive about your health, family relationships, or ancestry may be stressful or upsetting.
- People may make important decisions about disease treatment or prevention based on inaccurate, incomplete, or misunderstood information from their test results.
- There is currently little oversight or regulation of testing companies.

Common Screening and Diagnostic Tests

- Unproven or invalid tests can be misleading. There may not be enough scientific evidence to link a particular genetic variation with a given disease or trait.
- Genetic privacy may be compromised if testing companies use your genetic information in an unauthorized way or if your data is stolen.
- The results of genetic testing may impact your ability to obtain life, disability, or long-term care insurance.

Direct-to-consumer genetic testing provides only partial information about your health. Other genetic and environmental factors, lifestyle choices, and family medical history also affect the likelihood of developing many disorders. These factors would be discussed during a consultation with a doctor or genetic counselor, but in many cases they are not addressed when using at-home genetic tests.

Section 7.7 | Biomarkers

This section includes text excerpted from "A Painless Skin Patch Simplifies Diagnostic Tests," National Institute of Biomedical Imaging and Bioengineering (NIBIB), August 16, 2019.

Many diagnostic tests require blood, but the researchers funded by the National Institute of Biomedical Imaging and Bioengineering (NIBIB) have developed a skin patch with tiny needles that painlessly collect interstitial fluid (ISF) for testing. Diagnostic tests can measure trace amounts of essential proteins or hormones in the blood called "biomarkers." High or low levels of biomarkers are specific indicators for a disease. In the new test, a unique paper on the patch's backing stores small amounts ISF, where it remains for analysis. Researchers think the ISF patch will simplify diagnostic testing and enable the continuous monitoring of biomarkers. Monitoring biomarkers is crucial because doctors routinely use them to diagnose and monitor patients at risk for cancer, heart disease, and diabetes.

Interstitial fluid fills the space between cells throughout the body and contains most of the same biomarkers found in the blood. ISF lacks cells and clotting agents, which can complicate blood analysis, thereby making it an attractive target for diagnostic testing. Many groups have started using ISF for diagnostic testing, but Mark Prausnitz, Ph.D., a Regents' professor of chemical and biomolecular engineering at the Georgia Institute of Technology, thought the procedure for analyzing ISF could be simplified.

Prausnitz and his team, in collaboration with Srikanth Singamaneni, Ph.D., a professor of mechanical engineering and materials science at Washington

University, used surface-enhanced Raman scattering (SERS) to speed up the analysis. This technique measures the amount of molecules by detecting a unique light-scattering pattern. Negatively charged gold nanorods are incorporated into the paper on the patch's backing and trap the positively charged biomarker of interest in the ISF.

Their research results, published in *ACS Sensors*, show that the nanorods successfully attracted a positively charged molecule that researchers had injected into rats' bloodstream that is absorbed in their ISF. The interaction between the nanorods and the trapped molecules amplified the Raman scattering so they could analyze it with SERS with enhanced sensitivity. The researchers reported the new procedure to be as sensitive as the previous multistep methods.

Prausnitz said, "As a next step, we can adapt the methods we use to trap molecules in ISF to be more selective, using antibodies specific to a certain biomarker. In the future, we could create capture methods for multiple biomarkers all in the same patch." The researchers say the patch can speed diagnostic testing, is designed to take less effort than previous methods, and can be produced in mass quantities at low cost.

"This is an excellent example of how rethinking common medical tests can lead to a new technology that may accelerate healthcare, especially the continuous monitoring of important biomarkers," said Tiffani Lash, Ph.D., director of the NIBIB programs in Point-of-Care Technologies and Connected Health (mHealth and Telehealth).

Chapter 8 | **After Your Diagnosis: Finding Information and Support**

TAKE THE TIME YOU NEED
A Diagnosis Can Change Your Life in an Instant

Like so many other people in your situation, you might be feeling one or more of the following emotions after getting your diagnosis:

- Afraid
- Alone
- Angry
- Anxious
- Ashamed
- Confused
- Depressed
- Helpless
- In denial
- Numb
- Overwhelmed
- Panicky
- Powerless
- Relieved (that you finally know what is wrong)
- Sad
- Shocked
- Stressed

This chapter includes text excerpted from "Next Steps after Your Diagnosis," Agency for Healthcare Research and Quality (AHRQ), U.S. Department of Health and Human Services (HHS), July 2018.

It is perfectly normal to have these feelings. It is also normal, and very common, to have trouble taking in and understanding information after you receive the news—especially if the diagnosis was a surprise. And it can be even harder to make decisions about treating or managing your disease or condition.

Take Time to Make Your Decisions

No matter how the news of your diagnosis has affected you, do not rush into a decision. In most cases, you do not need to take action right away. Ask your doctor how much time you can safely take.

Taking the time you need to make decisions can help you:
- Feel less anxious and stressed
- Avoid depression
- Cope with your condition
- Feel more in control of your situation
- Play a key role in decisions about your treatment

GET THE SUPPORT YOU NEED
You Do Not Have to Go through It Alone

Sometimes the emotional side of illness can be just as hard to deal with as the physical side. You may have fears or concerns. You may feel overwhelmed. No matter what your situation, having other people to turn to will help you know you are not alone.

Here are the kinds of support you might want to seek.

Family and Friends

Talking to family and friends you feel close to can help you cope with your illness or condition. Just knowing that someone is there can be a comfort.

Sometimes it is hard to ask for help. And sometimes your family and friends want to help, but they do not want to intrude, or they do not know how to ask or what to offer. Think about specific ways people can help you. One idea is to ask someone to come with you to a doctor's appointment to help ask questions, take notes, and talk with you afterward.

Other People or Groups Who Can Provide Support

If you do not have family or friends who can provide support, other people or groups can.

Support or Self-Help Groups

Support groups are made up of people with the same disease or condition who get together to share information and concerns and to help one another.

Support groups may or may not be led by experts. Self-help groups are similar to support groups but usually are led by the participants. The names "support group" and "self-help group" sometimes are used to refer to either kind.

After Your Diagnosis: Finding Information and Support

Research on support groups shows that participants feel less anxious, experience less depression, have a better quality of life (QOL) and have more success in coping with their disease or condition. Similar findings have been reported for self-help groups.

Online Support or Self-Help Groups

The Internet has support or self-help groups for people whose concerns and situations may be similar to yours. You can also find "message boards" where you can post questions and get answers. These online communities can help you connect with people who can give you support and provide information. But, be careful. Not every idea or treatment you come across in these groups will be scientifically proven to be safe and effective. If you read about something interesting and new, check it out with your doctor.

Mental-Health Counselor or Therapist

A good mental-health counselor or therapist can help you cope with sadness, depression, and feelings of being overwhelmed. If you think this kind of help might be right for you, ask your doctor or other healthcare professional to recommend someone in your area.

People Like You

You might want to meet and talk with someone in your own situation. Someone who has "been there" can talk about the real-life outcomes of their treatment choices as well as how they have learned to live with their disease or condition. Some advocacy or support groups can help you make this kind of contact.

Part 2 | Working with Healthcare Providers and the Healthcare System

Chapter 9 | Talking with Your Healthcare Provider

Chapter Contents

Section 9.1 | Why Being Able to Talk with Your Doctor Matters

This section includes text excerpted from "Next Steps after Your Diagnosis," Agency for Healthcare Research and Quality (AHRQ), U.S. Department of Health and Human Services (HHS), July 2018.

YOUR DOCTOR IS YOUR PARTNER IN HEALTHCARE

You probably have many questions about your disease or condition. The first person to ask is your doctor. It is fine to seek more information from other sources; in fact, it is important to do so. But, consider your doctor your partner in healthcare—someone who can discuss your situation with you, explain your options, and help you make decisions that are right for you.

It is not always easy to feel comfortable around doctors. But, research has shown that good communication with your doctor can actually be good for your health. It can help you to:

- Feel more satisfied with the care you receive
- Have better outcomes (end results), such as reduced pain and better recovery from symptoms

Being an active member of your healthcare team also helps to reduce your chances of medical mistakes, and it helps you get high-quality care.

Of course, good communication is a two-way street. Here are some ways to help make the most of the time you spend with your doctor:

Prepare for Your Visit

- Think about what you want to get out of your appointment. Write down all your questions and concerns.
- Prepare and bring to your doctor to visit a list of all the medicines you take.
- Consider bringing along a trusted relative or friend. This person can help ask questions, take notes, and help you remember and understand everything once you leave the doctor's office.

Give Information to Your Doctor

- Do not wait to be asked.
- Tell your doctor everything she or he needs to know about your health—even the things that might make you feel embarrassed or uncomfortable.
- Tell your doctor how you are feeling—both physically and emotionally.
- Tell your doctor if you are feeling depressed or overwhelmed.

Get Information from Your Doctor

- Ask questions about anything that concerns you. Keep asking until you understand the answers. If you do not, your doctor may think you understand everything that is said.
- Ask your doctor to draw pictures if that will help you understand something.
- Take notes.
- Tape-record your doctor visit, if that will be helpful to you. But, first, ask your doctor if this is okay.
- Ask your doctor to recommend resources, such as websites, booklets, or tapes with more information about your disease or condition.

GET INFORMATION ABOUT NEXT STEPS

Get the results of any tests or procedures. Discuss the meaning of these results with your doctor. Make sure you understand what will happen if you need surgery. Talk with your doctor about which hospital is best for your healthcare needs. Finally, if you are not satisfied with your doctor, you can do two things:

- Talk with your doctor and try to work things out.
- Switch doctors, if you are able to.

It is very important to feel confident about your care.

Section 9.2 | How to Prepare for a Doctor's Appointment

This section includes text excerpted from "How to Prepare for a Doctor's Appointment," National Institute on Aging (NIA), National Institutes of Health (NIH), May 18, 2017.

A basic plan can help you make the most of your appointment, whether you are starting with a new doctor or continuing with the doctor you have seen for years. The following tips will make it easier for you and your doctor to cover everything you need to talk about.

LIST AND PRIORITIZE YOUR CONCERNS

Make a list of what you want to discuss. For example:

- Do you have a new symptom you want to ask the doctor about?
- Do you want to get a flu shot?
- Are you concerned about how a treatment is affecting your daily life?

Talking with Your Healthcare Provider

If you have more than a few items to discuss, put them in order and ask about the most important ones first. Do not put off the things that are really on your mind until the end of your appointment—bring them up right away!

TAKE INFORMATION WITH YOU

Some doctors suggest you put all your prescription drugs, over-the-counter (OTC) medicines, vitamins, and herbal remedies or supplements in a bag and bring them with you. Others recommend you bring a list of everything you take and the dose. You should also take your insurance cards, names and phone numbers of other doctors you see, and your medical records if the doctor does not already have them.

CONSIDER BRINGING A FAMILY MEMBER OR FRIEND

Sometimes it is helpful to bring a family member or close friend with you. Let your family member or friend know in advance what you want from your visit. Your companion can remind you what you planned to discuss with the doctor if you forget. She or he can take notes for you and can help you remember what the doctor said.

Tips: Getting Started with a New Doctor

Your first meeting is a good time to talk with the doctor and the office staff about some communication basics.

- **First name or last name.** When you see the doctor and office staff, introduce yourself and let them know by what name you prefer to be called. For example: "Hello, my name is Mrs. Martinez," or "Good morning, my name is Bob Smith. Please call me Bob."
- **Ask how the office runs.** Learn what days are busiest and what times are best to call. Ask what to do if there is an emergency, or if you need a doctor when the office is closed.
- **Share your medical history.** Tell the doctor about your illnesses, operations, medical conditions, and other doctors you see. You may want to ask the doctor to send you a copy of the medical history form before your visit so you can fill it out at home, where you have the time and information you need to complete it. If you have problems understanding how to fill out any of the forms, ask for help. Some community organizations provide this kind of help.
- **Share former doctors' names.** Give the new doctor all of your former doctors' names and addresses, especially if they are in a different city. This is to help your new doctor get copies of your medical records. Your doctor will ask you to sign a medical release form giving her or his permission to request your records.

BE SURE YOU CAN SEE AND HEAR AS WELL AS POSSIBLE

Many people use glasses or need aids for hearing. Remember to take your eyeglasses to the doctor's visit. If you have a hearing aid, make sure that it is working well and wear it. Let the doctor and staff know if you have a hard time seeing or hearing. For example, you may want to say: "My hearing makes it hard to understand everything you're saying. It helps a lot when you speak slowly."

PLAN TO UPDATE THE DOCTOR

Let your doctor know what has happened in your life since your last visit. If you have been treated in the emergency room or by a specialist, tell the doctor right away. Mention any changes you have noticed in your appetite, weight, sleep, or energy level. Also, tell the doctor about any recent changes in any medications you take or the effects they have had on you.

REQUEST AN INTERPRETER IF YOU KNOW YOU WILL NEED ONE

If the doctor you selected or were referred to does not speak your language, ask the doctor's office to provide an interpreter. Even though some English-speaking doctors know basic medical terms in Spanish or other languages, you may feel more comfortable speaking in your own language, especially when it comes to sensitive subjects, such as sexuality or depression. Call the doctor's office ahead of time, as they may need to plan for an interpreter to be available.

Always let the doctor, your interpreter, or the staff knows if you do not understand your diagnosis or the instructions the doctor gives you. Do not let language barriers stop you from asking questions or voicing your concerns.

How to Use an Interpreter

- **Keep the interpreter informed.** Consider telling your interpreter what you want to talk about with your doctor before the appointment. Make sure your interpreter understands your symptoms or condition so that she or he can correctly translate your message to the doctor. You do not want the doctor to prescribe the wrong medication!
- **Prefer using universal terms.** If your language is spoken in multiple countries, such as Spanish, and your interpreter does not come from the same country or background as you, use universal terms to describe your symptoms and communicate your concerns.
- **Never hesitate to clarify your doubts.** Do not be afraid to let your interpreter know if you did not understand something that was said, even if you need to ask that it be repeated several times.

Section 9.3 | Make the Most of Your Time at the Doctor's Office

This section contains text excerpted from the following sources: Text beginning with the heading "Be Honest" is excerpted from "5 Ways to Make the Most of Your Time at the Doctor's Office," National Institute on Aging (NIA), National Institutes of Health (NIH), May 18, 2017; Text under the heading "What You Need to Tell Your Doctor" is excerpted from "What Do I Need to Tell the Doctor?" National Institute on Aging (NIA), National Institutes of Health (NIH), May 18, 2017.

BE HONEST

It is tempting to say what you think the doctor wants to hear, for example, that you smoke less or eat a more balanced diet than you really do. While this is natural, it is not in your best interest. Your doctor can suggest the best treatment only if you say what is really going on. For instance, you might say: "I have been trying to quit smoking, as you recommended, but I am not making much headway."

DECIDE WHAT QUESTIONS ARE MOST IMPORTANT

Pick three or four questions or concerns that you most want to talk about with the doctor. You can tell them what they are at the beginning of the appointment, and then discuss each in turn. If you have time, you can then go on to other questions.

STICK TO THE POINT

Although your doctor might like to talk with you at length, each patient is given a limited amount of time. To make the best use of your time, stick to the point. For instance, give the doctor a brief description of the symptom, when it started, how often it happens, and if it is getting worse or better.

SHARE YOUR POINT OF VIEW ABOUT THE VISIT

Tell the doctor if you feel rushed, worried, or uncomfortable. If necessary, you can offer to return for a second visit to discuss your concerns. Try to voice your feelings in a positive way. For example, you could say something such as: "I know you have many patients to see, but I'm really worried about this. I'd feel much better if we could talk about it a little more."

REMEMBER, THE DOCTOR MAY NOT BE ABLE TO ANSWER ALL YOUR QUESTIONS

Even the best doctor may be unable to answer some questions. Most doctors will tell you when they do not have answers. They also may help you find the information you need or refer you to a specialist. If a doctor regularly brushes off your questions or symptoms, think about looking for another doctor.

WHAT YOU NEED TO TELL YOUR DOCTOR

Talking about your health means sharing information about how you feel physically, emotionally, and mentally. Knowing how to describe your symptoms and bring up other concerns will help you become a partner in your healthcare.

Share Any Symptoms

A symptom is evidence of a disease or disorder in the body. Examples of symptoms include pain, fever, a lump or bump, unexplained weight loss or gain, or having a hard time sleeping.

Be clear and concise when describing your symptoms. Your description helps the doctor identify the problem. A physical exam and medical tests provide valuable information, but your symptoms point the doctor in the right direction.

Your doctor will ask when your symptoms started, what time of day they happen, how long they last (seconds? days?), how often they occur, if they seem to be getting worse or better, and if they keep you from going out or doing your usual activities.

Take the time to make some notes about your symptoms before you call or visit the doctor. Worrying about your symptoms is not a sign of weakness. Being honest about what you are experiencing does not mean that you are complaining. The doctor needs to know how you feel.

Questions to ask yourself about your symptoms may include:
- What exactly are my symptoms?
- Are the symptoms constant? If not, when do I experience them?
- Does anything I do make the symptoms better? Or worse?
- Do the symptoms affect my daily activities? Which ones? How?

Give Information about Your Medications

It is possible for medicines to interact causing unpleasant, and sometimes dangerous side effects. Your doctor needs to know about all of the medicines you take, including over-the-counter (OTC) drugs and herbal remedies or supplements. Make a list or bring everything with you to your visit—do not forget about eye drops, vitamins, and laxatives. Tell the doctor how often you take each. Describe any drug allergies or reactions you have had. Say which medications work best for you. Be sure your doctor has the phone number of the pharmacy you use.

Tell Your Doctor about Your Habits

To provide the best care, your doctor must understand you as a person and know what your life is like. The doctor may ask about where you live, what you eat, how you sleep, what you do each day, what activities you enjoy, what your sex life is like, and if you smoke or drink. Be open and honest with your doctor. It will help them to understand your medical conditions fully and recommend the best treatment choices for you.

Voice Other Concerns

Your doctor may ask you how your life is going. This is not being impolite or nosy. Information about what is happening in your life may be useful medically.

Talking with Your Healthcare Provider

Let the doctor know about any major changes or stresses in your life, such as a divorce or the death of a loved one. You do not have to go into detail; you may want to say something such as: "It might be helpful for you to know that my sister passed away since my last visit with you," or "I recently had to sell my home and move in with my daughter."

Section 9.4 | Questions to Ask Your Doctor

This section includes text excerpted from "Questions to Ask Your Doctor," Agency for Healthcare Research and Quality (AHRQ), U.S. Department of Health and Human Services (HHS), September 2018.

Your health depends on good communication. Asking questions and providing information to your doctor and other care providers can improve your care. Talking with your doctor builds trust and leads to better results, quality, safety, and satisfaction.

Quality healthcare is a team effort. You play an important role. One of the best ways to communicate with your doctor and healthcare team is by asking questions. Because time is limited during medical appointments, you will feel less rushed if you prepare your questions before your appointment.

YOUR DOCTOR WANTS YOUR QUESTIONS

Doctors know a lot about a lot of things, but they do not always know everything about you or what is best for you. Your questions give your doctor and healthcare team important information about you, such as your most important healthcare concerns. That is why they need you to speak up.

Questions You Should Know

A simple question can help you feel better, let you take better care of yourself, or save your life. The questions below can get you started.
- What is the test for?
- How many times have you done this procedure?
- When will I get the results?
- Why do I need this treatment?
- Are there any alternatives?
- What are the possible complications?
- Which hospital is best for my needs?
- How do you spell the name of that drug?
- Are there any side effects?
- Will this medicine interact with medicines that I'm already taking?

Questions to Ask before Your Appointment

Asking questions about your diagnosis, treatments, and medicines can improve the quality, safety, and effectiveness of your healthcare. Taking steps before your medical appointments will help you to make the most of your time with your doctor and healthcare team.

Prepare Your Questions

Time is limited during doctor visits. Prepare for your appointment by thinking about what you want to do during your next visit. Do you want to:

- Talk about a health problem?
- Get or change a medicine?
- Get medical tests?
- Talk about surgery or treatment options?

Write down your questions to bring to your appointment. The answers can help you make better decisions, get good care, and feel better about your healthcare.

Questions to Ask during Your Appointment

During your appointment, make sure to ask the questions you prepared before your appointment. Start by asking the ones that are most important to you.

To get the most from your visit, tell the nurse or person at the front desk that you have questions for your doctor. If your doctor does not ask you if you have questions, ask your doctor when the best time would be to ask them.

Understand the Answers and Next Steps

Asking questions is important but so is making sure you hear—and understand— the answers you get. Take notes or bring someone to your appointment to help you understand and remember what you heard. If you do not understand or are confused, ask your doctor to explain the answer again.

It is very important to understand the plan or next steps that your doctor recommends. Ask questions to make sure you understand what your doctor wants you to do.

The questions you may want to ask will depend on whether your doctor gives you a diagnosis; recommends a treatment, medical tests, or surgery; or gives you a prescription for medicine.

Questions could include:

- What is my diagnosis?
- What are my treatment options? What are the benefits of each option? What are the side effects?
- Will I need a test? What is the test for? What will the results tell me?

Talking with Your Healthcare Provider

- What will the medicine you are prescribing do? How do I take it? Are there any side effects?
- Why do I need surgery? Are there other ways to treat my condition? How often do you perform this surgery?
- Do I need to change my daily routine?

Find out what you are to do next. Ask for written instructions, brochures, videos, or websites that may help you learn more.

Questions to Ask after Your Appointment

After you meet with your doctor, you will need to follow their instructions to keep your health on track.

Your doctor may have you fill a prescription or make another appointment for tests, lab work, or a follow-up visit. It is important for you to follow your doctor's instructions.

It also is important to call your doctor if you are unclear about any instructions or have more questions.

Prioritize Your Questions

Create a list of follow-up questions to ask if you:
- Have a health problem
- Need to get or change a medicine
- Need a medical test
- Need to have surgery
- Other times to call your doctor

There are other times when you should follow up on your care and call your doctor. Call your doctor:
- If you experience any side effects or other problems with your medicines
- If your symptoms get worse after seeing the doctor
- If you receive any new prescriptions or start taking any over-the-counter (OTC) medicines
- To get results of any tests you have had. Do not assume that no news is good news.
- To ask about test results you do not understand

Your questions help your doctor and healthcare team learn more about you. Your doctor's answers to your questions can help you make better decisions, receive a higher level of care, avoid medical harm, and feel better about your healthcare. Your questions can also lead to better results for your health.

Section 9.5 | Be More Involved in Your Healthcare

This section includes text excerpted from "Be More Involved in Your Healthcare," Agency for Healthcare Research and Quality (AHRQ), U.S. Department of Health and Human Services (HHS), August 2018.

This section gives you tips to use before, during, and after your medical appointment to make sure you get the best possible care. One way you can make sure you get good quality healthcare is to be an active member of your healthcare team. Patients who talk with their doctors tend to be happier with their care and have better medical results.

BEFORE YOUR APPOINTMENT

Bring all the medicines you take to your appointment. This includes:

- Prescription medicines
- Nonprescription medicines, such as aspirin or antacids
- Vitamins
- Dietary or herbal supplements

Write down the questions you have for the visit. Know your current medical conditions, past surgeries, and illnesses.

DURING YOUR APPOINTMENT

Explain your symptoms, health history, and any problems with medicines you have taken in the past. Ask questions to make sure you understand what your doctor tells you.

Let your doctor know if you are worried about being able to follow their instructions. If your doctor recommends a treatment, ask about options.

If you need a test, ask:

- How the test is done
- How it will feel
- What you need to do to get ready for it
- How you will get the results

If you need a prescription, tell your doctor if you are pregnant, are nursing, have reactions to medicines, or take vitamins or herbal supplements.

Find out what to do next. Ask for:

- Written instructions
- Brochures
- Videos
- Websites

Talking with Your Healthcare Provider

AFTER YOUR APPOINTMENT

Always follow your doctor's instructions. If you do not understand your instructions after you get home, call your doctor. Talk with your doctor or pharmacist before you stop taking any medicines that your doctor prescribed. Call your doctor if your symptoms get worse or if you have problems following the instructions.

Make appointments to have tests done or see a specialist if you need to. Call your doctor's office to find out test results. Ask what you should do about the results.

Chapter 10 | Making Decisions with Your Doctor

Giving and getting information are two important steps in talking with your doctor. The third big step is making decisions about your care.

FIND OUT ABOUT DIFFERENT TREATMENTS

You will benefit most from a treatment when you know what is happening and are involved in making decisions. Make sure you understand what your treatment involves and what it will or will not do. Have the doctor give you directions in writing and feel free to ask questions. For example: "What are the pros and cons of having surgery at this stage?" or "Do I have any other choices?"

If your doctor suggests a treatment that makes you uncomfortable, ask if there are other treatments that might work. If cost is a concern, ask the doctor if less expensive choices are available. The doctor can work with you to develop a treatment plan that meets your needs.

Here are some things to remember when deciding on a treatment:

- **Discuss choices.** There are different ways to manage many health conditions, especially chronic conditions such as high blood pressure and cholesterol. Ask what your options are.
- **Discuss risks and benefits.** Once you know your options, ask about the pros and cons of each one. Find out what side effects might occur, how long the treatment would continue, and how likely it is that the treatment will work for you.
- **Consider your own values and circumstances.** When thinking about the pros and cons of a treatment, do not forget to consider its impact on your overall life. For instance, will one of the side effects interfere with a regular activity that means a lot to you? Is one treatment choice expensive and not covered by your insurance? Doctors need to know

This chapter includes text excerpted from "A Guide for Older People—Talking with Your Doctor," National Institute on Aging (NIA), National Institutes of Health (NIH), December 2016. Reviewed December 2019.

about these practical matters so they can work with you to develop a treatment plan that meets your needs.

Questions to Ask about Treatment
- Are there any risks associated with the treatment?
- How soon should treatment start? How long will it last?
- Are there other treatments available?
- How much will the treatment cost? Will my insurance cover it?

LEARN ABOUT PREVENTION

Doctors and other health professionals may suggest you change your diet, activity level, or other aspects of your life to help you deal with medical conditions. Research has shown that these changes, particularly an increase in exercise, have positive effects on overall health.

Until recently, preventing disease in older people received little attention. But, things are changing. People do realize now know that it is never too late to stop smoking, improving their diet, or start exercising. Getting regular checkups and seeing other health professionals, such as dentists and eye specialists, helps promote good health. Even people who have chronic diseases, such as arthritis or diabetes, can prevent further disability and, in some cases, control the progress of the disease.

If a certain disease or health condition runs in your family, ask your doctor if there are steps you can take to help prevent it. If you have a chronic condition, ask how you can manage it and if there are things you can do to keep it from getting worse. If you want to discuss health and disease prevention with your doctor, say so when you make your next appointment. This lets the doctor plan to spend more time with you.

It is just as important to talk with your doctor about lifestyle changes as it is to talk about treatment. For example: "I know that you've told me to eat more dairy products, but they really disagree with me. Is there something else I could eat instead?" or "Maybe an exercise class would help, but I have no way to get to the senior center. Is there something else you could suggest?"

As with treatments, consider all the alternatives, look at pros and cons, and remember to take into account your own point of view. Tell your doctor if you feel her or his suggestions will not work for you and explain why. Keep talking with your doctor to come up with a plan that works.

Questions to Ask about Prevention
- Is there any way to prevent a condition that runs in my family—before it affects me?
- Are there ways to keep my condition from getting worse?
- How will making a change in my habits help me?

Making Decisions with Your Doctor

- Are there any risks in making this change?
- Are there support groups or community services that might help me?

TALKING ABOUT EXERCISE

Exercise is often "just what the doctor ordered!"

Exercise can:

- Help you have more energy to do the things you want to do
- Help maintain and improve your physical strength and fitness
- Help improve mood and reduce depression
- Help manage and prevent diseases, such as heart disease, diabetes, some types of cancer, osteoporosis, and disabilities as people grow older
- Help improve your balance and prevent falls

Many doctors now recommend that older people try to make physical activity a part of everyday life. When you are making your list of things to talk about with your doctor, add exercise. Ask how exercise would benefit you, if there are any activities you should avoid, and whether your doctor can recommend any specific kinds of exercise.

Start exercising with the National Institute on Aging's (NIA) exercise and physical activity campaign, *Go4Life*®. See how to stick with a safe, effective program of endurance, stretching, balance, and strength-training exercises. Visit www.nia.nih.gov/Go4Life or call toll-free: 800-222-2225 for information about the health benefits of exercise and physical activity, along with activities you can do to stay fit.

Chapter 11 | **Seek Out Information**

By knowing your treatment options, you can learn which ones are backed up by the best scientific evidence. "Evidence-based" information—that is, information that is based on a careful review of the latest scientific findings in medical journals—can help you make decisions about the best possible treatments for you.

EVIDENCE-BASED INFORMATION COMES FROM RESEARCH ON PEOPLE

Evidence-based information about treatments generally comes from two major types of scientific studies:

- **Clinical trials** are research studies on human volunteers to test new drugs or other treatments. Participants are randomly assigned to different treatment groups. Some get the research treatment, and others get a standard treatment or may be given a placebo (a medicine that has no effect), or no treatment. The results are compared to learn whether the new treatment is safe and effective.
- **Outcomes research** looks at the impact of treatments and other healthcare on health outcomes (end results) for patients and populations. End results include effects that people care about, such as changes in their quality of life (QOL).

TAKE ADVANTAGE OF THE EVIDENCE-BASED INFORMATION THAT IS AVAILABLE

Health information is everywhere—in books, newspapers, magazines, Internet, television, and radio. However, not all information is good information. Your best bets for sources of evidence-based information include the federal government, national nonprofit organizations, medical-specialty groups, medical schools, and university medical centers.

This chapter includes text excerpted from "Seek Out Information," Agency for Healthcare Research and Quality (AHRQ), U.S. Department of Health and Human Services (HHS), July 2018.

Information

Information about your disease or condition and its treatment are available from many sources. Here are some of the most reliable:

- **Healthfinder®.** The healthfinder® site—sponsored by the U.S. Department of Health and Human Services (HHS)—offers carefully selected health information websites from government agencies, clearinghouses, nonprofit groups, and universities.
- **Health information resource database.** Sponsored by the National Health Information Center (NHIC), this database includes 1,400 organizations and government offices that provide health information upon request.
- **MedlinePlus®.** MedlinePlus® has extensive information from the National Institutes of Health (NIH) and other trusted sources on over 650 diseases and conditions. The site includes many additional features.
- **National nonprofit groups,** such as the American Heart Association (AHA), American Cancer Society (ACS), and American Diabetes Association (ADA) can be valuable sources of reliable information. Many have chapters nationwide. Check your phone book for a local chapter in your community. The health information resource database can help you find national offices of nonprofit groups.
- **Health or medical libraries** run by government, hospitals, professional groups, and other reliable organizations often welcome consumers. For a list of libraries in your area, use the MedlinePlus® "Find a Library" feature.

Current Medical Research

You can find the latest medical research in medical journals at your local health or medical library, and in some cases, on the Internet. Here are two major online sources of medical articles:

- **MEDLINE®/PubMed®.** PubMed® is the National Library of Medicine's (NLM) database of references to more than 14 million articles published in 4,800 medical and scientific journals. All of the listings have information to help you find the articles at a health or medical library. Many listings also have short summaries of the article (abstracts), and some have links to the full article. The article might be free, or it might require a fee charged by the publisher.
- **PubMed Central.** PubMed Central is the NLM's database of journal articles that are available free of charge to users.

Clinical Trials

Perhaps you wonder whether there is a clinical trial that is right for you. Or you may want to learn about results from previous clinical trials that might be relevant to your situation. Here are two reliable resources:

Seek Out Information

- **ClinicalTrials.gov.** ClinicalTrials.gov provides regularly updated information about federally and privately supported clinical research on people who volunteer to participate. The site has information about a trial's purpose, who may participate, locations, and phone numbers for more details. The site also describes the clinical trial process and includes news about recent clinical trial results.
- **Cochrane Collaboration.** The Cochrane Collaboration writes summaries ("reviews") about evidence from clinical trials to help people make informed decisions. You can search and read the review abstracts free of charge.

Outcomes Research

Outcomes research provides research about benefits, risks, and outcomes (end results) of treatments so that patients and their doctors can make better-informed decisions. The Agency for Healthcare Research and Quality (AHRQ) supports improvements in health outcomes through research and sponsors products that result from research such as:

- **Guidelines and measures.** This AHRQ microsite, Guidelines, and Measures (GAM), was set up by AHRQ to provide users a place to find information about its legacy guidelines and measures clearinghouses, National Guideline Clearinghouse™ (NGC) and National Quality Measures Clearinghouse™ (NQMC).

STEER CLEAR OF DECEPTIVE ADVERTISEMENTS AND INFORMATION

While searching for information either on or off the Internet, beware of "miracle" treatments and cures. They can cost you money and your health, especially if you delay or refuse proper treatment. Here are some tip-offs that a product truly is too good to be true:

- Phrases, such as "scientific breakthrough," "miraculous cure," "exclusive product," "secret formula," or "ancient ingredient"
- Claims that the product treats a wide range of ailments
- Use of impressive-sounding medical terms. These often cover up a lack of good science behind the product.
- Case histories from consumers claiming "amazing" results
- Claims that the product is available from only one source, and for a limited time only
- Claims of a "money-back guarantee"
- Claims that others are trying to keep the product off the market
- Advertisements that fail to list the company's name, address, or other contact information

Chapter 12 | **Getting a Second Opinion**

A second opinion is when another doctor examines your medical records and gives her or his views about your condition and how it should be treated.

WHAT IS THE NEED FOR A SECOND OPINION?
You might want a second opinion to:
- Be clear about what you have
- Know all of your treatment choices
- Have another doctor look at your choices with you

It is not pushy or rude to want a second opinion. Most doctors will understand that you need more information before making important decisions about your health.

Check to see whether your health plan covers a second opinion. In some cases, health plans require second opinions.

FINDING A DOCTOR FOR A SECOND OPINION
Ask your doctor for the name of another doctor to see for a second opinion. Do not hesitate to ask—most doctors will encourage you to get a second opinion. You can also ask another doctor you trust to recommend a doctor for a second opinion.

Ask your local medical society for the names of doctors who treat your illness or injury. Your local library can help you find your local medical society.

Make sure the doctor giving the second opinion accepts Medicare. Find a doctor that accepts Medicare.

This chapter contains text excerpted from the following sources: Text in this chapter begins with excerpts from "Next Steps after Your Diagnosis," Agency for Healthcare Research and Quality (AHRQ), U.S. Department of Health and Human Services (HHS), June 2016. Reviewed December 2019; Text beginning with the heading "Finding a Doctor for a Second Opinion" is excerpted from "Get a Second Opinion before Surgery," Centers for Medicare & Medicaid Services (CMS), July 18, 2012. Reviewed December 2019.

WHAT TO DO WHEN YOU GET A SECOND OPINION

Before you visit the second doctor, you may want to:

- Ask your doctor to send your medical records to the doctor giving the second opinion. That way, you may not have to repeat any tests you already had. Also, call the second doctor's office and make sure they got your records.
- Write down a list of questions to take with you to the appointment
- Ask a friend or loved one to go to the appointment with you

During your visit with the second doctor, you may want to:

- Tell the doctor what treatment your first doctor recommended
- Tell the doctor what tests you already had
- Ask the questions you have on your list. Encourage your friend or loved one to ask any questions that she or he may have.

WHAT IF THE FIRST AND SECOND OPINIONS ARE DIFFERENT?

If the second doctor does not agree with the first, you may feel unsure what to do. In that case, you may want to:

- Talk more about your condition with your first doctor
- Talk to a third doctor. Medicare helps pay for a third opinion

Getting a second opinion does not mean you have to change doctors. You choose which doctor you want to get treated.

Chapter 13 | **Medical Specialties Overview**

This chapter provides definitions of medical specialties for physicians followed by a list of specialties for other clinicians. Please note that the specialties listed here are the specialties that the clinicians indicate when they enroll in Medicare.

PHYSICIAN SPECIALTIES

- **Addiction medicine.** Specialists in addiction medicine treat substance abuse and addiction.
- **Advanced heart failure and transplant cardiology.** Advanced heart failure and transplant cardiologists manage and treat advanced or complicated heart failure.
- **Allergy/immunology.** Specialists in allergy and immunology treat conditions that involve the immune system, such as allergies, immune deficiency diseases, and autoimmune diseases.
- **Anesthesiology.** Anesthesiologists provide anesthesia for patients who are having surgery or other procedures. They also treat pain and care for patients with critical illnesses or severe injuries.
- **Cardiac electrophysiology.** Cardiac electrophysiologists use technical procedures to evaluate heart rhythms.
- **Cardiac surgery.** Cardiac surgeons treat problems in the chest, including problems affecting the heart, lungs, or windpipe. This is related to thoracic surgery.
- **Cardiology.** Cardiologists treat diseases of the heart and blood vessels.
- **Chiropractic.** Chiropractors adjust specific parts of the body (often the spine) to prevent and treat diseases.
- **Colorectal surgery (proctology).** Colorectal surgeons treat diseases of the lower digestive tract.

This chapter includes text excerpted from "Physician Compare," Centers for Medicare & Medicaid Services (CMS), October 3, 2019.

- **Critical care (intensivists).** Intensivists treat critically ill or injured patients.
- **Dermatology.** Dermatologists treat skin conditions.
- **Diagnostic radiology.** Diagnostic radiologists use imaging, such as x-rays or ultrasound, to diagnose diseases.
- **Emergency medicine.** Emergency medicine specialists take care of patients with critical illnesses or injuries.
- **Endocrinology.** Endocrinologists treat diseases that involve the internal (endocrine) glands. Examples include diabetes and diseases of the thyroid, pituitary, or adrenal glands.
- **Family practice.** Family practitioners provide primary care for people of all ages. They treat illnesses, provide preventive care, and coordinate the care provided by other health clinicians.
- **Gastroenterology.** Gastroenterologists treat diseases of the digestive organs, including the stomach, bowels, liver, and gallbladder.
- **General practice.** General practitioners provide primary care. They treat illnesses, provide preventive care, and coordinate the care provided by other clinicians.
- **General surgery.** General surgeons take care of patients who may need surgery.
- **Geriatric medicine.** Geriatricians provide primary care for elderly patients.
- **Gynecological oncology.** Gynecological oncologists treat cancers of the female reproductive organs.
- **Hand surgery.** Hand surgeons perform surgery for patients with problems that affect the hand, wrist, or forearm.
- **Hematology.** Hematologists treat diseases of the blood, spleen, and lymph. Examples include anemia, sickle cell disease, hemophilia, and leukemia.
- **Hematology/oncology.** Hematologists treat diseases of the blood, spleen, and lymph. Examples include anemia, sickle cell disease (SCD), hemophilia, and leukemia. Oncologists treat cancer with chemotherapy, hormonal therapy, biological therapy, and targeted therapy. They may also coordinate cancer care given by other specialists.
- **Hematopoietic cell transplantation and cellular therapy.** Hematopoietic cell transplantation and cellular therapy specialists provide immune system treatment for patients with leukemia or other blood or bone marrow diseases.
- **Hospice and palliative care.** Hospice and palliative care physicians manage pain and other distressing symptoms of serious illnesses. "Hospice care" is palliative care for patients who are expected to have six months or less to live.
- **Hospitalist.** Hospitalists are physicians who provide general medical care to hospitalized patients.

Medical Specialties Overview

- **Infectious disease.** Infectious disease physicians treat patients with all types of infectious diseases.
- **Internal medicine.** Internists treat diseases of the internal organs that do not require surgery. They also provide primary care for teenagers, adults, and elderly people.
- **Interventional cardiology.** Interventional cardiologists are the heart and circulatory system specialists who use minimally invasive catheterization techniques to diagnose and treat coronary arteries, the peripheral vascular system, heart valves, and congenital heart defects (CHD).
- **Interventional pain management.** Interventional pain management specialists use special procedures to treat and manage pain. For example, they may use cryoablation (a procedure involving extreme cold) to stop a nerve from working for a long period of time.
- **Interventional radiology.** Interventional radiologists perform procedures guided by various types of imaging. For example, they may use imaging to find a clogged spot in an artery and to guide a procedure to unclog it.
- **Medical genetics and genomics.** Medical geneticists specialize in the interaction between genes and health. They evaluate, treat, and counsel patients with hereditary disorders.
- **Medical oncology.** Medical oncologists treat cancer with chemotherapy, hormonal therapy, biological therapy, and targeted therapy. They may also coordinate cancer care given by other specialists.
- **Medical toxicology.** Medical toxicologists specialize in the prevention and treatment of injury and illness from exposure to drugs and chemicals.
- **Nephrology.** Nephrologists treat disorders of the kidneys.
- **Neurology.** Neurologists treat diseases of the brain, spinal cord, and nerves.
- **Neuropsychiatry.** Neuropsychiatrists treat patients with behavioral disturbances related to nervous system problems.
- **Neurosurgery.** Neurosurgeons perform surgery to treat problems in the brain, spine, and nerves.
- **Nuclear medicine.** Nuclear medicine specialists use radioactive materials to diagnose and treat diseases.
- **Obstetrics/gynecology.** Obstetricians and gynecologists take care of women during pregnancy and childbirth (called "obstetrics"). They also treat disorders of the female reproductive system (called "gynecology").
- **Ophthalmology.** Ophthalmologists are physicians who specialize in the care of the eyes. They prescribe glasses and contact lenses, diagnose and treat eye conditions, and perform eye surgery.

- **Optometry.** Optometrists are eye care professionals who perform eye examinations, prescribe corrective lenses, and treat some eye diseases that do not require surgery.
- **Oral surgery.** Oral surgeons are dentists who use surgery to treat problems in the mouth and nearby areas.
- **Orthopedic surgery.** Orthopedic surgeons treat diseases, injuries, and deformities of the bones and muscles.
- **Osteopathic manipulative medicine.** Osteopathic physicians often use a treatment method called "OMT" This is a hands-on approach to make sure that the body is moving freely.
- **Otolaryngology.** Otolaryngologists treat conditions of the ears, nose, and throat (ENT) and related areas of the head and neck.
- **Pain management.** Pain management specialists take care of patients with pain.
- **Palliative care.** Palliative-care physicians manage pain and other distressing symptoms of serious illnesses. This is related to hospice care.
- **Pathology.** Pathologists examine body tissues and interpret laboratory test results.
- **Pediatric medicine.** Pediatricians provide primary care for infants, children, and teenagers.
- **Peripheral vascular disease (PVD).** PVD physicians treat diseases of the circulatory system other than those of the brain and heart.
- **Physical medicine and rehabilitation.** Physical medicine and rehabilitation specialists are physicians who treat patients with short- or long-term disabilities.
- **Plastic and reconstructive surgery.** Plastic and reconstructive surgeons perform procedures to improve the appearance or function of parts of the body.
- **Podiatry.** Podiatrists specialize in caring for the foot and treating foot diseases.
- **Preventive medicine.** Preventive medicine specialists work to promote the health and well-being of individuals or groups of people.
- **Primary care.** Primary-care physicians treat illnesses, provide preventive care, and coordinate the care provided by other clinicians. Physicians in family practice, general practice, geriatric medicine, and internal medicine provide primary care.
- **Psychiatry.** Psychiatrists treat mental, addictive, and emotional disorders.
- **Psychiatry (Geriatric).** Geriatric psychiatrists treat mental and emotional disorders in elderly people.
- **Pulmonary disease.** Pulmonologists treat diseases of the lungs and airways.

Medical Specialties Overview

- **Radiation oncology.** Radiation oncologists use radiation to treat cancer.
- **Rheumatology.** Rheumatologists treat problems involving the joints, muscles, bones, and tendons.
- **Sleep medicine.** Sleep medicine physicians treat problems related to sleep or sleep–wake cycle.
- **Sports medicine.** Sports medicine specialists treat problems related to participation in sports or exercise.
- **Surgical oncology.** Surgical oncologists specialize in the surgical diagnosis and treatment of cancer.
- **Thoracic surgery.** Thoracic surgeons treat problems in the chest, including problems affecting the heart, lungs, or windpipe. This is related to cardiac surgery.
- **Undersea and hyperbaric medicine.** Undersea and hyperbaric medicine physicians prevent and treat injury and illness from exposure to environments with increased pressure, such as in diving.
- **Urology.** Urologists treat problems in the male and female urinary tract and the male reproductive system.
- **Vascular surgery.** Vascular surgeons treat diseases of the circulatory system, other than the brain and heart.

OTHER CLINICIANS

- **Anesthesiologist assistant.** Anesthesiologist assistants work under the direction of an anesthesiologist as a part of the anesthesia care team.
- **Audiology.** Audiologists have advanced training and evaluate hearing or balance problems. They provide hearing aids and counsel people about how to cope with hearing loss.
- **Certified nurse-midwife (CNM).** CNMs are registered nurses who have earned a master's degree in nursing and met other requirements. They practice in hospitals and medical clinics. They may also deliver babies in birthing centers and attend home births.
- **Certified registered nurse anesthetist (CRNA).** CRNAs are registered nurses who have earned a master's degree in nursing and met other requirements. They provide anesthesia and work with other clinicians.
- **Clinical nurse specialist (CNS).** CNSs are registered nurses who have earned a master's degree in nursing and met other requirements. They handle a range of physical and mental-health problems.
- **Clinical psychologist.** Clinical psychologists have a doctorate in psychology and have advanced training in promoting mental health and helping people cope with problems.
- **Clinical social worker (CSW).** CSWs have earned a master's degree, and help people deal with life changes and challenges, including mental disorders.

- **Nurse practitioner (NP).** NPs are registered nurses who have earned a master's degree in nursing and met other requirements. They provide primary and preventive care, prescribe medicines, and treat common minor illnesses and injuries.
- **Occupational therapy.** Occupational therapists (OTs) help people who are recovering from injuries to regain skills. They also support people who are going through changes related to aging. They provide home assessments, teach people to use adaptive equipment (such as devices to help with bathing, dressing, or eating), and work with family members and caregivers. OTs are state-licensed and nationally certified to practice.
- **Physical therapy.** Physical therapists (PTs) provide rehabilitation to help people move, reduce pain, restore function, and prevent disability. PTs are state-licensed and nationally certified to practice.
- **Physician assistant (PA).** PAs are graduates of accredited PA educational programs. They are licensed to practice medicine with a physician's supervision. They examine patients, diagnose and treat illnesses, order lab tests, prescribe medicines, perform procedures, assist in surgery, and counsel patients.
- **Registered dietitian/nutrition professional.** RDs and other nutrition professionals are food and nutrition experts. They teach patients about nutrition. They also provide medical nutrition therapy.
- **Speech-language pathology.** Speech-language pathologists (SLP), sometimes called "speech therapists," treat communication and swallowing disorders. They are state-licensed and nationally certified in speech-language pathology.

Chapter 14 | Selecting a Complementary and Alternative Medicine Practitioner

CONSIDERING COMPLEMENTARY HEALTH APPROACH: WHAT YOU NEED TO KNOW

Millions of Americans use complementary health approaches. Like any decision concerning your health, decisions about whether to use complementary approaches are important. This chapter will assist you in your decision-making about complementary-health products and practices.

What Do "Complementary," Alternative," and "Integrative" Mean?

"Complementary and alternative medicine," "complementary medicine," "alternative medicine," "integrative medicine"—you may have seen these terms on the Internet and in marketing, but what do they really mean? While the terms are often used to mean the array of healthcare approaches with a history of use or origins outside of mainstream medicine, they are actually hard to define and may mean different things to different people.

The terms "complementary" and "integrative" refer to the use of nonmainstream approaches together with conventional medical approaches.

This chapter contains text excerpted from the following sources: Text under the heading "Considering Complementary Health Approach: What You Need to Know" is excerpted from "Are You Considering a Complementary Health Approach?" National Center for Complementary and Integrative Health (NCCIH), September 2016. Reviewed December 2019; Text under the heading "Things to Know When Selecting a Complementary-Health Practitioner" is excerpted from "6 Things to Know When Selecting a Complementary Health Practitioner," National Center for Complementary and Integrative Health (NCCIH), October 9, 2019; Text under the heading "Talk with Your Healthcare Providers about Complementary Health Approaches" is excerpted from "4 Tips: Start Talking with Your Healthcare Providers about Complementary Health Approaches," National Center for Complementary and Integrative Health (NCCIH), October 9, 2019.

"Alternative health approaches" refers to the use of nonmainstream products or practices in place of conventional medicine. The National Center for Complementary and Integrative Health (NCCIH) advises against using any product or practice that has not been proven safe and effective as a substitute for conventional medical treatment or as a reason to postpone seeing your healthcare provider about any health problem. In some instances, stopping—or not starting—conventional treatment can have serious consequences. Before making a decision not to use a proven conventional treatment, talk to your healthcare providers.

Are Complementary Health Approaches Safe?

As with any medical product or treatment, there can be risks with complementary approaches. These risks depend on the specific product or practice. Each needs to be considered on its own. However, if you are considering a specific product or practice, the following general suggestions can help you think about safety and minimize risks.

- Be aware that individuals respond differently to health products and practices, whether conventional or complementary. How you might respond to one depends on many things, including your state of health, how you use it, or your belief in it.
- Keep in mind that "natural" does not necessarily mean "safe." (Think of mushrooms that grow in the wild: some are safe to eat, while others are not.)
- Learn about factors that affect safety. For a practice that is administered by a practitioner, such as chiropractic, these factors include the training, skill, and experience of the practitioner. For a product such as a dietary supplement, the specific ingredients and the quality of the manufacturing process are important factors.
- If you decide to use a practice provided by a complementary-health practitioner, choose the practitioner as carefully as you would your primary-healthcare provider.
- If you decide to use a dietary supplement, such as an herbal product, be aware that some products may interact in harmful ways with medications (prescription or over-the-counter (OTC)) or other dietary supplements, and some may have side effects on their own.
- Tell all your healthcare providers about any complementary or integrative-health approaches you use. Give them a full picture of what you do to manage your health. This will help ensure coordinated and safe care.

Where Can I Get Reliable Information about a Complementary-Health Approach?

It is important to learn what scientific studies have discovered about the complementary-health approach you are considering. Evidence from research studies

Selecting a Complementary and Alternative Medicine Practitioner

is stronger and more reliable than something you have seen in an advertisement or on a website, or something someone told you about that worked for them.

Understanding a product's or practice's potential benefits, risks, and scientific evidence is critical to your health and safety. Scientific research on many complementary-health approaches is relatively new, so this kind of information may not be available for each one. However, many studies are underway, including those that NCCIH supports, and knowledge and understanding of complementary approaches are increasing all the time. Here are some ways to find reliable information:

- **Talk with your healthcare providers.** Tell them about the complementary-health approach you are considering and ask any questions you may have about safety, effectiveness, or interactions with medications (prescription or nonprescription) or dietary supplements.
- **Visit the NCCIH website.** The "Health Information" page has an A-to-Z list of complementary-health products and practices, which describes what the science says about them, and links to other objective sources of online information. The website also has contact information for the NCCIH Clearinghouse, where information specialists are available to assist you in searching the scientific literature and to suggest useful NCCIH publications.
- **Visit your local library or a medical library.** Ask the reference librarian to help you find scientific journals and trustworthy books with information on the product or practice that interests you.

How Can I Determine Whether Statements Made about the Effectiveness of a Complementary-Health Approach Are True?

Before you begin using a complementary-health approach, it is a good idea to ask the following questions:

- Is there scientific evidence (not just personal stories) to back up the statements?
- What is the source? Statements that manufacturers or other promoters of some complementary-health approaches may make about effectiveness and benefits can sound reasonable and promising. However, the statements may be based on a biased view of the available scientific evidence.
- Does the federal government have anything to report about the product or practice?
- Visit the NCCIH website or contact the NCCIH Clearinghouse to see if NCCIH has information about the product or practice.
- Visit the U.S. Food and Drug Administration (FDA) online at www.fda.gov to see if there is any information available about the product or practice.

- Information specifically about dietary supplements can be found on the FDA's website at www.fda.gov/Food/DietarySupplements and on the website of the National Institutes of Health's (NIH) Office of Dietary Supplements (ODS) at ods.od.nih.gov.
- Visit the FDA's webpage on recalls and safety alerts at www.fda.gov/Safety/Recalls. The FDA has a rapid public-notification system to provide information about tainted dietary supplements.
- Check with the Federal Trade Commission (FTC) at www.ftc.gov to see if there are any enforcement actions for deceptive advertising regarding the therapy. Also, visit the site's consumer information section at www.consumer.ftc.gov.
- How does the provider or manufacturer describe the approach?
- Beware of terms such as "scientific breakthrough," "miracle cure," "secret ingredient," or "ancient remedy."
- If you encounter claims of a "quick fix" that departs from previous research, keep in mind that science usually advances over time by small steps, slowly building an evidence base.

Remember. If it sounds too good to be true—for example, claims that a product or practice can cure a disease or work for a variety of ailments—it usually is.

Is That Health Website Trustworthy?

If you are visiting a health website for the first time, these five quick questions can help you decide whether the site is a helpful resource.
- **Who?** Who runs the website? Can you trust them?
- **What?** What does the site say? Do its claims seem too good to be true?
- **When?** When was the information posted or reviewed? Is it up-to-date?
- **Where?** Where did the information come from? Is it based on scientific research?
- **Why?** Why does the site exist? Is it selling something?

Are You Reading Real Online News or Just Advertising?

In April 2011, the FTC warned the public about fake online news sites promoting an acai berry weight-loss product. For example, one described an investigation in which a reporter used the product for several weeks, with "dramatic" results. The site looked real, but it was actually an advertisement. Everything was fake: there was no reporter, no news organization, and no investigation. The only real things were the links to a sales site that appeared in the story and elsewhere on the webpage. Similar fake news sites have promoted other products, including work-at-home opportunities and debt reduction plans.

You should suspect that a news site may be fake if it:
- Endorses a product. Real news organizations generally do not do this.

Selecting a Complementary and Alternative Medicine Practitioner

- Only quotes people who say good things about the product
- Presents research findings that seem too good to be true or fail to point out any limitations in research. (If something seems too good to be true, it usually is.)
- Contains links to a sales site
- Includes positive reader comments only, and you cannot add a comment of your own

How to Protect Yourself

If you suspect that a news site might be fake, look for a disclaimer somewhere on the page (often in small print) that indicates that the site is an advertisement. Also, do not rely on Internet news reports when making important decisions about your health. If you are considering a health product described in the news, discuss it with your healthcare provider.

Are Complementary-Health Approaches Tested to See If They Work?

While scientific evidence now exists regarding the effectiveness and safety of some complementary-health approaches, there remain many yet-to-be-answered questions about whether others are safe, whether they work for the diseases or medical conditions for which they are promoted, and how those approaches with health benefits may work. As the federal government's lead agency for scientific research on health interventions, practices, products, and disciplines that originate from outside mainstream medicine, NCCIH supports scientific research to answer these questions and determine who might benefit most from the use of specific approaches.

I Am Interested in an Approach That Involves Seeing a Complementary-Health Practitioner. How Do I Go about Selecting a Practitioner?

- Your primary-healthcare provider or local hospital may be able to recommend a complementary-health practitioner.
- The professional organization for the type of practitioner you are seeking may have helpful information, such as licensing and training requirements. Many states have regulatory agencies or licensing boards for certain types of complementary-health practitioners; they may be able to help you locate practitioners in your area.
- Make sure any practitioner you are considering is willing to work in collaboration with your other healthcare providers.

Can I Receive Treatment or Referral to a Complementary-Health Practitioner from NCCIH?

The NCCIH does not provide treatment or referrals to complementary-health practitioners.

THINGS TO KNOW WHEN SELECTING A COMPLEMENTARY-HEALTH PRACTITIONER

If you are looking for a complementary-health practitioner to help treat a medical problem, it is important to be as careful and thorough in your search as you are when looking for conventional care.

Here are some tips to help you in your search:

- **If you need names of practitioners in your area, first check with your doctor or other healthcare provider.** A nearby hospital or medical school, professional organizations, state regulatory agencies or licensing boards, or even your health-insurance provider may be helpful. Unfortunately, the NCCIH cannot refer you to practitioners.
- **Find out as much as you can about any potential practitioner, including education, training, licensing, and certifications.** The credentials required for complementary-health practitioners vary tremendously from state to state and from discipline to discipline.

Once you have found a possible practitioner, here are some tips about deciding whether she or he is right for you:

- **Find out whether the practitioner is willing to work together with your conventional healthcare providers.** For safe, coordinated care, it is important for all of the professionals involved in your health to communicate and cooperate.
- **Explain all of your health conditions to the practitioner, and find out about the practitioner's training and experience in working with people who have your conditions.** Choose a practitioner who understands how to work with people with your specific needs, even if general well-being is your goal. And, remember that health conditions can affect the safety of complementary approaches; for example, if you have glaucoma, some yoga poses may not be safe for you.
- **Do not assume that your health insurance will cover the practitioner's services.** Contact your health-insurance provider and ask. Insurance plans differ greatly in what complementary-health approaches they cover, and even if they cover a particular approach, restrictions may apply.
- **Tell all your healthcare providers about the complementary approaches you use and about all practitioners who are treating you.** Keeping your healthcare providers fully informed helps you to stay in control and effectively manage your health.

TALK WITH YOUR HEALTHCARE PROVIDERS ABOUT COMPLEMENTARY-HEALTH APPROACHES

When patients tell their providers about their use of complementary-health practices, they can better stay in control and more effectively manage their health. When providers ask their patients, they can ensure that they are fully informed and can help patients make wise healthcare decisions.

Find below a few tips to help you and your healthcare providers start talking:

- **List the complementary-health practices you use on your patient history form.** When completing the patient history form, be sure to include everything you use—from acupuncture to zinc. It is important to give healthcare providers a full picture of what you do to manage your health.
- **At each visit, be sure to tell your providers about what complementary-health approaches you are using.** Do not forget to include OTC and prescription medicines, as well as dietary and herbal supplements. Make a list in advance and take it with you. Your healthcare provider needs to know in advance if you are following any complementary-health approaches for some of them can have an effect on conventional medicine.
- **If you are considering a new complementary-health practice, ask questions.** Ask your healthcare provider about its safety, effectiveness, and possible interactions with medications (both prescription and nonprescription).
- **Do not wait for your providers to ask about any complementary-health practice you are using.** Be proactive. Start the conversation.

Chapter 15 | An Introduction to Clinical Studies

WHAT IS A CLINICAL STUDY?

A clinical study involves research using human volunteers (also called "participants") that is intended to add to medical knowledge. There are two main types of clinical studies: clinical trials (also called "interventional studies") and observational studies.

Clinical Trials

In a clinical trial, participants receive specific interventions according to the research plan or protocol created by the investigators. These interventions may be medical products, such as drugs or devices; procedures; or changes to participants' behavior, such as diet. Clinical trials may compare a new medical approach to a standard one that is already available, to a placebo that contains no active ingredients, or to no intervention. Some clinical trials compare interventions that are already available to each other. When a new product or approach is being studied, it is not usually known whether it will be helpful, harmful, or no different than available alternatives (including no intervention). The investigators try to determine the safety and efficacy of the intervention by measuring certain outcomes in the participants. For example, investigators may give a drug or treatment to participants who have high blood pressure to see whether their blood pressure decreases.

Clinical trials used in drug development are sometimes described by phase. These phases are defined by the U.S. Food and Drug Administration (FDA).

Some people who are not eligible to participate in a clinical trial may be able to get experimental drugs or devices outside of a clinical trial through expanded access.

This chapter includes text excerpted from "Learn about Clinical Studies," ClinicalTrials.gov, National Institutes of Health (NIH), March 2019.

Observational Studies

In an observational study, investigators assess health outcomes in groups of participants according to a research plan or protocol. Participants may receive interventions (which can include medical products, such as drugs or devices) or procedures as part of their routine medical care, but participants are not assigned to specific interventions by the investigator (as in a clinical trial). For example, investigators may observe a group of older adults to learn more about the effects of different lifestyles on cardiac health.

WHO CONDUCTS CLINICAL STUDIES?

Every clinical study is led by a principal investigator, who is often a medical doctor. Clinical studies also have a research team that may include doctors, nurses, social workers, and other healthcare professionals.

Clinical studies can be sponsored, or funded, by pharmaceutical companies, academic medical centers, voluntary groups, and other organizations, in addition to federal agencies, such as the National Institutes of Health (NIH), the U.S. Department of Defense (DOD), and the U.S. Department of Veterans Affairs (VA). Doctors, other healthcare providers, and other individuals can also sponsor clinical research.

WHERE ARE CLINICAL STUDIES CONDUCTED?

Clinical studies can take place in many locations, including hospitals, universities, doctors' offices, and community clinics. The location depends on who is conducting the study.

HOW LONG DO CLINICAL STUDIES LAST?

The length of a clinical study varies, depending on what is being studied. Participants are told how long the study will last before they enroll.

REASONS FOR CONDUCTING CLINICAL STUDIES

In general, clinical studies are designed to add to medical knowledge related to the treatment, diagnosis, and prevention of diseases or conditions. Some common reasons for conducting clinical studies include:

- Evaluating one or more interventions (for example, drugs, medical devices, approaches to surgery or radiation therapy) for treating a disease, syndrome, or condition
- Finding ways to prevent the initial development or recurrence of a disease or condition. These can include medicines, vaccines, or lifestyle changes, among other approaches.
- Evaluating one or more interventions aimed at identifying or diagnosing a particular disease or condition

- Examining methods for identifying a condition or the risk factors for that condition
- Exploring and measuring ways to improve the comfort and quality of life (QOL) through supportive care for people with a chronic illness

PARTICIPATING IN CLINICAL STUDIES

A clinical study is conducted according to a research plan known as the "protocol." The protocol is designed to answer specific research questions and safeguard the health of participants. It contains the following information:

- The reason for conducting the study
- Who may participate in the study (the eligibility criteria)?
- The number of participants needed
- The schedule of tests, procedures, or drugs and their dosages
- The length of the study
- What information will be gathered about the participants?

Who Can Participate in a Clinical Study?

Clinical studies have standards outlining who can participate. These standards are called "eligibility criteria" and are listed in the protocol. Some research studies seek participants who have illnesses or conditions that will be studied, other studies are looking for healthy participants, and some studies are limited to a predetermined group of people who are asked by researchers to enroll.

Eligibility. The factors that allow someone to participate in a clinical study are called "inclusion criteria," and the factors that disqualify someone from participating are called "exclusion criteria." They are based on characteristics, such as age, gender, the type and stage of a disease, previous treatment history, and other medical conditions.

How Are Participants Protected?

Informed consent is a process used by researchers to provide potential and enrolled participants with information about a clinical study. This information helps people decide whether they want to enroll or continue to participate in the study. The informed consent process is intended to protect participants and should provide enough information for a person to understand the risks of, potential benefits of, and alternatives to the study. In addition to the informed consent document, the process may involve recruitment materials, verbal instructions, question-and-answer sessions, and activities to measure participant understanding. In general, a person must sign an informed consent document before joining a study to show that she or he was given information on the risks, potential benefits, and alternatives and that she or he understands it. Signing the document and providing consent is not a contract. Participants may withdraw from a study at any time, even if the study is not over.

Institutional review boards (IRB). Each federally supported or conducted clinical study and each study of a drug, biological product, or medical device regulated by the FDA must be reviewed, approved, and monitored by an IRB. An IRB is made up of doctors, researchers, and members of the community. Its role is to make sure that the study is ethical and that the rights and welfare of participants are protected. This includes making sure that research risks are minimized and are reasonable in relation to any potential benefits, among other responsibilities. The IRB also reviews the informed consent document.

In addition to being monitored by an IRB, some clinical studies are also monitored by data monitoring committees (also called "data safety" and "monitoring boards").

Various federal agencies, including the Office of Human Subjects Research Protection (OHRP) and FDA, have the authority to determine whether sponsors of certain clinical studies are adequately protecting research participants.

Relationship to Usual Healthcare

Typically, participants continue to see their usual healthcare providers while enrolled in a clinical study. While most clinical studies provide participants with medical products or interventions related to the illness or condition being studied, they do not provide extended or complete healthcare. By having her or his usual healthcare provider work with the research team, a participant can make sure that the study protocol will not conflict with other medications or treatments that she or he receives.

Considerations for Participation

Participating in a clinical study contributes to medical knowledge. The results of these studies can make a difference in the care of future patients by providing information about the benefits and risks of therapeutic, preventative, or diagnostic products or interventions.

Clinical trials provide the basis for the development and marketing of new drugs, biological products, and medical devices. Sometimes, the safety and effectiveness of the experimental approach or use may not be fully known at the time of the trial. Some trials may provide participants with the prospect of receiving direct medical benefits, while others do not.

Most trials involve some risk of harm or injury to the participant, although it may not be greater than the risks related to routine medical care or disease progression. (For trials approved by IRBs, the IRB has decided that the risks of participation have been minimized and are reasonable in relation to anticipated benefits.)

An Introduction to Clinical Studies

Many trials require participants to undergo additional procedures, tests, and assessments based on the study protocol. These requirements will be described in the informed consent document. A potential participant should also discuss these issues with members of the research team and with her or his usual healthcare provider.

Questions to Ask

Anyone interested in participating in a clinical study should know as much as possible about the study and feel comfortable asking the research team questions about the study, the related procedures, and any expenses. The following questions may be helpful during such a discussion. Answers to some of these questions are provided in the informed consent document. Many of the questions are specific to clinical trials, but some also apply to observational studies.

- What is being studied?
- Why do researchers believe the intervention being tested might be effective? Why might it not be effective? Has it been tested before?
- What are the possible interventions that I might receive during the trial?
- How will it be determined which interventions I receive (for example, by chance)?
- Who will know which intervention I receive during the trial? Will I know? Will members of the research team know?
- How do the possible risks, side effects, and benefits of this trial compare with those of my current treatment?
- What should I do?
- What tests and procedures are involved?
- How often will I have to visit the hospital or clinic?
- Will hospitalization be required?
- How long will the study last?
- Who will pay for my participation?
- Will I be reimbursed for other expenses?
- What type of long-term follow-up care is part of this trial?
- If I benefit from the intervention, will I be allowed to continue receiving it after the trial ends?
- Will the results of the study be provided to me?
- Who will oversee my medical care while I am participating in the trial?
- What are my options if I am injured during the study?

Chapter 16 | **Clinical Trials: An Overview**

WHAT ARE CLINICAL TRIALS AND WHY DO PEOPLE PARTICIPATE?

Clinical research is medical research that involves people like you. When you volunteer to take part in clinical research, you help doctors and researchers learn more about the disease and improve healthcare for people in the future. Clinical research includes all research that involves people. Types of clinical research include:

- **Epidemiology,** which improves the understanding of a disease by studying patterns, causes, and effects of health and disease in specific groups
- **Behavioral,** which improves the understanding of human behavior and how it relates to health and disease
- **Health services,** which looks at how people access healthcare providers and healthcare services, how much care costs, and what happens to patients as a result of this care
- **Clinical trials,** which evaluate the effects of an intervention on health outcomes

WHAT ARE CLINICAL TRIALS AND WHY WOULD YOU WANT TO TAKE PART?

Clinical trials are part of clinical research and at the heart of all medical advances. Clinical trials look at new ways to prevent, detect, or treat disease. Clinical trials can study:

- New drugs or new combinations of drugs
- New ways of doing surgery
- New medical devices
- New ways to use existing treatments
- New ways to change behaviors to improve health

This chapter includes text excerpted from "The Basics," National Institutes of Health (NIH), October 20, 2017.

- New ways to improve the quality of life (QOL) for people with acute or chronic illnesses

The goal of clinical trials is to determine if these treatments, prevention, and behavior approaches are safe and effective. People take part in clinical trials for many reasons. Healthy volunteers say they take part to help others and to contribute to moving science forward. People with an illness or disease also participate to help others, but also to possibly receive the newest treatment and to have added (or extra) care and attention from the clinical trial staff. Clinical trials offer hope for many people and a chance to help researchers find better treatments for others in the future.

HOW DOES THE RESEARCH PROCESS WORK?

The idea for a clinical trial often starts in the lab. After researchers test new treatments or procedures in the lab and in animals, the most promising treatments are moved into clinical trials. As new treatments move through a series of steps called "phases," more information is gained about the treatment, its risks, and its effectiveness.

WHAT ARE CLINICAL TRIAL PROTOCOLS?

Clinical trials follow a plan known as a "protocol." The protocol is carefully designed to balance the potential benefits and risks to participants and answer specific research questions. A protocol describes the following:

- The goal of the study
- Who is eligible to take part in the trial
- Protections against risks to participants
- Details about tests, procedures, and treatments
- How long the trial is expected to last
- What information will be gathered

A clinical trial is led by a principal investigator (PI). Members of the research team regularly monitor the participants' health to determine the study's safety and effectiveness.

WHAT IS AN INSTITUTIONAL REVIEW BOARD?

Most, but not all, clinical trials in the United States are approved and monitored by an institutional review board (IRB) to ensure that the risks are reduced and are outweighed by potential benefits. IRBs are committees that are responsible for reviewing research in order to protect the rights and safety of people who take part in research, both before the research starts and as it proceeds. You should ask the sponsor or research coordinator whether the research you are thinking about joining was reviewed by an IRB.

WHAT IS A CLINICAL TRIAL SPONSOR?

Clinical trial sponsors may be people, institutions, companies, government agencies, or other organizations that are responsible for initiating, managing or financing the clinical trial, but do not conduct the research.

WHAT IS INFORMED CONSENT?

Informed consent is the process of providing you with key information about a research study before you decide whether to accept the offer to take part. The process of informed consent continues throughout the study.

To help you decide whether to take part, members of the research team explain the details of the study. If you do not understand English, a translator or interpreter may be provided. The research team provides an informed consent document that includes details about the study, such as its purpose, how long it is expected to last, tests or procedures that will be done as part of the research, and who to contact for further information. The informed consent document also explains risks and potential benefits. You can then decide whether to sign the document.

Taking part in a clinical trial is voluntary and you can leave the study at any time.

WHAT ARE THE TYPES OF CLINICAL TRIALS?

There are different types of clinical trials.

- **Prevention trials** look for better ways to prevent a disease in people who have never had the disease or to prevent the disease from returning. Approaches may include medicines, vaccines, or lifestyle changes.
- **Screening trials** test new ways of detecting diseases or health conditions.
- **Diagnostic trials** study or compare tests or procedures for diagnosing a particular disease or condition.
- **Treatment trials** test new treatments, new combinations of drugs, or new approaches to surgery or radiation therapy.
- **Behavioral trials** evaluate or compare ways to promote behavioral changes designed to improve health.
- **Quality of life trials** (or supportive care trials) explores and measure ways to improve the comfort and QOL of people with conditions or illnesses.

WHAT ARE THE PHASES OF CLINICAL TRIALS?

Clinical trials are conducted in a series of steps called "phases." Each phase has a different purpose and helps researchers answer different questions.

- **Phase I trials.** Researchers test a drug or treatment in a small group of people (20 to 80) for the first time. The purpose is to study the drug or treatment to learn about safety and identify side effects.
- **Phase II trials.** The new drug or treatment is given to a larger group of people (100 to 300) to determine its effectiveness and to further study its safety.
- **Phase III trials.** The new drug or treatment is given to large groups of people (1,000 to 3,000) to confirm its effectiveness, monitor side effects, compare it with standard or similar treatments, and collect information that will allow the new drug or treatment to be used safely.
- **Phase IV trials.** After a drug is approved by the U.S. Food and Drug Administration (FDA) and made available to the public, researchers track its safety in the general population, seeking more information about the benefits of a drug or a treatment, and optimal use.

WHAT DO THE TERMS "PLACEBO," "RANDOMIZATION," AND "BLINDED" MEAN IN CLINICAL TRIALS?

In clinical trials that compare a new product or therapy with another that already exists, researchers try to determine if the new one is as good, or better than the existing one. In some studies, you may be assigned to receive a placebo (an inactive product that resembles the test product, but without its treatment value).

Comparing a new product with a placebo can be the fastest and most reliable way to show the new product's effectiveness. However, placebos are not used if you would be put at risk—particularly in the study of treatments for serious illnesses—by not having effective therapy. You will be told if placebos are used in the study before entering a trial.

"Randomization" is the process by which treatments are assigned to participants by chance rather than by choice. This is done to avoid any bias in assigning volunteers to get one treatment or another. The effects of each treatment are compared at specific points during a trial. If one treatment is found superior, the trial is stopped so that most volunteers receive more beneficial treatment.

"Blinded" (or "masked") studies are designed to prevent members of the research team and study participants from influencing the results. Blinding allows the collection of scientifically accurate data. In single-blind ("single-masked") studies, you are not told what is being given, but the research team knows. In a double-blind study, neither you nor the research team is told what you are given; only the pharmacist knows. Members of the research team are not told which participants are receiving which treatment, in order to reduce bias. If medically necessary, however, it is always possible to find out which treatment you are receiving.

WHO DOES TAKE PART IN CLINICAL TRIALS?

Many different types of people take part in clinical trials. Some are healthy, while others may have illnesses. Research procedures with healthy volunteers are designed to develop new knowledge, not to provide direct benefit to those taking part. Healthy volunteers have always played an important role in research.

Healthy volunteers are needed for several reasons. When developing a new technique, such as a blood test or imaging device, healthy volunteers help define the limits of "normal." These volunteers are the baseline against which patient groups are compared and are often matched to patients on factors, such as age, gender, or family relationship. They receive the same tests, procedures, or drugs the patient group receives. Researchers learn about the disease process by comparing the patient group to healthy volunteers.

Factors such as how much of your time is needed, the discomfort you may feel, or the risk involved depend on the trial. While some require minimal amounts of time and effort, other studies may require a major commitment of your time and effort and may involve some discomfort. The research procedure(s) may also carry some risk. The informed consent process for healthy volunteers includes a detailed discussion of the study's procedures and tests and their risks.

A patient volunteer has a known health problem and takes part in research to better understand, diagnose, or treat that disease or condition. Research with a patient volunteer helps develop new knowledge. Depending on the stage of knowledge about the disease or condition, these procedures may or may not benefit the study participants.

Patients may volunteer for studies similar to those in which healthy volunteers take part. These studies involve drugs, devices, or treatments designed to prevent, or treat disease. Although these studies may provide direct benefit to patient volunteers, the main aim is to prove, by scientific means, the effects and limitations of the experimental treatment. Therefore, some patient groups may serve as a baseline for comparison by not taking the test drug, or by receiving test doses of the drug large enough only to show that it is present, but not at a level that can treat the condition.

Researchers follow clinical trial guidelines when deciding who can participate in a study. These guidelines are called "inclusion/exclusion criteria." Factors that allow you to take part in a clinical trial are called "inclusion criteria." Those that exclude or prevent participation are "exclusion criteria." These criteria are based on factors, such as age, gender, the type and stage of a disease, treatment history, and other medical conditions. Before joining a clinical trial, you must provide information that allows the research team to determine whether or not you can take part in the study safely. Some research studies seek participants with illnesses or conditions to be studied in the clinical trial, while others need healthy volunteers. Inclusion and exclusion criteria are not used to reject people personally.

Instead, the criteria are used to identify appropriate participants and keep them safe, and to help ensure that researchers can find new information they need.

TAKING PART IN A CLINICAL TRIAL
Risks and Potential Benefits
Clinical trials may involve risk, as can routine medical care and the activities of daily living. When weighing the risks of research, you can think about these important factors:
- The possible harms that could result from taking part in the study
- The level of harm
- The chance of any harm occurring

Most clinical trials pose the risk of minor discomfort, which lasts only a short time. However, some study participants experience complications that require medical attention. In rare cases, participants have been seriously injured or have died of complications resulting from their participation in trials of experimental treatments. The specific risks associated with a research protocol are described in detail in the informed consent document, which participants are asked to consider and sign before participating in research. Also, a member of the research team will explain the study and answer any questions about the study. Before deciding to participate, carefully consider risks and possible benefits.

Potential Benefits
Well-designed and well-executed clinical trials provide the best approach for you to:
- Help others by contributing to knowledge about new treatments or procedures
- Gain access to new research treatments before they are widely available
- Receive regular and careful medical attention from a research team that includes doctors and other health professionals

Risks
Risks of taking part in clinical trials include the following:
- There may be unpleasant, serious, or even life-threatening effects of experimental treatment.
- The study may require more time and attention than standard treatment would, including visits to the study site, more blood tests, more procedures, hospital stays, or complex dosage schedules.

WHAT QUESTIONS SHOULD YOU ASK IF OFFERED A CLINICAL TRIAL?
If you are thinking about taking part in a clinical trial, you should feel free to ask any questions or bring up any issues concerning the trial at any time.

Clinical Trials: An Overview

The following suggestions may give you some ideas as you think about your own questions.

The Study
- What is the purpose of the study?
- Why do researchers think the approach may be effective?
- Who will fund the study?
- Who has reviewed and approved the study?
- How are the study results and safety of participants being monitored?
- How long will the study last?
- What will my responsibilities be if I take part?
- Who will tell me about the results of the study and how will I be informed?

Risks and Possible Benefits
- What are my possible short-term benefits?
- What are my possible long-term benefits?
- What are my short-term risks, and side effects?
- What are my long-term risks?
- What other options are available?
- How do the risks and possible benefits of this trial compare with those options?

Participation and Care
- What kinds of therapies, procedures and/or tests will I have during the trial?
- Will they hurt, and if so, for how long?
- How do the tests in the study compare with those I would have outside of the trial?
- Will I be able to take my regular medications while taking part in a clinical trial?
- Where will I have my medical care?
- Who will be in charge of my care?

Personal Issues
- How could being in this study affect my daily life?
- Can I talk to other people in the study?

Cost Issues
- Will I have to pay for any part of the trial such as tests or the study drug?
- If so, what will the charges likely be?
- What is my health insurance likely to cover?

- Who can help answer any questions from my insurance company or health plan?
- Will there be any travel or child care costs that I need to consider while I am in the trial?

Tips for Asking Your Doctor about Trials

- Consider taking a family member or friend along for support and for help in asking questions or recording answers.
- Plan what to ask—but do not hesitate to ask any new questions.
- Write down questions in advance to remember them all.
- Write down the answers so that they are available when needed.
- Ask about bringing a tape recorder to make a taped record of what is said (even if you write down answers).

HOW IS YOUR SAFETY PROTECTED WHILE PARTICIPATING IN A CLINICAL TRIAL?
Ethical Guidelines

The goal of clinical research is to develop knowledge that improves human health or increases understanding of human biology. People who take part in clinical research make it possible for this to occur. The path to finding out if a new drug is safe or effective is to test it on patients in clinical trials. The purpose of ethical guidelines is both to protect patients and healthy volunteers and to preserve the integrity of the science.

Informed Consent

"Informed consent" is the process of learning the key facts about a clinical trial before deciding whether to participate. The process of providing information to participants continues throughout the study. To help you decide whether to take part, members of the research team explain the study. The research team provides an informed consent document, which includes such details about the study as its purpose, duration, required procedures, and who to contact for various purposes. The informed consent document also explains risks and potential benefits.

If you decide to enroll in the trial, you will need to sign the informed consent document. You are free to withdraw from the study at any time.

Institutional Review Board Review

Most, but not all, clinical trials in the United States are approved and monitored by an IRB to ensure that the risks are minimal when compared with potential benefits. An IRB is an independent committee that consists of physicians, statisticians, and members of the community who ensure that clinical trials are ethical and that the rights of participants are protected. You should ask the sponsor or research coordinator whether the research you are considering participating in was reviewed by an IRB.

WHAT HAPPENS AFTER A CLINICAL TRIAL IS COMPLETED?

After a clinical trial is completed, the researchers carefully examine information collected during the study before making decisions about the meaning of the findings and about the need for further testing. After a phase I or II trial, the researchers decide whether to move on to the next phase or to stop testing the treatment or procedure because it was unsafe or not effective. When a phase III trial is completed, the researchers examine the information and decide whether the results have medical importance.

Results from clinical trials are often published in peer-reviewed scientific journals. Peer review is a process by which experts review the report before it is published to ensure that the analysis and conclusions are sound. If the results are particularly important, they may be featured in the news, and discussed at scientific meetings and by patient advocacy groups before or after they are published in a scientific journal. Once a new approach has been proven safe and effective in a clinical trial, it may become a new standard of medical practice.

Ask the research team members if the study results have been or will be published. Published study results are also available by searching for the study's official name or protocol ID number in the U.S. National Library of Medicine's (NLM) PubMed® database.

HOW DOES CLINICAL RESEARCH MAKE A DIFFERENCE TO YOU AND YOUR FAMILY?

Clinical research helps in gaining insights and answers about the safety and effectiveness of treatments and procedures. Groundbreaking scientific advances in the present and the past were possible only because of the participation of volunteers, both healthy and those with an illness, in clinical research.

Clinical research requires complex and rigorous testing in collaboration with communities that are affected by the disease. As research opens new doors to finding ways to diagnose, prevent, treat, or cure disease and disability, clinical trial participation is essential to find the answers.

Chapter 17 | Healthcare Quality Issues

Chapter Contents

Section 17.1 | Understanding Healthcare Quality

This section includes text excerpted from "Guide to Healthcare Quality," Agency for Healthcare Research and Quality (AHRQ), U.S. Department of Health and Human Services (HHS), September 2005. Reviewed December 2019.

YOU DESERVE QUALITY HEALTHCARE

Getting quality healthcare can help you stay healthy and recover faster when you become sick. However, often people do not get high-quality care. A 2004 study of 12 large U.S. communities found that just over half (54.9%) of people were receiving the care they needed.

What Exactly Is Healthcare Quality?

Quality means different things to different people. Some people think that getting quality healthcare means seeing the doctor right away, being treated courteously by the doctor's staff, or having the doctor spend a lot of time with them.

While these things are important to all of us, clinical quality of care is even more important. Think of it like this: getting quality healthcare is like taking your car to a mechanic. The people in the shop can be friendly and listen to your complaints, but the most important thing is whether they fix the problem with your car.

Healthcare providers, the government, and many other groups are working hard to improve healthcare quality. You also have a role to play to make sure you and your family members receive the best quality care possible.

BE ACTIVE: TAKE CHARGE OF YOUR HEALTHCARE

The single, most important thing you can do to ensure you get high-quality healthcare is to find and use health information, and take an active role in making decisions about your care.

Here are some steps you can take to improve your care:

- Work together with your doctor and other members of the healthcare team to make decisions about your care.
- Be sure to ask questions. (Select for examples of questions to ask your doctor.)
- Ask your doctor what the scientific evidence has to say about your condition.
- Do your homework; go online or to the library to find out more information about your condition.
- Find and use quality information in making healthcare choices. Be sure the information comes from a reliable source.

TALKING WITH YOUR DOCTOR

Here are some examples of questions to ask your doctor. It is not a complete list. You will probably have many other questions. You should keep asking questions until you understand what is wrong with you, and what you need to do to get better.

Understand your diagnosis:

- What is wrong with me?
- What do I need to do to get better?
- Where can I get more information about my condition?

If you need a lab test, an x-ray, or another kind of test, ask your doctor:

- How will the test be done?
- How accurate will the results be?
- What are the benefits and risks of the test?
- When and how will I receive the results?
- What should I do if I do not receive the results?

If you receive a prescription for a new medicine:

- What is the name of the medicine?
- What is it supposed to do?
- When should I take the medicine, and how much should I take?
- Does the medicine have any side effects?

If you need surgery:

- What kind of operation do I need?
- Why do I need an operation?
- What are the benefits and risks of the operation?
- How long will it take to recover?
- What will happen if I do not have the operation?
- Are there any other treatments I could have instead of an operation?
- Where can I get a second opinion?

UNDERSTANDING WHAT A QUALITY HEALTHCARE IS

Research has shown that science-based measures can be used to assess quality for various conditions and for specific types of care. For example, quality healthcare is:

- Doing the right thing (getting the healthcare services you need)
- At the right time (when you need them)
- In the right way (using the appropriate test or procedure)
- To achieve the best possible results

Healthcare Quality Issues

Providing quality healthcare also means striking the right balance of services by:

- Avoiding underuse (for example, not screening a person for high blood pressure)
- Avoiding overuse (for example, performing tests that a patient does not need)
- Eliminating misuse (for example, providing medications that may have dangerous interactions)

It is usually believed that every doctor, nurse, pharmacist, hospital, and other provider gives high-quality care, but the fact is not always the case. Quality varies depending on where you live. Quality can vary from one state to another, and it can vary from one doctor's office across the street to another. Healthcare quality varies widely and for many reasons.

For example, timely receipt of clot-busting drugs can save lives for patients suffering heart attacks. The national standard for providing clot-busting drugs is within 30 minutes of a patient's arrival at the hospital. But, this varies widely across states, from a low of 20 minutes in 1 state to a high of 140 minutes in another.

EFFORTS TO IMPROVE HEALTHCARE QUALITY

Improving healthcare quality is a team effort, and it is ongoing on many levels. To succeed, every part of the healthcare system must become involved, including government and nongovernment organizations, doctors, nurses, pharmacists, hospitals, other providers, and you, the patient.

One way to assess and track quality of care is by using measures that are based on the latest scientific evidence. A healthcare measure clearly defines which healthcare services should be provided to patients who have or are at risk for certain conditions. Measures also set standards for screening, immunizations, and other preventive care.

There are two types of measures: clinical measures and consumer ratings. Because measures are intended to set general standards for a broad population, they may or may not apply to you. Always check with your doctor about your level of risk for a particular condition, and which types of screening and tests you should have.

CLINICAL MEASURES

Clinical measures can be used to assess the quality of care and patient satisfaction. Examples provided here are of measures that can be used to assess care quality for three of the most common conditions: diabetes, heart disease, and cancer.

Diabetes

More than six percent of all Americans have diabetes. Diabetes is the leading cause of blindness, leg amputation not resulting from trauma, and kidney disease. Diabetes increases the risk of complications in pregnant women, and it is a risk factor for heart disease and stroke. People who have diabetes are two to four times as likely to die from heart disease or stroke as those without diabetes.

The following five measures can be used to assess the quality of care for diabetes. If you have diabetes, you should receive the following tests and exams:
- Regular hemoglobin A1c (blood glucose) testing
- Regular cholesterol testing
- Annual retinal eye exam
- Annual foot exam
- Flu shot each year

Heart Disease

Heart disease—or cardiovascular disease (CVD)—is a collection of diseases of the heart and blood vessels that includes heart attack, stroke, and heart failure. About 64 million Americans are living with heart disease.

Heart disease is the number one cause of death in the United States. Maintaining control of blood pressure and cholesterol can help you prevent heart attack and stroke.

The following are examples of measures that can be used to assess care for heart disease.

For adults age 18 and older:
- Blood pressure measurement
- Cholesterol testing

In general:
- If you smoke, being advised to stop smoking
- If you suffer a heart attack, receiving aspirin within 24 hours of hospital admission and being prescribed beta-blocker therapy at hospital discharge

Cancer

In the United States, cancer is the second leading cause of death, after heart disease. Each year, more than one million new cases of cancer are diagnosed. Four cancers, lung, colorectal, breast, and prostate, account for over half of the new cases reported each year.

Screening to permit early detection holds the most promise for successful cancer treatment. Talk to your doctor about screening tests for all of these cancers, especially if other members of your family have had these cancers or if you smoke.

The following are examples of quality measures for cancer screening.

For breast and cervical cancer:

- Mammography exam for women age 40 and older
- Pap smear testing for women age 18 and older

For colorectal cancer, men and women age 50 and older should receive the following tests:

- Fecal occult blood testing (a test to detect blood in the stool)
- Flexible sigmoidoscopy/colonoscopy exam. Check with your doctor about how often you should have this screening.

FINDING QUALITY INFORMATION

A great deal of information about healthcare quality, both online and in print is available. New tools and resources for assessing and improving healthcare quality are being developed.

Report Cards

Reports cards and other quality reports include consumer ratings, clinical performance measures, or both. They can help you select the right treatment and the right healthcare provider based on what is most important to you. You may be able to get quality reports from:

- **Your employer.** Ask your personnel office for information on health plans.
- **Health plans.** Ask the plan's customer service office about quality reports.
- **Other healthcare providers.** Hospitals, nursing homes, and community health clinics may have quality reports.

Several government agencies publish quality reports and other types of quality information. For example, the U.S. Department of Health and Human Services (HHS) has a quality tool that helps you compare the care provided by hospitals in your area. This tool is available online (www.hospitalcompare.hhs.gov). Another website (www.medicare.gov/NHCompare/home.asp) provided by the Centers for Medicare & Medicaid Services (CMS) has detailed information on the past performance of every Medicare- and Medicaid-certified nursing home in the country.

Accreditation

Accreditation is another indicator that can be used to judge quality. Accreditation is a "seal of approval" given by a private, independent group. Healthcare organizations—such as hospitals—must meet national standards, including clinical performance measures, in order to be accredited.

Accreditation reports present quality information on hospitals, nursing homes, and other healthcare facilities. For example, the Joint Commission on Accreditation of Healthcare Organizations (JCAHO) prepares a performance report on each hospital that it surveys. Another group, the National Committee for Quality Assurance (NCQA), rates health plans such as HMOs. The NCQA's Health Plan Report Card presents accreditation results for hundreds of health plans across the country.

If you need help in finding quality reports, accreditation reports, or other types of quality information, check with your local library or your local or state health department. You can find your state health department listed in the blue pages of your phone book.

Consumer Ratings

Consumer ratings tell you what other people like you think about their healthcare. Some consumer ratings focus on health plans. For example, a survey called "CAHPS®" asks people about the quality of care in their own health plans. Their answers can help you decide whether you want to join one of those plans.

Hospital CAHPS (HCAHPS®) will ask patients about their experiences with hospital care.

CHOOSING QUALITY HEALTHCARE

Here are some tips for making quality a key factor in the healthcare decisions you make about health plans, doctors, treatments, hospitals, and long-term care.

Look for a health plan that:
- Has been given high ratings by its members on the things that are important to you
- Has the doctors and hospitals you want or need
- Provides the benefits (covered services) you need
- Provides services where and when you need them
- Has a documented history of doing a good job of preventing and treating illness

Look for a doctor who:
- Has received high ratings for quality of care
- Has the training and experience to meet your needs
- Will work with you to make decisions about your healthcare

If you become ill, make sure you understand:
- Your diagnosis
- How soon you need to be treated

- Your treatment choices, including the benefits and risks of each treatment
- How much experience your doctor has in treating your condition

Look for a hospital that:
- Is accredited by the JCAHO
- Is rated highly by the state and by consumer groups or other organizations
- Has a lot of experience and success in treating your condition
- Monitors quality of care and works to improve quality

In choosing a nursing home or other long-term care facility, look for one that:
- Has been found by state agencies and other groups to provide quality care
- Provides a level of care, including staff and services, that will meet your needs

Section 17.2 | Identifying Quality Laboratory Services

This section includes text excerpted from "Laboratory Quality Assurance and Standardization Programs," Centers for Disease Control and Prevention (CDC), July 25, 2017.

More than a billion laboratory tests that identify and measure chemicals, such as lead or cholesterol, are performed each year in the United States. The test results have a significant influence on medical decisions.

Given the importance of laboratory test results, the Centers for Disease Control and Prevention's (CDC) National Center for Environmental Health (NCEH) has programs to help assure the quality of these data so patients and healthcare providers (as well as researchers and public-health officials) can be confident that laboratory test results they receive are accurate. These CDC programs focus specifically on laboratory tests that are related to chronic diseases (Cardiovascular Disease Biomarker Standardization Programs and Hormone Standardization Program), newborn screening disorders (Newborn Screening Quality Assurance Program), nutritional status (Vitamin A Laboratory-External Quality Assurance and Vitamin D Standardization Program), and environmental exposures (Ensuring Quality of Urinary Iodine Procedures, Lead and Multielement Proficiency Program, and Proficiency of Arsenic Speciation).

QUALITY ASSURANCE AND STANDARDIZATION PROGRAMS
Cardiovascular Disease Biomarker Standardization Programs

Cardiovascular (or heart) disease is the leading killer of Americans, accounting for approximately 960,000 deaths each year. People with high cholesterol have about twice the risk of heart disease than people with lower levels. At least 50 million U.S. adults have levels of cholesterol in their blood that require medical advice and treatment.

The CDC's Reference Laboratory and Clinical Standardization Programs improve the detection and diagnosis of cardiovascular diseases by ensuring laboratory measurements that test patients' blood for cholesterol levels are accurate and reliable. Standardization is an activity in which the accuracy, precision, and other analytical performance parameters of a laboratory test are assessed against analytical performance goals. This assessment is done by an independent, impartial, and competent organization. A standardized laboratory test has demonstrated (through an independent and impartial assessment) an analytical performance (such as accuracy and precision testing) that meets specific analytical performance goals.

Approximately 71 million American adults have high low-density lipoprotein (LDL), or "bad," cholesterol. The CDC's Cardiovascular Disease Biomarker Standardization programs help ensure tests used to identify these people are accurate and reliable. Once identified they can be treated to reduce their risk of death from heart disease.

Cholesterol Reference Method Laboratory Network

The Cholesterol Reference Method Laboratory Network (CRMLN) is a network of highly specialized laboratories that work directly with manufacturers and laboratories to assess the analytical accuracy and precision of their tests. CRMLN provides reference measurement services to laboratories for measuring total cholesterol (TC), HDL-cholesterol (HDL-C), LDL-cholesterol (LDL-C), and total glycerides (TG). CRMLN laboratories have to meet stringent analytical performance criteria to ensure their measurements are sufficiently accurate and precise for evaluating these tests.

Network laboratories assess tests produced by manufacturers and laboratories for their analytical accuracy and precision. Tests and laboratories meeting established criteria for accuracy and precision are considered "CDC-certified," and sufficiently accurate and precise for use in patient care. Lists of the clinical diagnostic products that have been certified through this process are updated regularly.

The U.S. Food and Drug Administration (FDA) has recognized the value of the CDC's Standardization Programs and work performed through CRMLN, and encourages manufacturers to be standardized to the CDC.

Hormone and Vitamin D Standardization Programs

The CDC Hormone and Vitamin D Standardization Programs improve the diagnosis of polycystic ovary syndrome (PCOS), certain cancers, and other diseases of hormone excess and deficiency. The program assists in providing more accurate and precise hormone measurements used in patient care and research, specifically testosterone, 25-hydroxyvitamin D, and estradiol.

The Clinical Chemistry Branch, Division of Laboratory Sciences (DLS) conducts this voluntary program. The program is nonregulatory, and it helps clinical, research, and public-health laboratories maintain and enhance the quality and comparability of measurement results obtained from steroid hormone and vitamin D tests.

Newborn Screening Quality Assurance Program

Newborn screening identifies conditions that can affect a child's long-term health or survival. The CDC's Newborn Screening and Molecular Biology Branch (NSMBB) manages the Newborn Screening Quality Assurance Program (NSQAP) to enhance and maintain the quality and accuracy of newborn screening results. The program provides training, consultation, proficiency testing, guidelines, and materials to state public-health laboratories and other laboratories responsible for newborn screening in the U.S. and many other countries.

Vitamin A Laboratory—External Quality Assurance

The Vitamin A Laboratory—External Quality Assurance (VITAL—EQA) program is a standardization program designed to provide labs measuring nutritional markers in serum with an independent assessment of their analytical performance. The program assists labs in monitoring the degree of variability and bias in their assays.

Ensuring the Quality of Urinary Iodine Procedures

Iodine deficiency disorders are thought to affect more than a billion people worldwide. Accurate laboratory tests can detect iodine deficiency. Urinary iodine (UI) analysis is the most common method used, worldwide, for assessing the iodine status of a population. Ensuring the Quality of Iodine Procedures (EQUIP) is a standardization program that addresses laboratory quality-assurance issues related to testing for iodine deficiency. The CDC's EQUIP program currently assists more than 126 iodine laboratories in more than 60 countries.

Lead and Multielement Proficiency Program

The CDC's Lead and Multielement Proficiency (LAMP) program is a voluntary laboratory standardization program that focuses on whole blood multianalyte quality-assurance. More than 100 laboratories, including 30 international labs, participate in LAMP. Each quarter, these laboratories are required to analyze a CDC-provided set of blood samples and return those results to the CDC.

Proficiency of Arsenic Speciation

The CDC established the proficiency in arsenic speciation program to help laboratories worldwide assess the accuracy of their arsenic analysis and provide them with technical support.

Arsenic in drinking water has been recognized for many decades in some regions of the world. People in these areas use groundwater as their drinking water source. This water can become contaminated from naturally-occurring sources of arsenic and/or human activities.

Accurate laboratory tests that can detect arsenic contamination are essential. The urinary arsenic analysis is the most common method used worldwide for assessing the arsenic contamination of a population.

Vitamin D Standardization–Certification Program

Osteoporosis and other bone diseases affect millions of U.S. residents and are a major cause of disability. Half of all women and as many as a quarter of men age 50 years and older will have an osteoporosis-related fracture in their lifetime.

Vitamin D is an essential nutrient long-known for its role in maintaining bone health. People who are deficient in vitamin D are at higher risk for osteoporosis. Laboratory tests for vitamin D are used to determine a person's vitamin D status, and to identify persons with vitamin D deficiency. These tests must be accurate to ensure the correct diagnosis and treatment of patients with vitamin D deficiency.

LABORATORY QUALITY ASSURANCE AND STANDARDIZATION PROGRAMS
Quality Assurance

Laboratory quality assurance (QA) encompasses a range of activities that enable laboratories to achieve and maintain high levels of accuracy and proficiency despite changes in test methods and the volume of specimens tested. A good QA system does these four things:

- It establishes standard operating procedures (SOPs) for each step of the laboratory testing process, ranging from specimen handling to instrument performance validation.
- It defines administrative requirements, such as mandatory recordkeeping, data evaluation, and internal audits to monitor adherence to SOPs.
- It specifies corrective actions, documentation, and the persons responsible for carrying out corrective actions when problems are identified.
- It sustains high-quality employee performance.

Laboratory Standardization

Laboratory standardization is achieved when test results have the same analytical accuracy and precision across measurement systems, laboratories, and over time. The CDC's standardization programs consist of three main steps:

- **Reference system** consisting of reference methods and reference materials with target values assigned by the reference methods
- **Traceability procedure** in which participants use the reference materials created in the previous step to calibrate their tests or to verify the analytical accuracy and precision of their testing system
- **Verification procedure** in which the analytical accuracy and precision of the test calibrated in the previous step is being assessed under routine testing conditions

Well-executed standardization programs greatly improve the quality of laboratory measurements that are used to detect signs of illnesses and to guide interventions to prevent or treat illnesses. Standardization also ensures the production of credible and comparable data across laboratories—a boon to epidemiologists and researchers who may need to pool data from multiple sources.

Section 17.3 | Patient Safety in Ambulatory Care

This section includes text excerpted from "Ambulatory Care Safety," Agency for Healthcare Research and Quality (AHRQ), U.S. Department of Health and Human Services (HHS), September 2019.

Despite the fact that the vast majority of healthcare takes place in the outpatient or ambulatory care setting, efforts to improve safety have mostly focused on the inpatient setting. However, a body of research dedicated to patient safety in ambulatory care has emerged over the past few years. These efforts have identified and characterized factors that influence safety in office practice, the types of errors commonly encountered in ambulatory care, and potential strategies for improving ambulatory safety.

FACTORS INFLUENCING SAFETY IN AMBULATORY CARE

Ensuring patient safety outside of the hospital setting poses unique challenges for both providers and patients. One article proposed a model for patient safety in chronic disease management, modified from the original Chronic Care Model (CCM). This model broadly encompasses three concepts that influence safety in ambulatory care:

- The role of patient and caregiver behaviors

- The role of provider—patient interactions
- The role of the community and health system

Specific types of errors can be linked to each of these three concepts.

TYPES OF SAFETY EVENTS IN AMBULATORY CARE

Since face-to-face interactions between providers and patients in the ambulatory setting are limited and occur weeks to months apart, patients must assume a much greater role in and responsibility for managing their own health. This elevates the importance of including the patient as a partner and ensuring that patients understand their illnesses and treatments. The need for outpatients to self-manage their own chronic diseases requires that they monitor their symptoms and, in some cases, adjust their own lifestyle or medications. For example, a patient with diabetes must measure her own blood sugars and perhaps adjust her/his insulin dose based on blood sugar values and dietary intake. A patient's inability or failure to perform such activities may compromise safety in the short term and clinical outcomes in the long term. Patients must also understand how and when to contact their caregivers outside of routine appointments, and they must often play a role in ensuring their own care coordination (e.g., by keeping an updated list of medications).

The nature of interactions between patients and providers—and between different providers—may also be a source of adverse events. Patients consistently voice concerns about coordination of care, particularly when one patient sees multiple physicians, and indeed communication between physicians in the outpatient setting is often suboptimal. Poorly handled care transitions (e.g., when a patient is discharged from the hospital or when care is transferred from one physician to another) also place patients at high risk for preventable adverse events. When a clinician is not immediately available—for example, after-hours—patients may have to rely on telephone advice for acute illnesses, an everyday practice that has its own inherent risks.

Underlying health system flaws have been documented to increase the risk for medical errors, particularly medication errors and diagnostic errors, issues that are certainly germane to ambulatory safety. Medication errors are very common in ambulatory care, with one landmark study finding that more than 4.5 million ambulatory care visits occur every year due to adverse drug events. Likewise, prescribing errors are startlingly common in ambulatory practice. Because the likelihood of a medication error is linked to a patient's understanding of the indication, dosage schedule, proper administration, and potential adverse effects, low health literacy and poor patient education contribute to elevated error risk.

The fragmentation of ambulatory care in outpatient settings increases the challenge of making a timely and accurate diagnosis. Indeed, a study estimated that five percent of adults in the United States experience a missed or delayed diagnosis each year. Data suggests that timely information availability and managing test results contribute to delayed and missed diagnoses in outpatient care. Although use of electronic health records (EHRs) in the ambulatory setting is growing, many practices still lack reliable systems for following up on test results—a problem that has been implicated in missed and delayed diagnoses.

Finally, while an increasing amount of attention has been devoted to measuring and improving the culture of safety in acute care settings, less is known about safety culture in office practice. Burnout and work dissatisfaction, particularly among primary-care physicians, may adversely affect the quality of care. The Agency for Healthcare Research and Quality's (AHRQ) Medical Office Survey on Patient Safety Culture is designed to assess safety culture in ambulatory care, and its comparative database (which includes data from more than 900 participating practices) is freely available from AHRQ.

IMPROVING SAFETY IN AMBULATORY CARE

Improving outpatient safety will require both structural reform of office practice functions as well as the engagement of patients in their own safety. While EHRs hold great promise for reducing medication errors and tracking test results, these systems have yet to reach their full potential. Coordinating care between different physicians remains a significant challenge, especially if the doctors do not work in the same office or share the same medical record system. Efforts are being made to increase the use of EHRs in ambulatory care, and physicians believe that the use of EHRs leads to higher quality and improved safety.

Patient engagement in outpatient safety involves two related concepts:

- **Educating patients** about their illnesses and medications, using methods that require patients to demonstrate understanding (such as "teach-back")
- **Empowering patients** and caregivers to act as a safety "double-check" by providing access to advise and test results and encouraging patients to ask questions about their care

Success has been achieved in this area for patients taking high-risk medications, even in patients with low health literacy at baseline.

Although efforts to improve safety have largely focused on hospital care, the Joint Commission now publishes National Patient Safety Goals® (NPSGs) focused on ambulatory care. The AHRQ is also leading efforts to improve ambulatory quality and safety through programs and research funding. A 2016 systematic review commissioned by the World Health Organization (WHO) identified missed and delayed diagnoses and medication errors as the chief safety priorities in ambulatory care, and it highlighted the need to develop clear and consistent definitions for patient safety incidents in primary care.

Chapter 18 | **Hospitalization**

Chapter Contents

Section 18.1 | Choosing a Hospital

This section includes text excerpted from "Guide to Choosing a Hospital," Centers for Medicare & Medicaid Services (CMS), December 15, 2017.

When you are sick, you may go to the closest hospital or the hospital where your doctor practices. But, which hospital is the best for your individual needs? Research shows that some hospitals do a better job taking care of patients with certain conditions than other hospitals. When you have a life-threatening emergency, always go to the nearest hospital. Understanding your choices will help you have a more informed discussion with your doctor or other healthcare providers.

BEFORE YOU GET STARTED

Make the most of your appointments with your doctor or other healthcare provider to learn about your condition and healthcare needs:

- Before your appointment, make a list of things you want to talk to your doctor or healthcare provider about (such as recent symptoms, drug side effects, or other general health questions). Bring this list to your appointment.
- Bring any prescription drugs, over-the-counter (OTC) drugs, vitamins, and supplements to your appointment and review them with your doctor or healthcare provider.
- Take notes during your appointment. Then, take a moment to repeat back to the doctor or healthcare provider what they told you. Ask any questions you may have.
- Bring along a trusted family member or friend.
- Ask if there is any written information about your condition that you can take with you.
- Call the office if you have questions when you get home.

STEPS TO CHOOSING A HOSPITAL CHECKLIST
Step 1: Learn about the Care You Need and Your Hospital Choices

Talk to your doctors or healthcare providers.

- Find out which hospitals they work with.
- Ask which hospitals they think give the best care for your condition (for example, have enough staffing, coordinate care, promote medication safety, and prevent infection).
- Ask how well these hospitals check and improve their quality of care.
- Ask if the hospitals participate in Medicare or in the network of your Medicare Advantage Plan (such as a health maintenance organization

127

(HMO) or preferred provider organization (PPO) or other Medicare health plan, if you have one.

Based on your condition, ask your doctors or healthcare providers:
- If you should consider a specialty hospital, teaching hospital (usually part of a university), community hospital, or one that does research or has clinical trials related to your condition
- If you need a surgeon or other type of specialist, what is their experience and success treating your condition?
- Who will be responsible for your overall care while you are in the hospital?
- Will you need care after leaving the hospital and, if so, what kind of care? Who will arrange this care?
- Are there any alternatives to hospital care?

Step 2: Think about Your Personal and Financial Needs

Think about your preferences.
- Do you want a hospital located near family members or friends?
- Does the hospital have convenient visiting hours and other rules that are important to you (for example, can a relative or someone helping with your care stay overnight in the room with you)?

Step 3: Find and Compare Hospitals Based on Your Condition and Needs

Visit Hospital Compare at Medicare.gov/hospitalcompare to:
- Find hospitals by name, city, state, or ZIP code
- Check the results of patient surveys (what patients said about their hospital experience)
- Compare the results of certain measures of quality that show how well these hospitals treat patients with certain conditions

You can also call 800-MEDICARE (800-633-4227). TTY users can call 877-486-2048.

Search online for other sources to compare the quality of the hospitals you are considering. Some states have laws that require hospitals to report data about the quality and cost of their care and post the data online

Step 4: Discuss Your Hospital Options and Choose a Hospital

- Talk with family members or friends about the hospitals you are comparing.
- Talk to your doctor or healthcare provider about how the hospital information you gathered applies to you.
- Considering all the above factors, choose the hospital that is best for you.

HOSPITAL QUALITY QUICK CHECK

Here is a quick summary of what to look for when comparing hospitals. Look for a hospital that:

- Has the best experience with your condition
- Checks and improves the quality of its care
- Performs well on measures of quality, including a national patient survey
- Participates in Medicare (and your Medicare health plan, if you have one)
- Meets your needs in terms of location and other factors, such as visiting hours
- Is covered by your Medicare health plan

Section 18.2 | Medicare and Hospital Expenses

This section includes text excerpted from "Are You a Hospital Inpatient or Outpatient?" Centers for Medicare & Medicaid Services (CMS), August 15, 2018.

Did you know that even if you stay in a hospital overnight, you might still be considered an "outpatient?" Your hospital status (whether the hospital considers you an "inpatient" or "outpatient") affects how much you pay for hospital services (such as x-rays, drugs, and lab tests) and may also affect whether Medicare will cover care you get in a skilled nursing facility (SNF) following your hospital stay.

- You are an inpatient starting when you are formally admitted to a hospital with a doctor's order. The day before you are discharged is your last inpatient day.
- You are an outpatient if you are getting emergency department services, observation services, outpatient surgery, lab tests, x-rays, or any other hospital services, and the doctor has not written an order to admit you to a hospital as an inpatient. In these cases, you are an outpatient, even if you spend the night at the hospital.

Note: Observation services are hospital outpatient services given to help the doctor decide if you need to be admitted as an inpatient or can be discharged.

Observation services may be given in the emergency department or another area of the hospital.

The decision for inpatient hospital admission is a complex medical decision based on your doctor's judgment and your need for medically necessary hospital care. An inpatient admission is generally appropriate for payment under

Medicare Part A when you are expected to need two or more midnight of medically necessary hospital care, but your doctor must order this admission and the hospital must formally admit you for you to become an inpatient.

If you have a Medicare Advantage Plan (such as an HMO or PPO), your costs and coverage may be different. Check with your plan.

WHAT DO YOU PAY AS AN INPATIENT?

Medicare Part A (hospital insurance) covers inpatient hospital services. Generally, this means you pay a one-time deductible for all of your hospital services for the first 60 days you are in a hospital.

Medicare Part B (medical insurance) covers most of your doctor services when you are an inpatient. You pay 20 percent of the Medicare-approved amount for doctor services after paying the Part B deductible.

WHAT DO YOU PAY AS AN OUTPATIENT?

Part B covers outpatient hospital services. Generally, this means you pay a copayment for each outpatient hospital service. This amount may vary by service.

Note: The copayment for a single outpatient hospital service cannot be more than the inpatient hospital deductible. However, your total copayment for all outpatient services may be more than the inpatient hospital deductible.

Part B also covers most of your doctor services when you are a hospital outpatient. You pay 20 percent of the Medicare-approved amount after you pay the Part B deductible.

Generally, prescription and over-the-counter (OTC) drugs you get in an outpatient setting (such as an emergency department), sometimes called "self-administered drugs," are not covered by Part B. Also, for safety reasons, many hospitals have policies that do not allow patients to bring prescription or other drugs from home. If you have Medicare prescription drug coverage (Part D), these drugs may be covered under certain circumstances. You will likely need to pay out-of-pocket for these drugs and submit a claim to your drug plan for a refund. Call your drug plan for more information.

SOME COMMON HOSPITAL SITUATIONS AND HOW MEDICARE WILL PAY

Note. Remember, you pay deductibles, coinsurance, and copayments.

Table 18.1. How Medicare Pays for Various Situations

Situation	Inpatient or Outpatient	Part A Pays	Part B Pays
You are in the emergency department (ED) (also known as the "emergency room" or "ER") and then you are formally admitted to the hospital with a doctor's order	Outpatient until you are formally admitted as an inpatient based on your doctor's order. Inpatient after your admission.	Your inpatient hospital stay and all related outpatient services provided during the three days before your admission date.	Your doctor services
You come to the ED with chest pain and the hospital keeps you for two nights. One night is spent in observation and the doctor writes an order for inpatient admission on the second day.	Outpatient until you are formally admitted as an inpatient based on your doctor's order. Inpatient after your admission.	Your inpatient hospital stay and all related outpatient services provided during the three days before your admission date.	Your doctor services
You go to a hospital for outpatient surgery, but they keep you overnight for high blood pressure. Your doctor does not write an order to admit you as an inpatient. You go home the next day	Outpatient	Nothing	Doctor services and hospital outpatient services (for example, surgery, lab tests, or intravenous medicines)
Your doctor writes an order for you to be admitted as an inpatient, and the hospital later tells you it is changing your hospital status to outpatient. Your doctor must agree, and the hospital must tell you in writing—while you are still a hospital patient before you are discharged—that your hospital status changed from inpatient to outpatient.	Outpatient	Nothing	Doctor services and hospital outpatient services

Remember. Even if you stay overnight in a regular hospital bed, you might be an outpatient. Ask the doctor or hospital.

HOW WOULD YOUR HOSPITAL STATUS AFFECT THE WAY MEDICARE COVERS YOUR CARE IN A SKILLED NURSING FACILITY?

Medicare will only cover care you get in a skilled nursing facility (SNF) if you first have a "qualifying inpatient hospital stay."

- A qualifying inpatient hospital stay means you have been a hospital inpatient (you were formally admitted to the hospital after your doctor wrote an inpatient admission order) for at least three days in a row (counting the day you were admitted as an inpatient, but not counting the day of your discharge).
- If you do not have a three-day inpatient hospital stay and you need care after your discharge from the hospital, ask if you can get care in other settings (such as home healthcare) or if any other programs (such as Medicaid or veterans' benefits) can cover your SNF care. Always ask your doctor or hospital staff if Medicare will cover your SNF stay.

HOW WOULD HOSPITAL OBSERVATION SERVICES AFFECT YOUR SKILLED NURSING FACILITY COVERAGE?

Your doctor may order "observation services" to help decide whether you need to be admitted to a hospital as an inpatient or can be discharged. During the time you are getting observation services in a hospital, you are considered an outpatient. This means Medicare will not count this time towards the three-day inpatient hospital stay needed for Medicare to cover your SNF stay.

If you have a Medicare Advantage Plan (such as an HMO or PPO), your costs and coverage may be different. Check with your plan. Table 18.2 describes some common hospital situations that may affect your SNF coverage.

Remember. Any days you spend in a hospital as an outpatient (before you are formally admitted as an inpatient based on the doctor's order) are not counted as inpatient days. An inpatient stay begins on the day you are formally admitted to a hospital as an inpatient with a doctor's order. That is your first inpatient day. The day of discharge does not count as an inpatient day.

WHAT ARE YOUR RIGHTS UNDER MEDICARE COVERAGE?

No matter what type of Medicare coverage you have, you have certain guaranteed rights. As a person with Medicare, you have the right to all of these:

- Have your questions about Medicare answered.
- Learn about all of your treatment choices and participate in treatment decisions.
- Get a decision about healthcare payment or services, or prescription drug coverage.

Hospitalization

Table 18.2. Common Hospital Situations That May Affect Your SNF Coverage

Situation	Is Your Skilled Nursing Facility Stay Covered?
You came to the ED and were formally admitted to the hospital with a doctor's order and spent three days in the hospital as an inpatient after admission. You were discharged on the fourth day.	Yes, if all other coverage requirements are met. You met the three-day inpatient hospital stay requirement for a covered SNF stay.
You came to the ED and spent one day getting observation services. Then, you were formally admitted to the hospital as an inpatient for two more days.	No. Even though you spent three days in the hospital, you were considered an outpatient while getting ED and observation services. These days do not count toward the three-day inpatient hospital stay requirement.

- Get a review (appeal) certain decisions about healthcare payment, coverage of services, or prescription drug coverage.
- File complaints (sometimes called "grievances"), including complaints about the quality of your care.

WHERE CAN YOU GET MORE HELP?

If you need help understanding your hospital status, talk to your doctor or someone from the hospital's utilization or discharge planning department.

- For more information on Part A and Part B coverage, read your "Medicare and You" handbook, visit Medicare.gov, or call 800-MEDICARE (800-633-4227). (Toll-free TTY: 877-486-2048).
- For more information about coverage of self-administered drugs, visit Medicare.gov to view the publication "How Medicare Covers Self-administered Drugs Given in Hospital Outpatient Settings," or call 800-MEDICARE (800-633-4227).
- To ask questions or report complaints about the quality of care of a Medicare-covered service, call your Quality Improvement Organization (QIO).
- To ask questions or report complaints about your care in a nursing home, call your state survey agency.

Section 18.3 | Caregivers and Their Role during a Hospital Stay

This section includes text excerpted from "Going to the Hospital: Tips for Dementia Caregivers," National Institute on Aging (NIA), National Institutes of Health (NIH), May 18, 2017.

A trip to the hospital can be stressful for most people and their caregivers. Being prepared for an emergency and planned hospital visits can relieve some of that stress.

HOSPITAL EMERGENCIES: WHAT YOU CAN DO

A trip to the emergency room (ER) can tire and frighten a person with a disease. Here are some ways to cope:

- Ask a friend or family member to go with you or meet you in the ER. She or he can stay with the person while you answer questions.
- Be ready to explain the symptoms and events leading up to the ER visit—possibly more than once to different staff members.
- Explain how best to talk with the person.
- Comfort the person. Stay calm and positive. How you are feeling will get absorbed by others.
- Be patient. It could be a long wait if the reason for your visit is not life-threatening.
- Recognize that results from the lab take time.
- Realize that just because you do not see staff at work does not mean they are not working.
- Be aware that ER staff may have limited training in a disease, so try to help them better understand the person with the disease.
- Encourage hospital staff to see the person with the disease as an individual and not just another patient with a disease.
- Do not assume the person will be admitted to the hospital.
- If the person must stay overnight in the hospital, try to have a friend or family member stay with her or him.

Do not leave the ER without a plan. If you are sent home, make sure you understand all instructions for follow-up care.

WHAT TO PACK

An emergency bag with the following items, packed ahead of time, can make a visit to the ER go more smoothly:

- Health insurance cards
- Lists of current medical conditions, medicines being taken, and allergies

Hospitalization

- Healthcare providers' names and phone numbers
- Copies of healthcare advance directives
- "Personal information sheet" stating the person's preferred name and language; contact information for key family members and friends; the need for glasses, dentures, or hearing aids; behaviors of concern; how the person communicates needs and expresses emotions; and living situation
- Snacks and bottles of water
- Incontinence briefs, if usually worn, moist wipes, and plastic bags
- Comforting objects or music player with earphones
- A change of clothing, toiletries, and personal medications for yourself
- Pain medicine, such as ibuprofen, acetaminophen, or aspirin—a trip to the ER may take longer than you think, and stress can lead to a headache or other symptoms
- A pad of paper and pen to write down information and directions given to you by hospital staff
- A small amount of cash
- A note on the outside of the emergency bag to remind you to take your cell phone and charger with you

By taking these steps in advance, you can reduce the stress and confusion that often accompany a hospital visit, particularly if the visit is an unplanned trip to the ER.

BEFORE A PLANNED HOSPITAL STAY

It is wise to accept that hospitalization is a "when" and not an "if" event. Due to the nature of any disease, it is very probable that, at some point, the person you are caring for may be hospitalized. Preparation can make all the difference. Here are some tips.

- Think about and discuss hospitalization before it happens and as the disease progresses. Hospitalization is a choice. Talk about when hospice may be a better and more appropriate alternative.
- Build a care team of family, friends, and/or professional caregivers to support the person during the hospital stay. Do not try to do it all alone.
- Ask the doctor if the procedure can be done during an outpatient visit. If not, ask if tests can be done before admission to the hospital to shorten the hospital stay.
- Ask questions about anesthesia, catheters, and IVs. General anesthesia can have side effects, so see if local anesthesia is an option.
- Ask if regular medications can be continued during the hospital stay.

- Ask for a private room, with a reclining chair or bed, if insurance will cover it. It will be calmer than a shared room.
- Involve the person with the disease in the planning process as much as possible.
- Do not talk about the hospital stay in front of the person as if she or he is not there. This can be upsetting and embarrassing.
- Shortly before leaving home, tell the person with disease that the two of you are going to spend a short time in the hospital.

DURING THE HOSPITAL STAY

While the person with the disease is in the hospital:

- Ask doctors to limit questions to the person, who may not be able to answer accurately. Instead, talk with the doctor in private, outside the person's room.
- Help hospital staff understand the person's normal functioning and behavior. Ask them to avoid using physical restraints or medications to control behaviors.
- Have a family member, trusted friend, or hired caregiver stay with the person at all times if possible—even during medical tests. This may be hard to do, but it will help keep the person calm and less frightened, making the hospital stay easier.
- Tell the doctor immediately if the person seems suddenly worse or different. Medical problems, such as fever, infection, medication side effects, and dehydration can cause delirium, a state of extreme confusion and disorientation.
- Ask friends and family to make calls, or use e-mail or online tools to keep others informed about the person's progress.
- Help the person fill out menu requests. Open food containers and remove trays. Assist with eating as needed.
- Remind the person to drink fluids. Offer fluids regularly and have her or him make frequent trips to the bathroom.
- Assume the person will experience difficulty finding the bathroom and/ or using a call button, bed adjustment buttons, or the phone.
- Communicate with the person in the way she or he will best understand and respond.
- Recognize that an unfamiliar place, medicines, invasive tests, and surgery will make a person with dementia more confused. She or he will likely need more assistance with personal care.
- Take deep breaths and schedule breaks for yourself!

Hospitalization

If anxiety or agitation occurs, try the following:

- Remove personal clothes from sight; they may remind the person of getting dressed and going home.
- Post reminders or cues, such as a sign labeling the bathroom door, if this comforts the person.
- Turn off the television, telephone ringer, and intercom. Minimize background noise to prevent over-stimulation.
- Talk in a calm voice and offer reassurance. Repeat answers to questions when needed.
- Provide a comforting touch or distract the person with offers of snacks and beverages.
- Consider "unexpressed pain" (i.e., furrowed brow, clenched teeth or fists, kicking). Assume the person has pain if the condition or procedure is normally associated with pain. Ask for pain evaluation and treatment every four hours—especially if the person has labored breathing, loud moaning, crying or grimacing, or if you are unable to console or distract her or him.
- Listen to soothing music or try comforting rituals, such as reading, praying, singing, or reminiscing.
- Slow down; try not to rush the person.
- Avoid talking about subjects or events that may upset the person.

WORKING WITH HOSPITAL STAFF

Remember that not everyone in the hospital knows the same basic facts about a disease. You may need to help teach hospital staff what approach works best with the person, what distresses or upsets her or him, and ways to reduce this distress.

You can help the staff by providing them with a personal information sheet that includes the person's normal routine, how she or he prefers to be addressed (e.g., Miss Minnie, Dr. James, Jane, Mr. Miller, etc.), personal habits, likes and dislikes, possible behaviors (what might trigger them and how best to respond), and nonverbal signs of pain or discomfort.

Help staff understands what the person's "baseline" is (prior level of functioning).

You should:

- Place a copy of the personal information sheet with the chart in the hospital room and at the nurse's station
- Decide, with the hospital staff, who will do what for the person. For example, you may want to be the one who helps with bathing, eating, or using the bathroom.
- Inform the staff about any hearing difficulties and/or other communication problems, and offer ideas for what works best in those instances

- Make sure the person is safe. Tell the staff about any previous issues with wandering, getting lost, falls, suspicious and/or delusional behavior.
- Not assume the staff knows the person's needs. Inform them in a polite and calm manner.
- Ask questions when you do not understand certain hospital procedures and tests or when you have any concerns. Do not be afraid to be an advocate.
- Plan early for discharge. Ask the hospital discharge planner about eligibility for home health services, equipment, or other long-term care options. Prepare for an increased level of caregiving.
- Realize that hospital staff are providing care for many people. Practice the art of patience.

Chapter 19 | Surgery

Chapter Contents

Section 19.1 | What You Need to Know about Surgery

This section contains text excerpted from the following sources: Text in this section begins with excerpts from "Surgery," MedlinePlus, National Institutes of Health (NIH), October 31, 2016. Reviewed December 2019; Text under the heading "What You Should Know before Your Surgery" is excerpted from "What You Should Know before Your Surgery," Centers for Disease Control and Prevention (CDC), March 14, 2016. Reviewed December 2019.

There are many reasons to have surgery. Some operations can relieve or prevent pain. Others can reduce the symptom of a problem or improve some body functions. Some surgeries are done to find a problem. For example, a surgeon may do a biopsy, which involves removing a piece of tissue to examine under a microscope. Some surgeries, such as heart surgery, can save your life.

Some operations that once needed large incisions (cuts in the body) can now be done using much smaller cuts. This is called "laparoscopic surgery." Surgeons insert a thin tube with a camera to see and use small tools to do the surgery.

After surgery, there can be a risk of complications, including infection, too much bleeding, reaction to anesthesia, or accidental injury. There is almost always some pain with surgery.

WHAT YOU SHOULD KNOW BEFORE YOUR SURGERY

Protect yourself and your loved ones from infections related to surgery.

Having any type of surgery can be stressful. You might be asking yourself:

- What is the recovery process? How long will I be out of work?
- What do I do after leaving the hospital or surgery center?

An important question you might not have thought of is: How do I avoid getting a surgical site infection?

An SSI is an infection patient can get during or after surgery. SSIs can happen on any part of the body where the surgery takes place and can sometimes involve only the skin. Other SSIs are more serious and can involve tissues under the skin, organs, or implanted material.

These infections can make recovery from surgery more difficult because they can cause additional complications, stress, and medical cost. It is important that healthcare providers, patients, and loved ones work together to prevent these infections.

What Can Healthcare Providers Do to Ensure That the Surgical Site Is Clean?

- Clean their hands and arms up to the elbows with an antiseptic agent just before the surgery
- Wear hair covers, masks, gowns, and gloves during surgery to keep the surgery area clean

- Give you antibiotics before surgery starts when indicated
- Clean the skin at the surgery site with a special soap that kills germs

How Can You and Your Loved Ones Prevent Surgical Site Infections?

- Before your surgery, discuss other health problems, such as diabetes, with your doctor. These issues can affect your surgery and your treatment.
- Quit smoking. Patients who smoke get more infections.
- Follow your doctor's instructions for cleaning your skin before your surgery. For example, if your doctor recommends using a special soap before surgery, make sure you do so.
- Avoid shaving near where you will have surgery. Shaving with a razor can irritate your skin and make it easier to develop an infection. If someone tries to shave you before surgery, ask why this is necessary.

After Surgery, Be Sure to Follow the Recommendations below to Protect against Surgical Site Infection

- Ask your healthcare provider to clean their hands before they examine you or check your wound.
- Do not allow visitors to touch the surgical wound or dressings.
- Ask family and friends to clean their hands before and after visiting you.
- Make sure you understand how to care for your wound before you leave the medical facility.
- Always clean your hands before and after caring for your wound.
- Make sure you know who to contact if you have questions or problems after you get home.
- If you have any symptoms of an infection, such as redness and pain at the surgery site, drainage, or fever, call your doctor immediately.

Section 19.2 | Anesthesia Basics

This section includes text excerpted from "Anesthesia," National Institute of General Medical Sciences (NIGMS), September 2017.

Anesthesia is a medical treatment that prevents patients from feeling pain during surgery. It allows people to have procedures that lead to healthier and longer lives.

To produce anesthesia, doctors use drugs called "anesthetics." Scientists have developed a collection of anesthetic drugs with different effects. These drugs include general, regional, and local anesthetics. General anesthetics put patients to sleep during the procedure. Local and regional anesthetics just numb part of the body and allow patients to remain awake during the procedure.

Depending on the type of pain relief needed, doctors deliver anesthetics by injection, inhalation, topical lotion, spray, eye drops, or skin patch.

WHAT IS GENERAL ANESTHESIA?

General anesthesia affects the whole body, making patients unconscious and unable to move. Surgeons use it when they operate on internal organs and for other invasive or time-consuming procedures such as back surgery. Without general anesthesia, many major, life-saving procedures would not be possible, including open-heart surgery, brain surgery, and organ transplants.

Doctors provide general anesthetics either directly into the bloodstream (intravenously) or as an inhaled gas. General anesthesia delivered intravenously will act quickly and disappear rapidly from the body. This allows patients to go home sooner after surgery. Inhaled anesthetics may take longer to wear off.

General anesthetics typically are very safe. But they can pose risks for some patients, such as the elderly or people with chronic illnesses such as diabetes. Also, side effects may linger for several days in some patients, especially the elderly and children.

Serious side effects—such as dangerously low blood pressure—are much less common than they once were. Still, as with any medical procedure, some risks exist. To minimize these risks, specialized doctors called "anesthesiologists" carefully monitor unconscious patients and can adjust the amount of anesthetic they receive.

WHAT ARE LOCAL AND REGIONAL ANESTHESIA?

Doctors use local and regional anesthetics to block pain in a part of the body. With these anesthetics, patients stay conscious and comfortable. Usually, patients may go home soon after surgery.

Local anesthetics affect a small part of the body, such as a single tooth. They are often used in dentistry, for eye surgeries such as cataract removal, and to remove small skin growths including warts and moles.

Regional anesthetics affect larger areas, such as an arm, a leg, or everything below the waist. For example, this sort of anesthesia is used for hand and joint surgeries, to ease the pain of childbirth, or during a C-section delivery.

HOW DOES ANESTHESIA WORK?

Until, we knew very little about how anesthetics work. Scientists are now able to study how the drugs affect specific molecules within cells. Most researchers agree that the drugs target proteins in the membranes around nerve cells. Because inhaled anesthetics have different effects than intravenous ones, scientists suspect that the two different types of drugs target different sets of proteins.

WHAT DO ANESTHESIOLOGISTS DO?

Anesthesiologists are doctors who carefully monitor patients throughout surgery and during recovery. They use highly advanced electronic devices that constantly display patients' blood pressure, blood oxygen levels, heart function, and breathing patterns. These devices have dramatically improved the safety of general anesthesia. They also make it possible to operate on many patients who used to be considered too sick to have surgery.

Anesthesiologists also provide pain relief for less invasive procedures, such as those used to examine blood vessels and internal organs (endoscopy) and during labor and delivery.

As experts in pain management, anesthesiologists may advise patients and their doctors on how to manage pain.

HOW ARE ANESTHESIOLOGISTS TRAINED?

Like all medical doctors, anesthesiologists earn a college degree, often in a life sciences field, then a medical degree (M.D. or D.O.). After that, they complete a four-year residency program in anesthesiology. Many also train for an additional year or more in a specialty, such as pain management, pediatric anesthesiology, or critical care medicine.

WHAT DOES THE FUTURE HOLD FOR ANESTHESIOLOGY?

Scientists are learning more about how anesthetics work at the most basic level. They are also studying the short- and long-term effects of these drugs on specific groups of people, such as the elderly and cancer survivors. These studies will reveal whether certain anesthetics are better than others for members of those groups.

Research on how a person's genetic makeup affects how she or he responds to anesthetics will allow doctors to further tailor drugs for each patient. In the future, scientists hope to design anesthetics that are safer, more effective, and more personalized.

Knowing how anesthetics affect pain and consciousness could also lead to new treatments for conditions that affect consciousness, such as epilepsy or coma. Studies of anesthesia may even help us better understand the nature of consciousness itself.

Section 19.3 | **Robotic Interventions**

This section contains text excerpted from the following sources: Text beginning with the heading "What Are Image-Guided Robotic Interventions?" is excerpted from "Image-Guided Robotic Interventions," National Institute of Biomedical Imaging and Bioengineering (NIBIB), October 2018; Text beginning with the heading "What Are Computer-Assisted Surgical Systems?" is excerpted from "Computer-Assisted Surgical Systems," U.S. Food and Drug Administration (FDA), March 13, 2019.

WHAT ARE IMAGE-GUIDED ROBOTIC INTERVENTIONS?

Image-guided robotic interventions are medical procedures that integrate sophisticated robotic and imaging technologies, primarily to perform minimally invasive surgery. This integrated technology approach offers distinct advantages for both patients and physicians.

Imaging

In image-guided procedures, the surgeon is guided by images from various techniques, including magnetic resonance (MR) and ultrasound. Images can also be obtained using tiny cameras attached to probes that are small enough to fit into a minimal incision. The camera allows the surgery to be performed using a much smaller incision than in traditional surgery.

Robotics

The surgeon's hands and traditional surgical tools are too large for small incisions. Instead, thin, finger-like robotic tools are used to perform the surgery. As the surgeon watches the image on the screen, she uses a tele-manipulator to transmit and direct hand and finger movements to a robot, which can be controlled by hydraulic, electronic, or mechanical means.

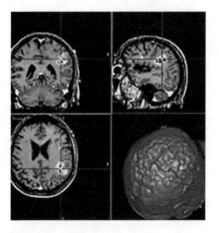

Figure 19.1. Images Help Target the Exact Site of Intervention

Robotic tools can also be controlled by computers. One advantage of a computerized system is that a surgeon could potentially perform the surgery from anywhere in the world. This type of long-distance surgery is currently in the experimental phase. The experiments illustrate the life-saving potential for such surgeries when a delicate operation requires a specially trained surgeon who is in a distant location.

WHAT ARE THE ADVANTAGES OF MINIMALLY INVASIVE PROCEDURES?

Minimally invasive surgery can reduce the damage to surrounding healthy tissues, thus decreasing the need for pain medication and reducing patients' recovery time. For surgeons, image-guided interventions using robots also have the advantage of reducing fatigue during long operations, allowing the surgeon to perform the procedure while seated.

WHAT ARE SOME EXAMPLES OF IMAGE-GUIDED ROBOTIC INTERVENTIONS AND HOW ARE THEY USED?

Robotic Prostatectomy

Complete prostate removal is performed through a series of small incisions, compared with a single large incision of four to five inches in traditional surgery. The small incisions result in a shorter postoperative recovery, less scarring, and a faster return to normal activities.

Ablation Techniques for Early Cancers

Patients with early kidney cancer can be treated with minimally invasive procedures to destroy small tumors. Cryoablation uses cold energy to destroy the tumors. Doctors use a computed tomography (CT) and ultrasound imaging to position a needle-like probe within each kidney tumor. Once in position, the tip of the probe is super-cooled to encase the tumor in a ball of ice. Alternate freeze/thaw cycles kill the tumor cells. Other minimally invasive methods of destroying early kidney cancers include heating the tumor cells, and surgical removal using a robotic device. Many patients can go home the same day and are able to perform regular activities in several days.

Orthopedics

Image-guided robotic procedures are improving the precision and outcome of a number of orthopedic procedures. For example, partial knee resurfacing surgeries aim to target only the damaged sections of the knee joint. Orthopedic surgeons are combining the use of a robotic surgical arm and fiber-optic cameras in such procedures, which results in patients retaining more of their normal healthy tissue. Image-guided robotic procedures also improve total knee replacements, allowing precise alignment and positioning of knee implants. The result is more natural knee function, a better range of motion, and improved balance for patients.

RESEARCH IN THE AREA OF IMAGE-GUIDED ROBOTIC INTERVENTIONS TO IMPROVE MEDICAL CARE

Portable Robot Uses 3D Near-Infrared Imaging to Guide Needle Insertion into Veins

Drawing blood and inserting IV lines are the most commonly performed medical procedures in hospitals and clinics. However, for many patients it can be difficult to find veins and accurately insert the needle, resulting in patient injury. The National Institute of Biomedical Imaging and Bioengineering (NIBIB)-funded scientists are developing a portable, lightweight medical robot to help perform these procedures. The device uses 3D near-infrared imaging to identify an appropriate vein for the robot to insert the needle. The current goal is to integrate the imaging system and software into a miniaturized version of the prototype robot. The outcome will be a compact, low-cost system that will greatly improve the safety and accuracy of accessing veins.

Robot-Assisted Needle Guidance Aids Removal of Liver Tumors

Radiofrequency ablation (RFA) is a minimally invasive treatment that kills tumors with heat and can be a life-saving option for patients who are not eligible for surgery. However, broad use of RFA has been limited because the straight paths taken by the needles that carry tumor-killing electrodes may damage lung or other sensitive organs. Also, large tumors require multiple needle insertions, which increases bleeding risk. To address the problem of tissue damage using straight needles, NIBIB-funded scientists are developing highly flexible needles that can be guided along controlled, curved paths through tissue, allowing the removal of tumors that are not accessible by a straight-line path. The technology combines needle flexibility with a 3D ultrasound guidance system that allows the doctor to correct the path of the needle to avoid unexpected obstacles as the needle advances toward the tumor. The device will ultimately increase the accuracy and reduce the damage to healthy tissue during tumor removal resulting in wider use of the technology for better patient outcomes.

Swallowable Capsule Identifies and Biopsies Abnormal Tissue in the Esophagus

Barrett's esophagus is a precancerous condition that requires repeated biopsies to monitor abnormal tissue. The NIBIB-funded researchers are developing a pill-sized device that can be swallowed to improve the management and treatment of this condition. The unsedated patient can easily swallow the pill, which is attached to a thin tether made of cable and optic fiber. The device detects microscopic areas of the esophagus that may show evidence of disease, and uses a laser to collect samples from the suspicious tissue—a technology known as "laser capture micro-dissection." The physician then retrieves the device from the patient without discomfort and the collected micro-samples are examined for visual evidence of disease, as well as genetic analysis. This minimally invasive device improves patient comfort and provides a precise molecular profile of the biopsied regions, which helps the physician to better monitor and treat the disorder.

WHAT ARE COMPUTER-ASSISTED SURGICAL SYSTEMS?

Different types of computer-assisted surgical systems can be used for preoperative planning, surgical navigation and to assist in performing surgical procedures. Robotically-assisted surgical (RAS) devices are one type of computer-assisted surgical system. Sometimes referred to as robotic surgery, RAS devices enable the surgeon to use computer and software technology to control and move surgical instruments through one or more tiny incisions in the patient's body (minimally invasive) for a variety of surgical procedures.

The benefits of a RAS device may include its ability to facilitate minimally invasive surgery and assist with complex tasks in confined areas of the body. The device is not actually a robot because it cannot perform surgery without direct human control.

Robotically-assisted surgical devices generally have several components, which may include:

- A **console**, where the surgeon sits during surgery. The console is the control center of the device and allows the surgeon to view the surgical field through a 3D endoscope and control movement of the surgical instruments
- The **bedside cart** that includes three or four hinged mechanical arms, camera (endoscope) and surgical instruments that the surgeon controls during surgical procedures
- A **separate cart** that contains supporting hardware and software components, such as an electrosurgical unit (ESU), suction/irrigation pumps, and light source for the endoscope

Most surgeons use multiple surgical instruments and accessories with the RAS device, such as scalpels, forceps, graspers, dissectors, cautery, scissors, retractors and suction irrigators.

COMMON USES OF ROBOTICALLY-ASSISTED SURGICAL DEVICES

The U.S. Food and Drug Administration (FDA) has cleared RAS devices for use by trained physicians in an operating room environment for laparoscopic surgical procedures in general surgery cardiac, colorectal, gynecologic, head and neck, thoracic and urologic surgical procedures. Some common procedures that may involve RAS devices are gall-bladder removal, hysterectomy, and prostatectomy (removal of the prostate).

RECOMMENDATIONS FOR PATIENTS AND HEALTHCARE PROVIDERS ABOUT ROBOTICALLY-ASSISTED SURGERY
Healthcare Providers

Robotically-assisted surgery is an important treatment option that is safe and effective when used appropriately and with proper training. The FDA does not regulate the practice of medicine, and therefore, does not supervise or provide accreditation for physician training nor does it oversee training and education related to legally marketed medical devices. Instead, training development and implementation is the responsibility of the manufacturer, physicians, and healthcare facilities. In some cases, professional societies and specialty board certification organizations may also develop and support training for their specialty physicians. Specialty boards also maintain certification status of their specialty physicians.

Physicians, hospitals and facilities that use RAS devices should ensure that proper training is completed and that surgeons have appropriate credentials to perform surgical procedures with these devices. Device users should ensure they maintain their credentialing. Hospitals and facilities should also ensure that other surgical staff that use these devices complete proper training.

Users of the device should realize that there are several different models of robotically-assisted surgical devices. Each model may operate differently and may not have the same functions. Users should know the differences between the models and make sure to get appropriate training on each model.

If you suspect a problem or complications associated with the use of RAS devices, the FDA encourages you to file a voluntary report through MedWatch, the FDA's Safety Information and Adverse Event Reporting program. Healthcare personnel employed by facilities that are subject to FDA's user facility reporting requirements should follow the reporting procedures established by their facilities. Prompt reporting of adverse events can help the FDA identify and better understand the risks associated with medical devices.

Patients

Robotically-assisted surgery is an important treatment option but may not be appropriate in all situations. Talk to your physician about the risks and benefits of RASs, as well as the risks and benefits of other treatment options.

Patients who are considering treatment with RASs should discuss the options for these devices with their healthcare provider, and feel free to inquire about their surgeon's training and experience with these devices.

Section 19.4 | Wrong-Site, Wrong-Procedure, and Wrong-Patient Surgery

This section includes text excerpted from "Wrong-Site, Wrong-Procedure, and Wrong-Patient Surgery," Agency for Healthcare Research and Quality (AHRQ), U.S. Department of Health and Human Services (HHS), September 2019.

Few medical errors are as vivid and terrifying as those that involve patients who have undergone surgery on the wrong body part, undergone the incorrect procedure, or had a procedure intended for another patient. These "wrong-site, wrong-procedure, wrong-patient errors" (WSPEs) are rightly termed "never events"—errors that should never occur and indicate serious underlying safety problems.

Wrong-site surgery may involve operating on the wrong side, as in the case of a patient who had the right side of her vulva removed when the cancerous lesion was on the left, or the incorrect body site. One example of surgery on the incorrect site is operating on the wrong level of the spine, a surprisingly common issue for neurosurgeons. A classic case of wrong-patient surgery involved a patient who underwent a cardiac procedure intended for another patient with a similar last name.

While much publicity has been given to these high-profile cases of WSPEs, these errors are in fact relatively rare. A seminal study estimated that such errors occur in approximately 1 of 112,000 surgical procedures, infrequent enough that an individual hospital would only experience one such error every 5 to 10 years. However, this estimate only included procedures performed in the operating room; if procedures performed in other settings (for example, ambulatory surgery or interventional radiology) are included, the rate of such errors may be significantly higher. One study using the U.S. Department of Veterans Affairs (VA) data found that fully half of WSPEs occurred during procedures outside of the operating room.

PREVENTING WRONG-SITE, WRONG-PROCEDURE, AND WRONG-PATIENT SURGERY

Early efforts to prevent WSPEs focused on developing redundant mechanisms for identifying the correct site, procedure, and patient, such as "sign your site" initiatives, that instructed surgeons to mark the operative site in an unambiguous fashion. However, it soon became clear that even this seemingly simple intervention was problematic. An analysis of the United Kingdom's (UK) efforts to prevent WSPEs found that, although dissemination of a site-marking protocol did increase the use of preoperative site marking, implementation and adherence to the protocol differed significantly across surgical specialties and hospitals, and many clinicians voiced concerns about unintended consequences of the protocol. In some cases, there was even confusion over whether the marked site indicates the area to be operated on or the area to be avoided. Site marking remains a core component of the Joint Commission's Universal Protocol to prevent WSPEs.

Root cause analyses of WSPEs consistently reveal communication issues as a prominent underlying factor. The concept of the surgical timeout—a planned pause before beginning the procedure in order to review important aspects of the procedure with all involved personnel—was developed to improve communication in the operating room and prevent WSPEs. The Universal Protocol also specifies the use of a timeout prior to all procedures. Although initially designed for operating room procedures, timeouts are now required before any invasive procedure. Comprehensive efforts to improve surgical safety have incorporated timeout principles into surgical safety checklists; while these checklists have been proven to improve surgical and postoperative safety, the low baseline incidence of WSPEs makes it difficult to establish that a single intervention can reduce or eliminate WSPEs.

It is worth noting, however, that many cases of WSPEs would still occur despite full adherence to the Universal Protocol. Errors may happen well before the patient reaches the operating room, a timeout may be rushed or otherwise ineffective, and production pressures may contribute to errors during the procedure itself. Ultimately, preventing WSPEs depends on the combination of system solutions, strong teamwork and safety culture, and individual vigilance.

CURRENT CONTEXT

Wrong-patient, wrong-site, and wrong-procedure errors are all considered never events by the National Quality Forum (NQP) and are considered sentinel events by the Joint Commission. In February 2009, the Centers for Medicare & Medicaid Services (CMS) announced that hospitals will not be reimbursed for any costs associated with WSPEs. (CMS has not reimbursed hospitals for additional costs associated with many preventable errors since 2007.)

Chapter 20 | **Preventive Care: Everyone Needs an Ounce of Prevention**

Preventive healthcare can help you stay healthier throughout your life. For many people, certain preventive healthcare is now free, with no copays or deductibles. This chapter will help you to have a better understanding of the preventive care that you and your loved ones need and to ask your healthcare provider what healthcare you need to stay healthy.

WHAT IS PREVENTIVE CARE?

Preventive care includes health services such as screenings, checkups, and patient counseling that are used to prevent illnesses, disease, and other health problems, or to detect illness at an early stage when treatment is likely to work best.

Getting recommended preventive services and making healthy lifestyle choices are key steps to good health and well-being.

The recommendations discussed in this chapter come from the U.S. Preventive Services Task Force (USPSTF).

WHAT ARE CHILD PREVENTIVE SERVICES?

A report from the Centers for Disease Control and Prevention (CDC) indicates that millions of infants, children, and adolescents in the U.S. did not receive selected clinical-preventive services. Increased use of preventive services could improve the health of infants, children, and adolescents and promote healthy lifestyles that will enable them to achieve their full potential.

Many insurance plans provide these services at no cost, without charging copays or deductible payments. Talk with your child's doctor about getting all of the preventive care that is recommended for your child's age.

This chapter includes text excerpted from "Prevention," Centers for Disease Control and Prevention (CDC), May 31, 2017.

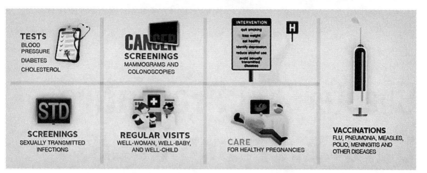

Figure 20.1. What Preventive Care Includes

Get Physical Exams on Schedule
Children need regular checkups. Talk to your child's doctor about when checkups are needed. Doctors commonly recommend checkups every year for children who are three years of age and older. For children under three years of age, more frequent checkups are needed. The doctor or nurse will check to make sure your child is healthy and developing on schedule.

Get Your Child's Vaccines on Schedule
Check with your child's doctor to find out which vaccines your child needs.

Get Your Child's Blood Pressure Checked
If your child is three years of age or older, request that the doctor measure your child's blood pressure during regular checkups.

Get Screened for Depression
Ask your child's doctor to screen him or her for depression, even if you do not see signs of a problem. This is recommended for children at least 12 years of age and above.

Follow Development with Monitoring and Screening
Watch your child's development and talk with your child's doctor at every checkup about how your child plays, learns, speaks, acts, and moves. Ask your child's doctor about developmental screening when your child is 9, 18, and either 24 or 30 months of age, and about autism screening at 18 and either 24 or 30 months of age or whenever there is a concern.

Get Your Child Tested for Lead Exposure
There are usually no signs or symptoms of lead poisoning. A lead test is the only way to know for sure if your child has lead poisoning. Talk with your child's doctor about this simple blood lead test. This is recommended for children

under six years of age who live in older housing (built before 1978), according to state or local requirements.

WHAT PREVENTIVE-CARE SERVICES ARE AVAILABLE FOR WOMEN?
Get Your Well-woman Visit Every Year

If you are above 65 years of age, you should see a doctor or nurse for a checkup once a year.

Get a Bone Density Test

Get your bone density tested starting at age 65.

Get Tested for Cancer

Talk with a doctor if breast or ovarian cancer run in your family. Get a mammogram every 2 years. Women who are 50 years of age and above can consider this recommendation. Get a Pap test every 3 years. If you are of age 30 or above, then get a Pap test and human papillomavirus (HPV) test, but you can get screened every 5 years instead.

WHAT PREVENTIVE-CARE SERVICES ARE AVAILABLE FOR ADULTS?

Many insurance plans provide these services at no cost, without charging copays or deductible payments.

Talk to Your Doctor about Abdominal Aortic Aneurysm

If you have ever smoked, talk with your doctor about abdominal aortic aneurysm (AAA). It is recommended for men who are of ages between 65 and 75 and those who have ever smoked tobacco.

Talk to Your Doctor about Your Alcohol Use

If you are concerned about your drinking, ask your doctor about screening and counselling. It is recommended for adults in general.

Talk to Your Doctor about Taking Aspirin Every Day

Talk to your doctor about taking an aspirin every day to help lower your risk of heart attack or stroke. Men who are of between the ages of 45 and 79 and women between the ages of 55 and 79 should have this conversation with their doctor.

Get Your Blood Pressure Checked

Get your blood pressure checked at least once every one to two years. Ask your doctor how often you need to get tested. It is recommended for adults in general.

Get Your Cholesterol Checked

Get your cholesterol checked once every 5 years. Men who are 35 and above and men and women age 20 and above who are at high risk of elevated cholesterol should get their cholesterol checked.

Get Tested for Colorectal Cancer

Talk with your doctor about options for getting tested. It is recommended for adults who are between 50 and 75 years of age.

Get Tested for Chlamydia, Gonorrhea, and Syphilis

Talk with your doctor to find out if you need to be tested for chlamydia, gonorrhea, or syphilis. It is recommended for adults who have had sex or are at high risk for a sexually transmitted infection.

Talk to Your Doctor about Depression

Talk with your doctor about how you are feeling if you have been feeling sad, down, or hopeless. It is recommended for adults in general.

Take Steps to Prevent Type 2 Diabetes

If you have high blood pressure, ask your doctor whether you need to get screened for type 2 diabetes. It is recommended for adults with high blood pressure.

Get Help with Healthy Eating

If your doctor has told you that you are at risk for heart disease or diabetes, ask about dietary counseling. It is recommended for adults with high cholesterol or at risk for heart disease or diabetes.

Talk to Your Doctor about Preventing Falls

If you are worried about falls, ask how exercise, physical therapy, and vitamin D supplements might help you prevent falls. It is recommended for adults who are above 65 years of age.

Get Tested for Hepatitis C

Get tested for hepatitis C at least once if you were born between 1945 and 1965.

Get Tested for Human Immunodeficiency Virus

Get tested for human immunodeficiency virus (HIV) at least once. You may need to get tested more often, depending on your risk. This is recommended for all adults.

Get Screened for Lung Cancer

Ask your doctor about screening for lung cancer if you have a history of heavy smoking and you smoke now or have quit within the past 15 years. An example of heavy smoking is smoking 1 pack of cigarettes a day for 30 years or 2 packs a day for 15 years. This is recommended for adults who are between the age of 55 and 80 and those who have smoked heavily.

Watch Your Weight

Adults, in general, should ask their doctor if they are at a healthy weight.

Talk to Your Doctor about Skin Cancer

If you have fair (pale) skin, talk to your doctor about how to reduce your risk for skin cancer. This is recommended for adults who are under 24 years of age and have fair skin.

Get Help to Quit Tobacco

If you use tobacco, ask your doctor about services to help you quit.

Get a Vaccine

Ask your doctor for a pneumonia vaccine is you are above 65 years of age. Get a flu vaccine every year to protect yourself and others from the flu.

Part 3 | Health Literacy and Making Informed Health Decisions

Chapter 21 | **Understanding Health Literacy**

WHAT IS HEALTH LITERACY?

The Patient Protection and Affordable Care Act of 2010, Title V, defines "health literacy" as the degree to which an individual has the capacity to obtain, communicate, process, and understand basic health information and services to make appropriate health decisions.

Health Literacy Capacity and Skills

Capacity is the potential a person has to do or accomplish something. Health literacy skills are those people use to realize their potential in health situations. They apply these skills either to make sense of health information and services or provide health information and services to others.

Anyone who needs health information and services also needs health literacy skills to:

- Find information and services
- Communicate their needs and preferences and respond to information and services
- Process the meaning and usefulness of the information and services
- Understand the choices, consequences, and context of the information and services
- Decide which information and services match their needs and preferences so they can act

Anyone who provides health information and services to others, such as a doctor, nurse, dentist, pharmacist, or public-health worker, also needs health literacy skills to:

- Help people find information and services

This chapter includes text excerpted from "What Is Health Literacy?" Centers for Disease Control and Prevention (CDC), October 23, 2019.

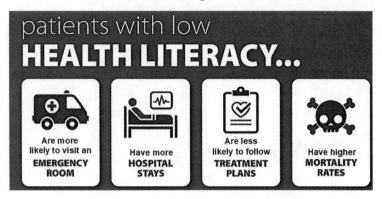

Figure 21.1. Risk for Patients with Low Health Literacy *(Source: "Infographic— Health Literacy," Centers for Disease Control and Prevention (CDC))*

- Communicate about health and healthcare
- Process what people are explicitly and implicitly asking for
- Understand how to provide useful information and services
- Decide which information and services work best for different situations and people so they can act

Researchers can choose from many different types of health literacy skill measures.

IMPORTANCE OF HEALTH LITERACY
Health Literacy Affects Everyone

Health literacy is important for everyone because, at some point in our lives, we all need to be able to find, understand, and use health information and services.

Taking care of our health is part of everyday life, not just when we visit a doctor, clinic, or hospital. Health literacy can help us prevent health problems and protect our health, as well as better manage those problems and unexpected situations that happen.

Even people who read well and are comfortable using numbers can face health literacy issues when:

- They are not familiar with medical terms or how their bodies work
- They have to interpret statistics and evaluate risks and benefits that affect their health and safety
- They are diagnosed with a serious illness and are scared and confused
- They have health conditions that require complicated self-care
- They are voting on an issue affecting the community's health and relying on unfamiliar technical information

Reasons for Health Literacy Problem in the United States

When organizations or people create and give others health information that is too difficult for them to understand, it creates a health literacy problem. When they are expected to figure out health services with many unfamiliar, confusing or even conflicting steps, that also creates a health literacy problem.

What Can Be Done to Improve Health Literacy among People?

People can use the health literacy skills they have through:

- Create and provide information and services people can understand and use most effectively with the skills they have
- Educators and others who can help them become more familiar with health information and services and build their health literacy skills over time
- Developing their own skills as communicators of health information

Limited Health Literacy Reports and Evidence

People need information they can understand and use to make the best decisions for their health. Limited health literacy happens when people's literacy and numeracy skills are poorly matched with the technical, complex, and unfamiliar information that organizations make available, or health services are too complex and difficult to understand and use effectively.

Several reports document that limited health literacy affects many types of health conditions, diseases, situations, and outcomes, including health status and costs.

The U.S. Department of Education (ED) published *The Health Literacy of America's Adults: Results from the 2003 National Assessment of Adult Literacy*, the only national data on health literacy skills in 2006. The study found that adults who self-report the worst health also have the most limited literacy, numeracy, and health literacy skills.

Are Limited Health Literacy and Limited Literacy the Same Problem?

No, but they are related. People's reading, writing, and numbers skills are only a part of health literacy. People do need strong literacy and numeracy skills to make it easier to understand and use health information and services. But, research shows that many health and healthcare activities are unfamiliar, complicated, and technical to most people.

UNDERSTANDING LITERACY AND NUMERACY

Literacy, numeracy, and technology skills are increasingly important in nowadays information-rich environments. What people know and what they do with what they know has a major impact on their life chances. For example, people with lower literacy proficiency are more likely than those with better literacy skills to report poor health.

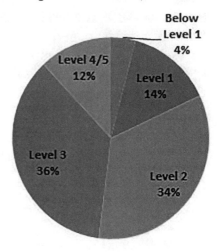

Figure 21.2. Percentage of the U.S. Adults Age 16 to 65 at Each Level of Proficiency on the PIAAC Literacy Scale

What Are Adult Literacy and Numeracy?

The ED defines "adult literacy" and "numeracy" in terms of skills that help people accomplish tasks and realize their purposes. Researchers can measure literacy and numeracy skills, but skills are not static. People can build their skills, and even adults with limited skills can get better results when their environments accommodate the skills they have.

- Literacy is understanding, evaluating, using, and engaging with written texts to participate in society, to achieve one's goals and to develop one's knowledge and potential.
- Numeracy is the ability to access, use, interpret, and communicate mathematical information and ideas, to engage in and manage the mathematical demands of a range of situations in adult life.

Population Measures of Literacy, Numeracy, Health Literacy Skills, and Technology Use
Adult Health Literacy Skills

The ED collects and reports data adult literacy and numeracy skills. In 2006, they published the only national data on health literacy skills. These studies found that adults who self-report the worst health also have the most limited literacy, numeracy, and health literacy skills.

Youth Literacy Skills

The ED also collects and reports data on school-aged children and youth. Elementary-school children with weak literacy and numeracy skills often struggle

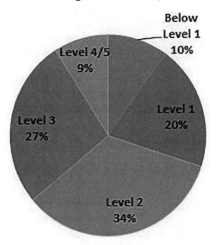

Figure 21.3. Percentage of the U.S. Adults Age 16 to 65 at Each Level of Proficiency on the PIAAC Numeracy Scale

academically through the middle and high-school years. Research shows that academic success, risky behaviors, and health status are linked.

Data on Adults' Literacy and Numeracy Skills

The most current adult literacy data come from the Program for the International Assessment of Adult Competencies (PIAAC), a 23-country comparative study. This study assessed adults' proficiency in three domains: literacy, numeracy, and problem-solving in technology-rich environments.

In each of these domains, adults perform tasks with different levels of complexity. Their skills with these tasks are quantified and categorized into "proficiency levels." The proficiency level "below level 1" is the lowest level and "level 5" is the highest proficiency level. If they can perform the most complex tasks, they are rated as having proficient skills.

Only 12 percent of U.S. adults scored in the highest literacy proficiency levels, and only 9 percent scored in the highest numeracy levels.

Chapter 22 | **The Importance of Health Communication and Health Information Technology**

THE NATIONAL ACTION PLAN TO IMPROVE HEALTH LITERACY

The National Action Plan to Improve Health Literacy (NAPIHL) seeks to engage organizations, professionals, policymakers, communities, individuals, and families in a linked, multisector effort to improve health literacy. The action plan is based on two core principles:

- All people have the right to health information that helps them make informed decisions.
- Health services should be delivered in ways that are easy to understand and that improve health, longevity, and quality of life (QOL).

The action plan contains seven goals that will improve health literacy and strategies for achieving them.

- Develop and disseminate health and safety information that is accurate, accessible, and actionable.
- Promote changes in the healthcare system that improve health information, communication, informed decision-making, and access to health services.

This chapter contains text excerpted from the following sources: Text under the heading "The National Action Plan to Improve Health Literacy" is excerpted from "National Action Plan to Improve Health Literacy," Office of Disease Prevention and Health Promotion (ODPHP), U.S. Department of Health and Human Services (HHS), October 30, 2019; Text beginning with the heading "Information Technology Plays a Key Role in Health Communication" is excerpted from "Health Communication and Health Information Technology," Office of Disease Prevention and Health Promotion (ODPHP), U.S. Department of Health and Human Services (HHS), October 30, 2019.

- Incorporate accurate, standards-based, and developmentally appropriate health and science information and curricula in child care and education through the university level.
- Support and expand local efforts to provide adult education, English language instruction, and culturally and linguistically appropriate health information services in the community.
- Build partnerships, develop guidance, and change policies.
- Increase basic research and the development, implementation, and evaluation of practices and interventions to improve health literacy.
- Increase the dissemination and use of evidence-based health literacy practices and interventions.

Many of the strategies highlight actions that particular organizations or professions can take to further these goals. It will take everyone working together in a linked and coordinated manner to improve access to accurate and actionable health information and usable health services. By focusing on health literacy issues and working together, accessibility, quality, and safety of healthcare; reduce costs can be improved and thereby improve the health and QOL of millions of people in the United States.

INFORMATION TECHNOLOGY PLAYS A KEY ROLE IN HEALTH COMMUNICATION

Ideas about health and behaviors are shaped by communication, information, and technology that people interact with every day. Health communication and health information technology (IT) are central to healthcare, public health, and the way our society views health. These processes make up the ways and the context in which professionals and the public search for, understand, and use health information, significantly impacting their health decisions and actions.

The ways in which health communication and health IT can have a positive impact on health, healthcare, and health equity include:
- Supporting shared decision-making between patients and providers
- Providing personalized self-management tools and resources
- Building social support networks
- Delivering accurate, accessible, and actionable health information that is targeted or tailored
- Facilitating the meaningful use of health IT and exchange of health information among healthcare and public health professionals
- Enabling quick and informed responses to health risks and public health emergencies
- Increasing health literacy skills
- Providing new opportunities to connect with culturally diverse and hard-to-reach populations

- Providing sound principles in the design of programs and interventions that result in healthier behaviors.
- Increasing Internet and mobile access

WHY ARE HEALTH COMMUNICATION AND HEALTH INFORMATION TECHNOLOGY IMPORTANT?

Effective use of communication and technology by healthcare and public-health professionals can bring about an age of patient- and public-centered health information and services. By strategically combining health IT tools and effective health communication processes, there is the potential to:

- Improve healthcare quality and safety
- Increase the efficiency of healthcare and public health service delivery
- Improve the public health information infrastructure
- Support care in the community and at home
- Facilitate clinical and consumer decision-making
- Build health skills and knowledge

UNDERSTANDING HEALTH COMMUNICATION AND HEALTH INFORMATION TECHNOLOGY

All people have some ability to manage their health and the health of those they care for. However, with the increasing complexity of health information and healthcare settings, most people need additional information, skills, and supportive relationships to meet their health needs.

Disparities in access to health information, services, and technology can result in lower usage rates of preventive services, less knowledge of chronic disease management (CDM), higher rates of hospitalization, and poorer reported health status.

Both public and private institutions are increasingly using the Internet and other technologies to streamline the delivery of health information and services. This results in an even greater need for health professionals to develop additional skills in the understanding and use of consumer health information.

The increase in online health information and services challenges users with limited literacy skills or limited experience using the Internet. For many of these users, the Internet is stressful and overwhelming—even inaccessible. Much of this stress can be reduced through the application of evidence-based best practices in user-centered design.

In addition, despite increased access to technology, other forms of communication are essential to ensuring that everyone, including nonweb users, is able to obtain, process, and understand health information to make good health decisions. These include printed materials, media campaigns, community outreach, and interpersonal communication.

EMERGING ISSUES IN HEALTH COMMUNICATION AND HEALTH INFORMATION TECHNOLOGY

During the coming decade, the speed, scope, and scale of adoption of health IT will only increase. Social media and emerging technologies promise to blur the line between expert and peer health information. Monitoring and assessing the impact of these new media, including mobile health, on public health will be challenging.

Equally challenging will be helping health professionals and the public adapt to the changes in healthcare quality and efficiency due to the creative use of health communication and health IT. Continual feedback, productive interactions, and access to evidence on the effectiveness of treatments and interventions will likely transform the traditional patient–provider relationship. It will also change the way people receive, process, and evaluate health information. Capturing the scope and impact of these changes—and the role of health communication and health IT in facilitating them—will require multidisciplinary models and data systems.

Such systems will be critical to expanding the collection of data to better understand the effects of health communication and health IT on population health outcomes, healthcare quality, and health disparities.

Chapter 23 | eHealth Literacy

Chapter Contents

Section 23.1 | What Is eHealth Literacy?

This section contains text excerpted from the following sources: Text in this section begins with excerpts from "Tackling eHealth Literacy," Centers for Disease Control and Prevention (CDC), March 5, 2018; Text under the heading "Need for eHealth Literacy" is excerpted from "eHealth Literacy, Online Help-Seeking Behavior, and Willingness to Participate in mHealth Chronic Disease Research among African Americans, Florida, 2014–2015," Centers for Disease Control and Prevention (CDC), November 17, 2016. Reviewed December 2019.

These days it seems as if everyone has a smartphone. Health services are increasingly being delivered through web-based and mobile resources. Examples of electronic health (eHealth) services include:

- Electronic communication between patients and healthcare providers
- Electronic medical records (EMRs)
- Patient portals
- Personal-health records

Mobile health (mHealth), a subcategory of eHealth, includes using tablets and phones to access apps and wearable tracking devices.

NEED FOR EHEALTH LITERACY

Searching online for health information is an easy and affordable way for Americans to learn more about their health, self-diagnose an illness, and manage a health condition. Approximately 6 in 10 American adults search online for

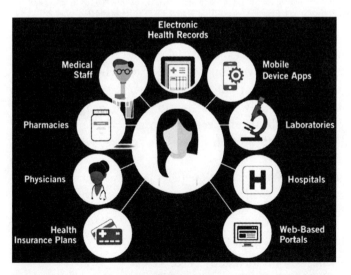

Figure 23.1. Your Rights to Your Health Information *(Source: "Your Health Information, Your Rights," HealthIT.gov, Office of the National Coordinator for Health Information Technology (ONC))*

8 in 10 individuals who have viewed their medical record online considered the information useful

27% of individuals were unaware or did not believe they had a right to an electronic copy of their medical record

41% of Americans have never seen their health information

HIPPA gives us the right to access our health information

Figure 23.2. Facts about Health Information Awareness and Your Rights *(Source: "Your Health Information, Your Rights," HealthIT.gov, Office of the National Coordinator for Health Information Technology (ONC))*

health information, and the trend is expected to increase as ownership of mobile devices grows and access to high-speed Internet expands.

Section 23.2 | What Is an eHealth Record?

This section contains text excerpted from the following sources: Text in this section begins with excerpts from "What Is an Electronic Health Record (EHR)?" HealthIT.gov, Office of the National Coordinator for Health Information Technology (ONC), September 10, 2019; Text under the heading "Electronic Health Records Foster Patient Participation" is excerpted from "Increase Patient Participation in Their Care," HealthIT.gov, Office of the National Coordinator for Health Information Technology (ONC), September 26, 2018; Text under the heading "Keeping Your Electronic Health Information Secure" is excerpted from "Privacy, Security, and Electronic Health Records," U.S. Department of Health and Human Services (HHS), March 17, 2013. Reviewed December 2019.

The world has been radically transformed by digital technology—smartphones, tablets, and web-enabled devices have transformed our daily lives and the way we communicate. Medicine is an information-rich enterprise.

A greater and more seamless flow of information within a digital healthcare infrastructure, created by electronic health records (EHRs), encompasses and leverages digital progress and can transform the way care is delivered and compensated.

An EHR is a digital version of a patient's paper chart. EHRs are real-time, patient-centered records that make information available instantly and securely to authorized users.

WHAT INFORMATION DOES AN eHEALTH RECORD CONTAIN?

An EHR contains patient health information, such as:

- Administrative and billing data
- Patient demographics

- Progress notes
- Vital signs
- Medical histories
- Diagnoses
- Medications
- Immunization dates
- Allergies
- Radiology images
- Lab and test results

While an EHR does contain the medical and treatment histories of patients, an EHR system is built to go beyond standard clinical data collected in a healthcare provider's office and can be inclusive of a broader view of a patient's care. EHRs are a vital part of health IT and can:

- Allow access to evidence-based tools that healthcare providers can use to make decisions about a patient's care
- Automate and streamline healthcare provider workflow

One of the key features of an EHR is that health information can be created and managed by authorized healthcare providers in a digital format capable of being shared with other healthcare providers across more than one healthcare organization. EHRs are built to share information with other healthcare providers and organizations—such as laboratories, specialists, medical imaging facilities, pharmacies, emergency facilities, and school and workplace clinics—so they contain information from all the clinicians involved in a patient's care.

BENEFITS OF ELECTRONIC HEALTH RECORDS

Electronic health records are real-time, patient-centered records that make information available instantly and securely to authorized users. While an EHR does contain the medical and treatment histories of patients, an EHR system is built to go beyond standard clinical data collected in a healthcare provider's office and can be inclusive of a broader view of a patient's care.

Electronic health records can:

- Contain a patient's medical history, diagnoses, medications, treatment plans, immunization dates, allergies, radiology images, and laboratory and test results
- Allow access to evidence-based tools that healthcare providers can use to make decisions about a patient's care
- Automate and streamline healthcare provider workflow

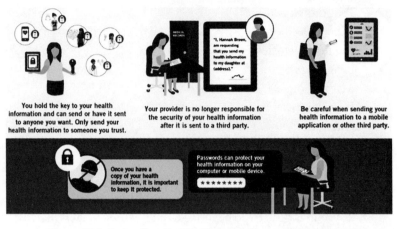

Figure 23.3. Protect Your Health Information *(Source: "Your Health Information, Your Rights," HealthIT.gov, Office of the National Coordinator for Health Information Technology (ONC))*

ELECTRONIC HEALTH RECORDS FOSTER PATIENT PARTICIPATION

Providers and patients who share access to electronic health information can collaborate in informed decision making. Patient participation is especially important in managing and treating chronic conditions such as asthma, diabetes, and obesity.

Electronic health records can help healthcare providers by:

- Ensuring high-quality care. With EHRs, healthcare providers can give patients full and accurate information about all of their medical evaluations. They can also offer follow-up information, such as self-care instructions, reminders for other follow-up care, and links to web resources, after an office visit or a hospital stay.

- Creating an avenue for communication with their patients. With EHRs, healthcare providers can manage appointment schedules electronically and exchange e-mail with their patients. Quick and easy communication between patients and healthcare providers may help the latter identify symptoms earlier. And it can position providers to be more proactive by reaching out to patients. Healthcare providers can also provide information to their patients through patient portals tied into their EHR system.

KEEPING YOUR ELECTRONIC HEALTH INFORMATION SECURE

Most of us feel that our health information is private and should be protected. The federal government put in place the Health Insurance Portability and Accountability Act (HIPAA) of 1996 Privacy Rule to ensure you have rights over your own health information, no matter what form it is in. The government also created the HIPAA Security Rule to require specific protections be in place in order to safeguard your electronic health information. A few possible measures that can be built into EHR systems include:

- "Access control" tools, such as passwords and PIN numbers, to help limit access to your information to authorized individuals
- "Encrypting" your stored information. This means your health information cannot be read or understood except by those using a system that can "decrypt" it with a "key."
- An "audit trail" feature, which records who accessed your information, what changes were made, and when

Finally, federal law requires doctors, hospitals, and other healthcare providers to notify you of a security "breach." The law also requires the healthcare provider to notify the Secretary of the U.S. Department of Health and Human Services (HHS). If a security breach affects more than 500 residents of a state or jurisdiction, the healthcare provider must also notify prominent media outlets serving the state or jurisdiction. This requirement helps patients know if something has gone wrong with the protection of their information and helps keep providers accountable for EHR protection.

Chapter 24 | **Patient Rights and Responsibilities**

Chapter Contents

Section 24.1 | Your Healthcare Rights and Responsibilities

This section contains text excerpted from the following sources: Text under the heading "What Are Your Healthcare Rights and Responsibilities?" is excerpted from "What Are My Healthcare Rights and Responsibilities?" U.S. Department of Health and Human Services (HHS), August 11, 2014. Reviewed December 2019; Text under the heading "Health Insurance Rights and Protections" is excerpted from "Health Insurance Rights and Protections—Rights and Protections," Centers for Medicare & Medicaid Services (CMS), November 21, 2015. Reviewed December 2019; Text under the heading "Your Health Information Rights" is excerpted from "Your Health Information Rights," HealthIT.gov, Office of the National Coordinator for Health Information Technology (ONC), September 7, 2017.

WHAT ARE YOUR HEALTHCARE RIGHTS AND RESPONSIBILITIES?

As a patient, you have certain rights. Some are guaranteed by federal law, such as the right to get a copy of your medical records, and the right to keep them private. Many states have additional laws protecting patients, and healthcare facilities often have a patient bill of rights.

An important patient right is informed consent. This means that if you need a treatment, your healthcare provider must give you the information you need to make a decision.

Many hospitals have patient advocates who can help you if you have problems. Many states have an ombudsman office for problems with long term care. Your state's department of health may also be able to help.

HEALTH INSURANCE RIGHTS AND PROTECTIONS

The healthcare law offers rights and protections that make coverage fair and easy to understand. Some rights and protections apply to plans in the Health Insurance Marketplace or other individual insurance, some apply to job-based plans, and some apply to all health coverage. The protections outlined below may not apply to grandfathered health insurance plans.

The Healthcare Law Protects You

- The healthcare law requires insurance plans to cover people with preexisting health conditions, including pregnancy, without charging more.
- It provides free preventive care.
- It gives young adults more coverage options.
- It ends lifetime and yearly dollar limits on coverage of essential health benefits.
- It helps you understand the coverage you are getting.
- It holds insurance companies accountable for rate increases.
- It makes it illegal for health insurance companies to cancel your health insurance just because you get sick.

- It protects your choice of doctors.
- It protects you from employer retaliation.

YOUR HEALTH INFORMATION RIGHTS
Do I Have the Right to See and Get a Copy of My Health Records?

Yes. The Health Insurance Portability and Accountability Act (HIPAA) Privacy Rule gives you the right to inspect, review, and receive a copy of your health and billing records that are held by health plans and healthcare providers covered under HIPAA.

In a few special cases, you may not be able to get all of your information. For example, your doctor may decide that something in your file could physically endanger you or someone else and may not have to give this information to you.

In most cases, your copies must be given to you within 30 days. However, if your health information is not maintained or accessible on-site, your healthcare provider or health plan can take up to 60 days to respond to your request. If, for some reason, they cannot take action by these deadlines, your provider or plan it may extend the deadline by another 30 days if they give you a reason for the delay in writing and tell you when to expect your copies.

The provider cannot charge a fee for searching for or retrieving your information, but you may have to pay for the cost of copying and mailing.

Your state may also have laws that give you rights to see and copy your medical records. If there is a difference between state and federal law, your provider must follow the law that gives you the most rights.

Do I Have a Right to Know When My Healthcare Provider Has Shared My Health Information with People Outside of Her or His Practice?

Yes. You have a right to receive an "accounting of disclosures," which is a list of certain instances when your healthcare provider or health plan has shared your health information with another person or organization. There are some major exceptions to this right. As of now, an accounting of disclosures does not include information about when your healthcare provider or health plan shares your information with another person or organization for treatment, payment, or healthcare operations.

Can I Ask to Correct the Information in My Health Records?

Yes. You can ask your healthcare provider or your health plan to correct your health record by adding information to it to make it more accurate or complete. This is called the "right to amend." For example, if you and your hospital agree that your record has the wrong result for a test, the hospital must change it. If you and your health provider or health plan do not agree that an amendment is necessary, you still have the right to have your disagreement noted in your record. In most cases, your record should be changed within 60 days, but the provider can take an extra 30 days if they provide you a reason.

Do I Have the Right to Receive a Notice That Tells Me How My Health Information Is Being Used and Shared?

Yes. You can learn how your health information is used and shared by your provider or health insurer. They must give you a notice that tells you how they legally may use and share your health information and how you can exercise your rights. In most cases, you should get this notice on your first visit to a provider or in the mail from your health plan, and you can ask for a copy at any time. This is the document that providers often ask for you to sign to indicate that you have received it.

Who Has to Follow the Parts of the HIPAA Privacy Rule That Give Me Rights with Respect to My Health Information?

- Most doctors, nurses, pharmacies, hospitals, clinics, nursing homes, and many other healthcare providers
- Health insurance companies, health maintenance organization (HMOs), and most employer group health plans
- Certain government programs that pay for healthcare, such as Medicare and Medicaid

Do I Have the Right to File a Complaint?

Yes. If you believe your information was used or shared in a way that is not allowed under the HIPAA Privacy Rule, or if you were not able to exercise your health information rights, you can file a complaint with your provider or health insurer. The privacy notice you receive from them will tell you how to file a complaint. You can also file a complaint with the U.S. Department of Health and Human Services' (HHS) Office for Civil Rights (OCR) or your state's Attorneys General Office.

Are State Governments Involved in Protecting Privacy Rights?

Yes. The HIPAA Privacy Rule sets a federal "floor" of privacy protections— a minimum level of privacy that healthcare providers and health plans must meet. Many states have health information privacy laws that have additional protections that are above this floor. In addition, even though HIPAA is a federal law, state Attorneys General have been given the authority to enforce HIPAA.

Section 24.2 | **Your Health Information Privacy Rights**

This section contains text excerpted from the following sources: Text in this section begins with excerpts from "Your Rights Under HIPAA," U.S. Department of Health and Human Services (HHS), February 1, 2017; Text beginning with the heading "What You Should Know about Your Health Information Privacy Rights" is excerpted from "Your Health Information Privacy Rights," U.S. Department of Health and Human Services (HHS), March 14, 2013. Reviewed December 2019; Text under the heading "Sharing Health Information with Family Members and Friends" is excerpted from "Sharing Health Information with Family Members and Friends," U.S. Department of Health and Human Services (HHS), March 14, 2013. Reviewed December 2019.

Most of us believe that our medical and other health information is private and should be protected, and we want to know who has this information. The Privacy Rule, a federal law, gives you rights over your health information and sets rules and limits on who can look at and receive your health information. The Privacy Rule applies to all forms of individuals' protected health information, whether electronic, written, or oral. The Security Rule is a federal law that requires security for health information in electronic form.

WHO MUST FOLLOW THESE LAWS?

The entities that must follow the Health Insurance Portability and Accountability Act (HIPAA) regulations is called "covered entities."

Covered entities include:

- Health plans, including health insurance companies, health maintenance organizations (HMOs), company health plans, and certain government programs that pay for healthcare, such as Medicare and Medicaid
- Healthcare providers—those that conduct certain business electronically, such as electronically billing your health insurance— including most doctors, clinics, hospitals, psychologists, chiropractors, nursing homes, pharmacies, and dentists
- Healthcare clearinghouses—entities that process nonstandard health information they receive from another entity into a standard (i.e., standard electronic format or data content), or vice versa

In addition, business associates of covered entities must follow parts of the HIPAA regulations.

Often, contractors, subcontractors, and other outside persons and companies that are not employees of a covered entity will need to have access to your health information when providing services to the covered entity. These entities are called "business associates." Examples of business associates include:

- Companies that help your doctors get paid for providing healthcare, including billing companies, and companies that process your healthcare claims

Patient Rights and Responsibilities

- Companies that help administer health plans
- People such as outside lawyers, accountants, and IT specialists
- Companies that store or destroy medical records

Covered entities must have contracts in place with their business associates, ensuring that they use and disclose your health information properly and safeguard it appropriately. Business associates must also have similar contracts with subcontractors. Business associates (including subcontractors) must follow the use and disclosure provisions of their contracts and the Privacy Rule, and the safeguard requirements of the Security Rule.

WHO IS NOT REQUIRED TO FOLLOW THESE LAWS?

Many organizations that have health information about you do not have to follow these laws.

Examples of organizations that do not have to follow the Privacy and Security Rules include:

- Life insurers
- Employers
- Workers compensation carriers
- Most schools and school districts
- Many state agencies, such as child protective service (CPS) agencies
- Most law enforcement agencies
- Many municipal offices

WHAT INFORMATION IS PROTECTED

The information protected by this law include:

- Information your doctors, nurses, and other healthcare providers put in your medical record
- Conversations your doctor has about your care or treatment with nurses and others
- Information about you in your health insurer's computer system
- Billing information about you at your clinic
- Most other health information about you held by those who must follow these laws

HOW THIS INFORMATION IS PROTECTED

According to the law:

- Covered entities must put in place safeguards to protect your health information and ensure they do not use or disclose your health information improperly
- Covered entities must reasonably limit uses and disclosures to the minimum necessary to accomplish their intended purpose

- Covered entities must have procedures in place to limit who can view and access your health information as well as implement training programs for employees about how to protect your health information
- Business associates also must put in place safeguards to protect you heal

WHAT RIGHTS DOES THE PRIVACY RULE GIVE YOU OVER YOUR HEALTH INFORMATION?

Health insurers and providers who are covered entities must comply with your right to:

- Ask to see and get a copy of your health records
- Have corrections added to your health information
- Receive a notice that tells you how your health information may be used and shared
- Decide if you want to give your permission before your health information can be used or shared for certain purposes, such as for marketing
- Get a report on when and why your health information was shared for certain purposes

If you believe your rights are being denied or your health information is not being protected, you can:

- File a complaint with your healthcare provider or health insurer
- File a complaint with U.S. Department of Health and Human Services (HHS)

You should get to know these important rights, which help you protect your health information. You can ask your healthcare provider or health insurer questions about your rights.

WHO CAN LOOK AT AND RECEIVE YOUR HEALTH INFORMATION?

The Privacy Rule sets rules and limits on who can look at and receive your health information to make sure that your health information is protected in a way that does not interfere with your healthcare, your information can be used and shared:

- For your treatment and care coordination
- To pay doctors and hospitals for your healthcare and to help run their businesses
- With your family, relatives, friends, or others you identify who are involved with your healthcare or your healthcare bills, unless you object
- To make sure doctors give good care and nursing homes are clean and safe

Patient Rights and Responsibilities

- To protect the public's health, such as by reporting when the flu is in your area
- To make required reports to the police, such as reporting gunshot wounds

Your health information cannot be used or shared without your written permission unless this law allows it. For example, without your authorization, your healthcare provider generally cannot:

- Give your information to your employer
- Use or share your information for marketing or advertising purposes or sell your information

WHAT YOU SHOULD KNOW ABOUT YOUR HEALTH INFORMATION PRIVACY RIGHTS

Most of us feel that our health information is private and should be protected. That is why there is a federal law that sets rules for healthcare providers and health insurance companies about who can look at and receive our health information. This law, (HIPAA), gives you rights over your health information, including the right to get a copy of your information, make sure it is correct, and know who has seen it.

Get It

You can ask to see or get a copy of your medical record and other health information. If you want a copy, you may have to put your request in writing and pay for the cost of copying and mailing. In most cases, your copies must be given to you within 30 days.

Check It

You can ask to change any wrong information in your file or add information to your file if you think something is missing or incomplete. For example, if you and your hospital agree that your file has the wrong result for a test, the hospital must change it. Even if the hospital believes the test result is correct, you still have the right to have your disagreement noted in your file. In most cases, the file should be updated within 60 days.

Know Who Has Seen It

By law, your health information can be used and shared for specific reasons not directly related to your care, such as making sure doctors give good care, making sure nursing homes are clean and safe, reporting when the flu is in your area, or reporting as required by state or federal law. In many of these cases, you can find out who has seen your health information.

You can:

- **Learn how your health information is used and shared by your doctor or health insurer.** Generally, your health information cannot be used for purposes not directly related to your care without your permission. For example, your doctor cannot give it to your employer, or share it for things such as marketing and advertising, without your written authorization. You probably received a notice telling you how your health information may be used on your first visit to a new healthcare provider or when you got new health insurance, but you can ask for another copy anytime.

- **Let your providers or health insurance companies know if there is information you do not want to share.** You can ask that your health information not be shared with certain people, groups, or companies. If you go to a clinic, for example, you can ask the doctor not to share your medical records with other doctors or nurses at the clinic. You can ask for other kinds of restrictions, but they do not always have to agree to do what you ask, particularly if it could affect your care. Finally, you can also ask your healthcare provider or pharmacy not to tell your health insurance company about the care you receive or drugs you take, if you pay for the care or drugs in full and the provider or pharmacy does not need to get paid by your insurance company.

- **Ask to be reached somewhere other than home.** You can make reasonable requests to be contacted at different places or in a different way. For example, you can ask to have a nurse call you at your office instead of your home or to send mail to you in an envelope instead of on a postcard.

If you think your rights are being denied or your health information is not being protected, you have the right to file a complaint with your provider, health insurer, or the HHS.

SHARING HEALTH INFORMATION WITH FAMILY MEMBERS AND FRIENDS

Health Insurance Portability and Accountability Act of 1996 sets rules for healthcare providers and health plans about who can look at and receive your health information, including those closest to you—your family members and friends. The HIPAA Privacy Rule ensures that you have rights over your health information, including the right to get your information, make sure it is correct, and know who has seen it.

What Happens If You Want to Share Health Information with a Family Member or a Friend

The HIPAA requires most doctors, nurses, hospitals, nursing homes, and other healthcare providers to protect the privacy of your health information. However,

Patient Rights and Responsibilities

if you do not object, a healthcare provider or health plan may share relevant information with family members or friends involved in your healthcare or payment for your healthcare in certain circumstances.

When Your Health Information Can Be Shared

Under HIPAA, your healthcare provider may share your information face-to-face, over the phone, or in writing. A healthcare provider or health plan may share relevant information if:

- You give your healthcare provider or plan permission to share the information
- You are present and do not object to sharing the information
- You are not present, and the healthcare provider determines, based on professional judgment, that it is in your best interest

Examples:

- An emergency room (ER) doctor may discuss your treatment in front of your friend when you ask your friend to come into the treatment room.
- Your hospital may discuss your bill with your daughter who is with you and has a question about the charges, if you do not object.
- Your doctor may discuss the drugs you need to take with your health aide who has come with you to your appointment.
- Your nurse may not discuss your condition with your brother if you tell her not to.
- The Health Insurance Portability and Accountability Act also allows healthcare providers to give prescription drugs, medical supplies, x-rays, and other healthcare items to a family member, friend, or other people you send to pick them up.

A healthcare provider or health plan may also share relevant information if you are not around or cannot give permission when a healthcare provider or plan representative believes, based on professional judgment, that sharing the information is in your best interest.

Examples:

- You had emergency surgery and are still unconscious. Your surgeon may tell your spouse about your condition, either in person or by phone, while you are unconscious.
- Your doctor may discuss your drugs with your caregiver who calls your doctor with a question about the right dosage.
- A doctor may not tell your friend about a past medical problem that is unrelated to your current condition.

Section 24.3 | How to Keep Your Health Information Private and Secure

This section contains text excerpted from the following sources: Text under the heading "Protecting the Privacy and Security of Your Health Information" is excerpted from "Protecting Your Privacy and Security," HealthIT. gov, Office of the National Coordinator for Health Information Technology (ONC), December 17, 2018; Text beginning with the heading "Health IT: How to Keep Your Health Information Private and Secure" is excerpted from "Health IT: How to Keep Your Health Information Private and Secure," HealthIT.gov, Office of the National Coordinator for Health Information Technology (ONC), September 17, 2013. Reviewed December 2019.

PROTECTING THE PRIVACY AND SECURITY OF YOUR HEALTH INFORMATION

The privacy and security of patient-health information is a top priority for patients and their families, healthcare providers and professionals, and the government. Federal laws require many of the key persons and organizations that handle health information to have policies and security safeguards in place to protect your health information—whether it is stored on paper or electronically.

The Health Insurance Portability and Accountability Act of 1996 (HIPAA) Privacy, Security, and Breach Notification Rules are the main federal laws that protect your health information. The Privacy Rule gives you rights with respect to your health information. The Privacy Rule also sets limits on how your health information can be used and shared with others. The Security Rule sets rules for how your health information must be kept secure with administrative, technical, and physical safeguards.

You may have additional protections and health information rights under your state's laws. There are also federal laws that protect specific types of health information, such as information related to federally-funded alcohol and substance-abuse treatment.

Your Privacy Rights

If you believe your health information privacy has been violated, the U.S. Department of Health and Human Services (HHS) has a division, the Office for Civil Rights (OCR), to educate you about your privacy rights, enforce the rules, and help you file a complaint.

Security

Healthcare providers and other key persons and organizations that handle your health information must protect it with passwords, encryption, and other technical safeguards. These are designed to make sure that only the right people have access to your information.

Be Responsible

While federal law can protect your health information, you should also use common sense to make sure that private information does not become public. If you access your health records online, make sure you use a strong password and keep it a secret. Keep in mind that if you post information online in a public forum, you cannot assume it is private or secure.

HEALTH IT: HOW TO KEEP YOUR HEALTH INFORMATION PRIVATE AND SECURE

There are laws that protect the privacy of your health information held by those who provide you healthcare services. But, as it becomes easier to get and share your own health information online, you need to take steps to protect it. This applies whether you are downloading a copy of your health information via Blue Button, e-mailing your doctor, taking an online health survey, or using a variety of digital apps or devices to monitor your health.

DOES THE HEALTH INSURANCE PORTABILITY AND ACCOUNTABILITY ACT PROTECT ALL HEALTH INFORMATION?

No. You may have heard about HIPPA, Privacy and Security Rules. These are federal laws that set national standards for protecting the privacy and security of health information. Health information that is kept by healthcare providers, health plans and organizations acting on their behalf is protected by these federal laws. However, you should know that there are many organizations that do not have to follow these laws. Some examples of health information that is not covered by HIPAA include health information that patients:

- Store in a mobile app or on a mobile device, such as a smartphone or table
- Share over social media websites or health-related online communities, such as message boards
- Store in a personal-health record (PHR) that is not offered through a health provider or health plan covered by HIPAA

KEEP YOUR ELECTRONIC HEALTH INFORMATION SECURE

There are a number of ways you can help protect your electronic-health information. Here are some tips to ensure your personal-health information is private and secure when accessing it electronically:

When Creating a Password

- Use a password or other function on your home computer or mobile. device so that you are the only one who can access your information.
- Use a strong password and update it often.
- Do not share your password with anyone.

When Using Social Media

- Think carefully before you post anything on the Internet that you do not want to be made public—do not assume that an online public forum is private or secure.

- If you decide to post health information on a social media platform, consider using the privacy setting to limit others' access.
- Be aware that information posted on the web may remain permanently.

When Using Mobile Devices

- Research mobile apps—software programs that perform one or more specific functions—before you download and install any of them. Be sure to use known app websites or trusted sources.
- Read the terms of service and privacy notice of the mobile app to verify that the app will perform only the functions you approve.
- Consider installing or using encryption software for your device. Encryption software is now widely available and increasingly affordable.
- Install and activate remote wiping and/or remote disabling on your mobile devices. The remote wipe feature allows you to permanently delete data stored on a lost or stolen mobile device. Remote disabling enables you to lock data stored on a lost or stolen mobile device, and unlock the data if the device is recovered.

Chapter 25 | Informed Consent

Informed consent is a process through which you learn details about the trial before deciding whether to take part. This includes learning about the trial's purpose and possible risks and benefits. This is a critical part of ensuring patient safety in research.

During the informed consent process, the research team, which is made up of doctors and nurses, first explains the trial to you. The team explains the trial's:

- Purpose
- Procedures
- Risks and benefits

They will also discuss your rights, including your right to:
- Make a decision about participating
- Leave the study at any time

Before agreeing to take part in a trial, you have the right to:
- Learn about all your treatment options
- Learn all that is involved in the trial, including all details about treatment, tests, and possible risks and benefits
- Discuss the trial with the principal investigator and other members of the research team
- Both hear and read the information in language you can understand

After discussing the study with you, the research team will give you an informed consent form to read. The form includes written details about the information that was discussed with you and describes the privacy of your medical

This chapter contains text excerpted from the following sources: Text in this chapter begins with excerpts from "Informed Consent," National Cancer Institute (NCI), June 22, 2016. Reviewed December 2019; Text under the heading "Tips for Informed Consent" is excerpted from "Informed Consent Tips (1993)," U.S. Department of Health and Human Services (HHS), March 18, 2016. Reviewed December 2019.

records. If you agree to take part in the study, you sign the form. But, even after you sign the consent form, you can leave the study at any time. You can always ask questions. And, as new information becomes available, the research team will inform you.

TIPS FOR INFORMED CONSENT

The process of obtaining informed consent must comply with the requirements of 45 CFR 46.116. The documentation of informed consent must comply with 45 CFR 46.117:

- Informed consent is a process, not just a form. Information must be presented to enable you to voluntarily decide whether or not to participate as a research subject. It is a fundamental mechanism to ensure respect for persons through provision of thoughtful consent for a voluntary act. The procedures used in obtaining informed consent should be designed to educate you in terms that you can understand. The written presentation of information is used to document the basis for consent and for your future reference.

- The document should describe the overall experience that you will be encountering. The document should explain the research activity, how it is experimental (e.g., a new drug, extra tests, separate research records, or nonstandard means of management, such as flipping a coin for random assignment or other design issues). It should inform the reasonably foreseeable harms, discomforts, inconvenience, and risks that are associated with the research activity.

- The document should describe the benefits that you may reasonably expect to encounter.

- Describe any alternatives to participating in the research project. For example, in drug studies the medication(s) may be available through your family doctor or clinic without the need to volunteer for the research activity.

- The regulations insist that you should be told the extent to which your personally identifiable private information will be held in confidence. For example, some studies require disclosure of information to other parties. Some studies inherently are in need of a Certificate of Confidentiality which protects the investigator from involuntary release (e.g., subpoena) of the names or other identifying characteristics of research subjects. The IRB will determine the level of adequate requirements for confidentiality in light of its mandate to ensure minimization of risk and determination that the residual risks warrant your involvement.

- If research-related injury (i.e., physical, psychological, social, financial, or otherwise) is possible in research that is more than minimal risk

Informed Consent

(45 CFR 46.102 [g]), an explanation must be given of whatever voluntary compensation and treatment will be provided. Note that the regulations do not limit injury to "physical injury." This is a common misinterpretation.

- The regulations prohibit waiving or appearing to waive any of your legal rights. You should not be given the impression that you have agreed to and are without recourse to seek satisfaction beyond the institution's voluntarily chosen limits.
- The regulations provide for the identification of contact persons who would be knowledgeable to answer your questions about the research, rights as a research subject, and research-related injuries. These three areas must be explicitly stated and addressed in the consent process and documentation. These questions could be addressed to the IRB, an ombudsman, an ethics committee, or other informed administrative body. Therefore, each consent document can be expected to have at least two names with local telephone numbers for contacts to answer questions in these specified areas.
- The statement regarding voluntary participation and the right to withdraw at any time can be taken almost verbatim from the regulations (45 CFR 46.116 [a][8]). It is important not to overlook the need to point out that no penalty or loss of benefits will occur as a result of both not participating or withdrawing at any time. It is equally important to alert you to any foreseeable consequences to you and that you should unilaterally withdraw while dependent on some intervention to maintain normal function.

Chapter 26 | **Personal Health Records and Patient Portals**

WHAT IS A PERSONAL HEALTH RECORD?

A personal health record, or PHR, is an electronic application through which patients can maintain and manage their health information (and that of others for whom they are authorized) in a private, secure, and confidential environment.

ARE THERE DIFFERENT TYPES OF PERSONAL HEALTH RECORDS?

Yes, there are two main kinds of PHRs.

- **Standalone PHRs.** With a standalone PHR, patients fill in information from their own records, and the information is stored on patients' computers or the Internet. In some cases, a standalone PHR can also accept data from external sources, including providers and laboratories. With a standalone PHR, patients could add diet or exercise information to track progress over time. Patients can decide whether to share the information with providers, family members, or anyone else involved in their care.
- **Tethered/connected PHRs.** A tethered, or connected, PHR is linked to a specific healthcare organization's electronic health record (EHR) system or to a health plan's information system. With a tethered PHR, patients can access their own records through a secure portal and

This chapter contains text excerpted from the following sources: Text under the heading "What Is a Personal Health Record?" is excerpted from "What Is a Personal Health Record?" HealthIT.gov, Office of the National Coordinator for Health Information Technology (ONC), May 2, 2016. Reviewed December 2019; Text under the heading "Are There Different Types of Personal Health Records?" is excerpted from "Are There Different Types of Personal Health Records (PHRs)?" HealthIT.gov, Office of the National Coordinator for Health Information Technology (ONC), July 30, 2019; Text under the heading "What Is a Patient Portal?" is excerpted from "What Is a Patient Portal?" HealthIT.gov, Office of the National Coordinator for Health Information Technology (ONC), September 29, 2017.

see, for example, the trend of their lab results over the last year, their immunization history, or due dates for screenings.

WHAT IS A PATIENT PORTAL?

A patient portal is a secure online website that gives patients convenient, 24-hour access to personal health information from anywhere with an Internet connection. Using a secure username and password, patients can view health information such as:

- Recent doctor visits
- Discharge summaries
- Medications
- Immunizations
- Allergies
- Lab results

Some patient portals also allow you to:
- Securely message your doctor
- Request prescription refills
- Schedule nonurgent appointments
- Check benefits and coverage
- Update contact information
- Make payments
- Download and complete forms
- View educational materials

With your patient portal, you can be in control of your health and care. Patient portals can also save your time, help you communicate with your doctor, and support care between visits.

Chapter 27 | Making Sense of Internet Health Information

Many people share a common concern: "How can I trust the health information I find on the Internet?"

There are thousands of medical websites. Some provide reliable health information. Some do not. Some of the medical news is current. Some of it is not. Choosing which websites to trust is an important step in gathering reliable health information is current. Some of it is not. Choosing which websites to trust is an important step in gathering reliable health information.

WHERE CAN YOU FIND RELIABLE HEALTH INFORMATION ONLINE?

The National Institutes of Health (NIH) website (www.nih.gov) is a good place to start for reliable health information.

As a rule, health websites sponsored by federal government agencies are good sources of information. You can reach all federal websites by visiting www.usa.gov. Large professional organizations and well-known medical schools may also be good sources of health information.

QUESTIONS TO ASK BEFORE TRUSTING A WEBSITE

As you search online, you are likely to find websites for many health agencies and organizations that are not well-known. By answering the following questions, you should be able to find more information about these websites. A lot of these details might be found in the website's "About Us" section.

Who Does Sponsor/Host the Website? Is That Information Easy to Find?

Websites cost money to create and update. Is the source of funding (sponsor) clear? Knowing who is funding the website may give you an insight into the mission or goal of the site. Sometimes, the website address (called a "uniform resource locator" (URL)) is helpful.

This chapter includes text excerpted from "Online Health Information: Is It Reliable?" National Institute on Aging (NIA), National Institutes of Health (NIH), October 31, 2018.

For example:
- .gov identifies a U.S. government agency
- .edu identifies an educational institution, such as a school, college, or university
- .org usually identifies nonprofit organizations (such as professional groups; scientific, medical, or research societies; advocacy groups)
- .com identifies commercial websites (such as businesses, pharmaceutical companies, and sometimes hospitals)

Who Did Write the Information? Who Did Review It?

Authors and contributors are often, but not always, identified. If the author is listed, ask yourself—is this person an expert in the field? Does this person work for an organization and, if so, what are the goals of the organization? A contributor's connection to the website, and any financial stake she or he has in the information on the website, should be clear.

Is the health information written or reviewed by a healthcare professional? Dependable websites will tell you where their health information came from and how and when it was reviewed.

Trustworthy websites will have contact information that you can use to reach the site's sponsor or authors. An e-mail address, phone number, and/or mailing address might be listed at the bottom of every page or on a separate "About Us" or "Contact Us" page.

Be careful about testimonials. Personal stories may be helpful and comforting, but not everyone experiences health problems the same way. Also, there is a big difference between a website, blog, or social media page developed by a single person interested in a topic and a website developed using strong scientific evidence (that is, information gathered from research).

No information should replace seeing a doctor or other health professional who can give you advice that caters to your specific situation.

When Was the Information Written?

Look for websites that stay current with their health information. You do not want to make decisions about your care based on out-of-date information. Often, the bottom of the page will have a date. Pages on the same site may be updated at different times—some may be updated more often than others. Older information is not useless, but using the most current, evidence-based information is best.

What Is the Purpose of the Site?

Why was the site created? Know the motive or goal of the website so you can better judge its content. Is the purpose of the site to inform or explain? Or is it trying to sell a product? Choose information based on scientific evidence rather than one person's opinion.

Is Your Privacy Protected? Does the Website Clearly State a Privacy Policy?

Read the website's privacy policy. It is usually at the bottom of the page or on a separate page titled "Privacy Policy" or "Our Policies." If a website says it uses "cookies," your information may not be private. While cookies may enhance your web experience, they can also compromise your online privacy—so it is important to read how the website will use your information. You can choose to disable the use of cookies through your Internet browser settings.

How Can You Protect Your Health Information?

If you are asked to share personal information, be sure to find out how the information will be used. Secure websites that collect personal information responsibly have an "s" after "http" in the start of their website address (https://) and often require that you create a username and password.

BE CAREFUL about sharing your Social Security number (SSN). Find out why your number is needed, how it will be used, and what will happen if you do not share this information. Only enter your SSN on secure websites. You might consider calling your doctor's office or health insurance company to give this information over the phone, rather than giving it online.

These precautions can help better protect your information:

- **Use common sense when browsing the Internet.** Do not open unexpected links. Hover your mouse over a link to confirm that clicking it will take you to a reputable website.
- **Use a strong password.** Include a variation of numbers, letters, and symbols. Change it frequently.
- **Use two-factor authentication when you can.** This requires the use of two different types of personal information to log into your mobile devices or accounts.
- **Do not enter sensitive information over public Wi-Fi that is not secure.** This includes Wi-Fi that is not password protected.
- **Be careful what information you share over social media sites.** This can include addresses, phone numbers, and e-mail addresses.

Does the Website Offer Quick and Easy Solutions to Your Health Problems? Are Miracle Cures Promised?

Be careful of websites or companies that claim any one remedy will cure a lot of different illnesses. Question dramatic writing or cures that seem too good to be true. Make sure you can find other websites with the same information. Even if the website links to a trustworthy source, it does not mean that the site has the other organization's endorsement or support.

HEALTH AND MEDICAL APPS

Mobile medical applications ("apps") are apps you can put on your smartphone. Health apps can help you track your eating habits, physical activity, test results, or other information. But, anyone can develop a health app—for any reason—and apps may include inaccurate or misleading information. Make sure you know who made any app you use.

When you download an app, it may ask for your location, your e-mail, or other information. Consider what the app is asking from you—make sure the questions are relevant to the app and that you feel comfortable sharing this information. Remember, there is a difference between sharing your personal information through your doctor's online health portal and posting on third-party social media or health sites.

SOCIAL MEDIA AND HEALTH INFORMATION

Social media sites, such as Facebook, Twitter, and Instagram, are online communities where people connect with friends, family, and strangers. Sometimes, you might find health information or health news on social media. Some of this information may be true, and some of it may not be. Recognize that just because a post is from a friend or colleague, it does not necessarily mean it is true or scientifically accurate.

Check the source of the information, and make sure the author is credible. Fact-checking websites can also help you figure out if a story is reliable.

TRUST YOURSELF AND TALK TO YOUR DOCTOR

Use common sense and good judgment when looking at health information online. There are websites on nearly every health topic, and many have no rules overseeing the quality of the information provided. Use the information you find online as one tool to become more informed. Do not count on anyone's website and check your sources. Discuss what you find with your doctor before making any changes to your healthcare.

Chapter 28 | Preventing Medical Errors

One in seven Medicare patients in hospitals experience a medical error. But medical errors can occur anywhere in the healthcare system; in hospitals, clinics, surgery centers, doctors' offices, nursing homes, pharmacies, and patients' homes. Errors can involve medicines, surgery, diagnosis, equipment, or lab reports.

Medical errors can happen even during the most routine tasks, such as when a hospital patient on a salt-free diet is given a high-salt meal. It results from

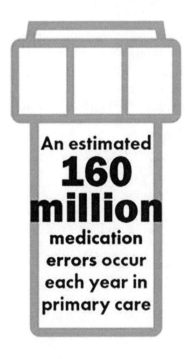

An estimated
**160
million**
medication
errors occur
each year in
primary care

Figure 28.1. Medication Errors in Primary Care
(Source: "Patient Safety Issues in Primary Care Are Real," Agency for Healthcare Research and Quality (AHRQ), U.S. Department of Health and Human Services (HHS))

This chapter includes text excerpted from "20 Tips to Help Prevent Medical Errors: Patient Fact Sheet," Agency for Healthcare Research and Quality (AHRQ), U.S. Department of Health and Human Services (HHS), August 2018.

problems created by the complex healthcare system. But errors also happen when doctors and patients have problems communicating. The tips provided in this chapter will help you in taking steps to get safer care.

WHAT YOU CAN DO TO STAY SAFE

The best way you can help to prevent errors is to be an active member of your healthcare team. That means taking part in every decision about your healthcare. Research shows that patients who are more involved with their care tend to get better results.

Medicines

- **Make sure that all of your doctors know about every medicine you are taking.** This includes prescription and over-the-counter (OTC) medicines and dietary supplements, such as vitamins and herbs.
- **Bring all of your medicines and supplements to your doctor visits.** "Brown bagging" your medicines can help you and your doctor talk about them and find out if there are any problems. It can also help your doctor keep your records up to date and help you get better quality care.
- **Make sure your doctor knows about any allergies and adverse reactions you have had to medicines.** This can help you to avoid getting a medicine that could harm you.
- **When your doctor writes a prescription for you, make sure you can read it.** If you cannot read your doctor's handwriting, your pharmacist might not be able to either.
- **Ask for information about your medicines in terms you can understand—both when your medicines are prescribed and when you get them:**
  - What is the medicine for?
  - How am I supposed to take it and for how long?
  - What side effects are likely? What do I do if they occur?
  - Is this medicine safe to take with other medicines or dietary supplements I am taking?
  - What food, drink, or activities should I avoid while taking this medicine?
- **When you pick up your medicine from the pharmacy, ask:** Is this the medicine that my doctor prescribed?
- **If you have any questions about the directions on your medicine labels, ask.** Medicine labels can be hard to understand. For example, ask if "four times daily" means taking a dose every six hours around the clock or just during regular waking hours.
- **Ask your pharmacist for the best device to measure your liquid medicine.** For example, many people use household teaspoons, which

often do not hold a true teaspoon of liquid. Special devices, such as marked syringes, help people measure the right dose.

- **Ask for written information about the side effects your medicine could cause.** If you know what might happen, you will be better prepared if it does or if something unexpected happens.

Hospital Stays

- **If you are in a hospital, consider asking all healthcare workers who will touch you whether they have washed their hands.** Handwashing can prevent the spread of infections in hospitals.
- **When you are being discharged from the hospital, ask your doctor to explain the treatment plan you will follow at home.** This includes learning about your new medicines, making sure you know when to schedule follow-up appointments, and finding out when you can get back to your regular activities.

It is important to know whether or not you should keep taking the medicines you were taking before your hospital stay. Getting clear instructions may help prevent an unexpected return trip to the hospital.

Surgery

- **If you are having surgery, make sure that you, your doctor, and your surgeon all agree on exactly what will be done.** Having surgery at the wrong site (for example, operating on the left knee instead of the right) is rare. But, even once is too often. The good news is that wrong-site surgery is 100 percent preventable. Surgeons are expected to sign their initials directly on the site to be operated on before the surgery.
- **If you have a choice, choose a hospital where many patients have had the procedure or surgery you need.** Research shows that patients tend to have better results when they are treated in hospitals that have a great deal of experience with their condition.

Other Steps

- **Speak up if you have questions or concerns.** You have a right to question anyone who is involved with your care.
- **Make sure that someone, such as your primary-care doctor, coordinates your care.** This is especially important if you have many health problems or are in the hospital.
- **Make sure that all your doctors have your important health information.** Do not assume that everyone has all the information they need.

- **Ask a family member or friend to go to appointments with you.** Even if you do not need help now, you might need it later.
- **Know that "more" is not always better.** It is a good idea to find out why a test or treatment is needed and how it can help you. You could be better off without it.
- **If you have a test, do not assume that no news is good news.** Ask how and when you will get the results.

Learn about your condition and treatments by asking your doctor and nurse and by using other reliable sources. For example, treatment options based on the latest scientific evidence are available on websites. Ask your doctor if your treatment is based on the latest evidence.

Chapter 29 | Healthcare Fraud Scams

A PERVASIVE PROBLEM[1]

Fraudulent products can cause serious injury. In the past few years, the U.S. Food and Drug Administration (FDA) laboratories have found more than 100 weight-loss products, illegally marketed as dietary supplements, that contained sibutramine, the active ingredient in the prescription weight-loss drug Meridia. In 2010, Meridia was withdrawn from the U.S. market after studies showed that it was associated with an increased risk of heart attack and stroke.

Fraudulent products marketed as "drugs" or "dietary supplements" are not the only health scams on the market. The FDA found a fraudulent and expensive light-therapy device with cure-all claims to treat fungal meningitis, Alzheimer disease (AD), skin cancer, concussions, and many other unrelated diseases. Generally, making health claims about a medical device without FDA clearance or approval of the device is illegal.

"Health fraud is a pervasive problem," says Gary Coody, R.Ph., the FDA's national health fraud coordinator, "especially when scammers sell online. It's difficult to track down the responsible parties. When we do find them and tell them their products are illegal, some will shut down their website. Unfortunately, these same products may reappear later on a different website, and sometimes may reappear with a different name."

WHAT ARE HEALTH FRAUD SCAMS?[2]

"Health fraud scams" refer to products that claim to prevent, treat, or cure diseases or other health conditions, but are not proven safe and effective for those

This chapter includes text excerpted from documents published by three public domain sources. Text under the headings marked 1 are excerpted from "6 Tip-Offs to Rip-Offs: Don't Fall for Health Fraud Scams," U.S. Food and Drug Administration (FDA), March 4, 2013. Reviewed December 2019; Text under the heading marked 2 is excerpted from "Health Fraud Scams," U.S. Food and Drug Administration (FDA), September 14, 2018; Text under the headings marked 3 are excerpted from "Health Fraud," MedlinePlus, National Institutes of Health (NIH), December 31, 2016. Reviewed December 2019.

uses. Health fraud scams waste money and can lead to delays in getting proper diagnosis and treatment. They can also cause serious or even fatal injuries.

WHAT DO HEALTH FRAUD SCAMS INVOLVE?[3]

Health fraud involves selling drugs, devices, foods, or cosmetics that have not been proven effective. Keep in mind—if it sounds too good to be true, it is probably a scam. At best, these scams do not work. At worst, they are dangerous. They also waste money, and they might keep you from getting the treatment you really need.

ARE HEALTH FRAUD SCAMS COMMON?[3]

Health fraud scams can be found everywhere, promising help for many common health issues, including weight loss, memory loss, sexual performance, and joint pain. They target people with serious conditions, such as cancer, diabetes, heart disease, human immunodeficiency virus (HIV)/acquired immunodeficiency syndrome (AIDS), arthritis, Addison disease, and many more.

TIPS TO PROTECT YOURSELF FROM HEALTHCARE FRAUD SCAMS[1]

The FDA offers some tip-offs to help you identify rip-offs.

- **One product does it all.** Be suspicious of products that claim to cure a wide range of diseases. A New York firm claimed its products marketed as dietary supplements could treat or cure senile dementia, brain atrophy, atherosclerosis, kidney dysfunction, gangrene, depression, osteoarthritis, dysuria, and lung, cervical and prostate cancer. In October 2012, at the FDA's request, U.S. marshals seized these products.
- **Personal testimonials.** Success stories, such as, "It cured my diabetes" or "My tumors are gone," are easy to make up and are not a substitute for scientific evidence.
- **Quick fixes. Few diseases or conditions can be treated quickly, even with legitimate products.** Beware of language such as, "Lose 30 pounds in 30 days" or "eliminates skin cancer in days."
- **"All natural."** Some plants found in nature (such as poisonous mushrooms) can kill when consumed. Moreover, the FDA has found numerous products promoted as "all natural" but that contain hidden and dangerously high doses of prescription drug ingredients or even untested active artificial ingredients.
- **"Miracle cure."** Alarms should go off when you see this claim or others like it such as, "new discovery," "scientific breakthrough" or "secret ingredient." If a real cure for a serious disease were discovered, it would be widely reported through the media and prescribed by health professionals—not buried in print ads, TV infomercials or on Internet sites.

- **Conspiracy theories.** Claims such as "The pharmaceutical industry and the government are working together to hide information about a miracle cure" are always untrue and unfounded. These statements are used to distract consumers from the obvious, common-sense questions about the so-called "miracle cure."

Even with these tips, fraudulent health products are not always easy to spot. If you are tempted to buy an unproven product or one with questionable claims, check with your doctor or other healthcare professional first.

Chapter 30 | Medical Identity Theft

A thief may use your name or health insurance numbers to see a doctor, get prescription drugs, file claims with your insurance provider, or get other care. If the thief's health information is mixed with yours, your treatment, insurance and payment records, and credit report may be affected.

If you see signs of medical identity theft, visit IdentityTheft.gov to report and recover from identity theft.

DETECTING MEDICAL IDENTITY THEFT

Read your medical and insurance statements regularly and completely. They can show warning signs of identity theft. Read the Explanation of Benefits (EOB) statement or Medicare Summary Notice that your health plan sends after treatment. Check the name of the healthcare provider, the date of service, and the service provided. Do the claims paid match the care you received? If you see a mistake, contact your health plan and report the problem.

Other signs of medical identity theft include:
- A bill for medical services you did not receive
- A call from a debt collector about a medical debt you do not owe
- Medical collection notices on your credit report that you do not recognize
- A notice from your health plan saying you reached your benefit limit
- A denial of insurance because your medical records show a condition you do not have

CORRECTING MISTAKES IN YOUR MEDICAL RECORDS
Get Copies of Your Medical Records

If you know a thief used your medical information, get copies of your records. Federal law gives you the right to know what is in your medical files. Check them for errors. Contact each doctor, clinic, hospital, pharmacy, laboratory,

This chapter includes text excerpted from "Medical Identity Theft," Federal Trade Commission (FTC), September 2018.

health plan, and location where a thief may have used your information. For example, if a thief got a prescription in your name, ask for records from the healthcare provider who wrote the prescription and the pharmacy that filled it.

You may need to pay for copies of your records. If you know when the thief used your information, ask for records from that time. Keep copies of your postal and e-mail correspondence, and a record of your phone calls, conversations, and activities with your health plan and medical providers.

A healthcare provider might refuse to give you copies of your medical or billing records because she or he thinks that would violate the identity thief's privacy rights. The fact is, you have the right to know what is in your file. If a healthcare provider denies your request for your records, you have a right to appeal. Contact the person the healthcare provider lists in its Notice of Privacy Practices, the patient representative, or the ombudsman. Explain the situation and ask for your file. If the healthcare provider refuses to provide your records within 30 days of your written request, you may complain to the U.S. Department of Health and Human Services' (HHS) Office for Civil Rights (OCR).

Get an Accounting of Disclosures

Ask each of your health plans and medical providers for a copy of the "accounting of disclosures" for your medical records. The accounting is a record of who got copies of your records from the healthcare provider. The law allows you to order one free copy of the accounting from each of your medical providers every 12 months.

The accounting includes details about:
- What medical information the provider sent
- When it sent the information
- Who got the information
- Why the information was sent

The accounting shows who has copies of your mistaken records and whom you need to contact. It may not have details about some routine disclosure of your information, such as those from your doctor's office to another doctor's office, or disclosure of payment information to an insurer.

Ask for Corrections

Write to your health plan and medical providers and explain which information is not accurate. Send copies of the documents that support your position. You can include a copy of your medical record and circle the disputed items. Ask the healthcare provider to correct or delete each error. Keep the original documents.

Medical Identity Theft

Send your letter by certified mail, and ask for a return receipt, so you have a record of what the plan or healthcare provider received. Keep copies of the letters and documents you sent.

The health plan or medical provider that made the mistakes in your files must change the information. It should also inform labs, other healthcare providers, and anyone else that might have gotten wrong information. If a health plan or medical provider will not make the changes you request, ask it to include a statement of your dispute in your record.

How to Correct Errors in Your Medical Records

- Contact each healthcare provider and ask for copies of your medical records.
- Complete the request form and pay any fees required to get copies of your records.
- If your provider refuses to give you copies of your records because it thinks that would violate the identity thief's privacy rights, you can appeal. Contact the person the provider lists in its Notice of Privacy Practices, the patient representative, or the ombudsman. Explain the situation and ask for your file. If the provider refuses to provide your records within 30 days of your written request, you may complain to the HHS's OCR.
- Review your medical records and report any errors to your healthcare provider.
- Write to your healthcare provider to report mistakes in your medical records.
- Include a copy of the medical record showing the mistake.
- Explain why this is a mistake and how to correct it.
- Include a copy of your police report or identity theft report.
- Send the letter by certified mail and ask for a return receipt. Your healthcare provider should respond to your letter within 30 days. It must fix the mistake and notify other healthcare providers who may have the same mistake in their records.
- Notify your health insurer and all three credit bureaus.
- Send copies of your police report or Identity Theft Report to your health insurer's fraud department and the three nationwide credit bureaus
- Order copies of your credit reports if you have not already.
- Consider placing a fraud alert or a security freeze on your credit reports.
- Update your files.
- Record the dates you made calls or sent letters.
- Keep copies of letters in your files.

PROTECTING YOUR MEDICAL INFORMATION

Your medical and insurance information are valuable to identity thieves.

Be wary if someone offers you "free" health services or products, but requires you to provide your health plan ID number. Medical identity thieves may pretend to work for an insurance company, doctor's offices, clinic, or pharmacy to try to trick you into revealing sensitive information.

Do not share medical or insurance information by phone or e-mail unless you initiated the contact and know who you are dealing with.

Keep paper and electronic copies of your medical and health insurance records in a safe place. Shred outdated health insurance forms, prescription and physician statements, and the labels from prescription bottles before you throw them out.

Before you provide sensitive personal information to a website that asks for your Social Security number, insurance account numbers, or details about your health, find out why it is needed, how it will be kept safe, whether it will be shared, and with whom. Read the Privacy Policy on the website.

If you decide to share your information online, look for a lock icon on the browser's status bar or a URL that begins with "https:" the "s" is for secure.

CHECKING FOR OTHER IDENTITY THEFT PROBLEMS

A thief that uses your name or health insurance information for medical care, may use it in other situations.

Credit Bureau Contact Information

Contact the national credit bureaus to request fraud alerts, credit freezes (also known as "security freezes"), and opt-outs from prescreened credit offers.

Equifax
Equifax.com/personal/credit-report-services
800-685-1111

Experian
Experian.com/help
888-397-3742

Transunion
TransUnion.com/credit-help
888-909-8872

Part 4 | Prescription and Over-the-Counter Medications

Chapter 31 | Understanding Medications and What They Do

Chapter Contents

Section 31.1 | About Medications and Their Categories

This section contains text excerpted from the following sources: Text in this section begins with excerpts from "Medicines," MedlinePlus, National Institutes of Health (NIH), December 1, 2014. Reviewed December 2019; Text beginning with the heading "What Are Prescription Drugs?" is excerpted from "Prescription Drugs and Over-the-Counter (OTC) Drugs: Questions and Answers," U.S. Food and Drug Administration (FDA), November 13, 2017; Text under the heading "How Are the Medicines Categorized?" is excerpted from "General Drug Categories," U.S. Food and Drug Administration (FDA), December 7, 2015. Reviewed December 2019.

Medicines, or drugs, or medication can treat diseases and improve your health. If you are similar to most people, you need to take medicine at some point in your life. You may need to take medicine every day, or you may only need to take medicine once in a while. Either way, you want to make sure that your medicines are safe, and that they will help you get better. The U.S. Food and Drug Administration (FDA) is in charge of ensuring that your prescription and over-the-counter (OTC) medicines are safe and effective.

WHAT ARE PRESCRIPTION DRUGS?

Prescription drugs are:
- Prescribed by a doctor
- Bought at a pharmacy
- Prescribed for and intended to be used by one person
- Regulated by the FDA through the New Drug Application (NDA) process. This is the formal step a drug sponsor takes to ask that the FDA consider approving a new drug for marketing in the United States. An NDA includes all animal and human data and analyses of the data, as well as information about how the drug behaves in the body and how it is manufactured.

WHAT ARE OVER-THE-COUNTER DRUGS?

Over-the-counter drugs are:
- Drugs that do NOT require a doctor's prescription
- Bought off-the-shelf in stores
- Regulated by the FDA through OTC drug monographs. OTC drug monographs are a kind of "recipe book" covering acceptable ingredients, doses, formulations, and labeling. Monographs will continually be updated adding additional ingredients and labeling as needed. Products conforming to a monograph may be marketed without further FDA clearance, while those that do not, must undergo separate review and approval through the "New Drug Approval System."

HOW ARE THE MEDICATIONS CATEGORIZED?

The medications are categorized as follows:

Analgesics. Drugs that relieve pain. There are two main types: nonnarcotic analgesics for mild pain, and narcotic analgesics for severe pain.

Antacids. Drugs that relieve indigestion and heartburn by neutralizing stomach acid.

Antianxiety drugs. Drugs that suppress anxiety and relax muscles (sometimes called "anxiolytics," "sedatives," or "minor tranquilizers").

Antiarrhythmics. Drugs used to control irregularities of a heartbeat.

Antibacterials. Drugs used to treat infections.

Antibiotics. Drugs made from naturally occurring and synthetic substances that combat bacterial infection. Some antibiotics are effective only against limited types of bacteria. Others, known as "broad-spectrum antibiotics," are effective against a wide range of bacteria.

Anticoagulants and thrombolytics. Anticoagulants prevent blood from clotting. Thrombolytics help dissolve and disperse blood clots and may be prescribed for patients with recent arterial or venous thrombosis.

Anticonvulsants. Drugs that prevent epileptic seizures.

Antidepressants. There are three main groups of mood-lifting antidepressants: tricyclics, monoamine oxidase inhibitors, and selective serotonin reuptake inhibitors (SSRIs).

Antidiarrheals. Drugs used for the relief of diarrhea. Two main types of antidiarrheal preparations are simple adsorbent substances and drugs that slow down the contractions of the bowel muscles so that the contents are propelled more slowly.

Antiemetics. Drugs used to treat nausea and vomiting.

Antifungals. Drugs used to treat fungal infections, the most common of which affect the hair, skin, nails, or mucous membranes.

Antihistamines. Drugs used primarily to counteract the effects of histamine, one of the chemicals involved in allergic reactions.

Antihypertensives. Drugs that lower blood pressure. The types of antihypertensives marketed include diuretics, beta-blockers, calcium channel blockers, angiotensin-converting enzyme (ACE) inhibitors, centrally acting antihypertensives and sympatholytics.

Antiinflammatories. Drugs used to reduce inflammation—the redness, heat, swelling, and increased blood flow found in infections and in many chronic noninfective diseases such as rheumatoid arthritis (RA) and gout.

Understanding Medications and What They Do

Antineoplastics. Drugs used to treat cancer.

Antipsychotics. Drugs used to treat symptoms of severe psychiatric disorders. These drugs are sometimes called "major tranquilizers."

Antipyretics. Drugs that reduce fever.

Antivirals. Drugs used to treat viral infections or to provide temporary protection against infections such as influenza.

Beta-blockers. Beta-adrenergic blocking agents, or beta-blockers for short, reduce the oxygen needs of the heart by reducing heartbeat rate.

Bronchodilators. Drugs that open up the bronchial tubes within the lungs when the tubes have become narrowed by muscle spasm. Bronchodilators ease breathing in diseases such as asthma.

Cold cures. Although there is no drug that can cure a cold, aches, pains, and fever that accompany a cold can be relieved by aspirin or acetaminophen often accompanied by a decongestant, antihistamine, and sometimes caffeine.

Corticosteroids. These hormonal preparations are used primarily as anti-inflammatories in arthritis or asthma or as immunosuppressives, but they are also useful for treating some malignancies or compensating for a deficiency of natural hormones in disorders such as Addison disease.

Cough suppressants. Simple cough medicines, which contain substances, such as honey, glycerin, or menthol, soothe throat irritation but do not actually suppress coughing. They are most soothing when taken as lozenges and dissolved in the mouth. As liquids, they are probably swallowed too quickly to be effective. A few drugs are actually cough suppressants. There are two groups of cough suppressants: those that alter the consistency or production of phlegm such as mucolytics and expectorants; and those that suppress the coughing reflex such as codeine (narcotic cough suppressants), antihistamines, dextromethorphan and isoproterenol (nonnarcotic cough suppressants).

Cytotoxics. Drugs that kill or damage cells. Cytotoxins are used as antineoplastics (drugs used to treat cancer) and also as immunosuppressives.

Decongestants. Drugs that reduce swelling of the mucous membranes that line the nose by constricting blood vessels, thus relieving nasal stuffiness.

Diuretics. Drugs that increase the quantity of urine produced by the kidneys and passed out of the body, thus ridding the body of excess fluid. Diuretics reduce waterlogging of the tissues caused by fluid retention in disorders of the heart, kidneys, and liver. They are useful in treating mild cases of high blood pressure.

Expectorant. A drug that stimulates the flow of saliva and promotes coughing to eliminate phlegm from the respiratory tract.

Hormones. Chemicals produced naturally by the endocrine glands (thyroid, adrenal, ovary, testis, pancreas, parathyroid). In some disorders, for example, diabetes mellitus, in which too little of a particular hormone is produced, synthetic equivalents or natural hormone extracts are prescribed to restore the deficiency. Such treatment is known as "hormone replacement therapy" (HRT).

Hypoglycemics (oral). Drugs that lower the level of glucose in the blood. Oral hypoglycemic drugs are used in diabetes mellitus if it cannot be controlled by diet alone, but does require treatment with injections of insulin.

Immunosuppressives. Drugs that prevent or reduce the body's normal reaction to invasion by disease or by foreign tissues. Immunosuppressives are used to treat autoimmune diseases (in which the body's defenses work abnormally and attack its own tissues) and to help prevent rejection of organ transplants.

Laxatives. Drugs that increase the frequency and ease of bowel movements, either by stimulating the bowel wall (stimulant laxative), by increasing the bulk of bowel contents (bulk laxative), or by lubricating them (stool-softeners, or bowel movement-softeners). Laxatives may be taken by mouth or directly into the lower bowel as suppositories or enemas. If laxatives are taken regularly, the bowels may ultimately become unable to work properly without them.

Muscle relaxants. Drugs that relieve muscle spasm in disorders such as backache. Antianxiety drugs (minor tranquilizers) that also have a muscle-relaxant action are used most commonly.

Sedatives. Same as Antianxiety drugs.

Sex hormones (female). There are two groups of these hormones (estrogens and progesterone), which are responsible for development of female secondary sexual characteristics. Small quantities are also produced in males. As drugs, female sex hormones are used to treat menstrual and menopausal disorders and are also used as oral contraceptives. Estrogen may be used to treat cancer of the breast or prostate, progestins (synthetic progesterone to treat endometriosis).

Sex hormones (male). Androgenic hormones, of which the most powerful is testosterone, are responsible for development of male secondary sexual characteristics. Small quantities are also produced in females. As drugs, male sex hormones are given to compensate for hormonal deficiency in hypopituitarism or disorders of the testes. They may be used to treat breast cancer in women, but either synthetic derivatives called "anabolic steroids," which have less marked side effects, or specific antiestrogens are often preferred. Anabolic steroids also have a "bodybuilding" effect that has led to their (usually nonsanctioned) use in competitive sports, for both men and women.

Understanding Medications and What They Do

Sleeping drugs. The two main groups of drugs that are used to induce sleep are benzodiazepines and barbiturates. All such drugs have a sedative effect in low doses and are effective sleeping medications in higher doses. Benzodiazepines drugs are used more widely than barbiturates because they are safer, the side-effects are less marked, and there is less risk of eventual physical dependence.

Tranquilizer. This is a term commonly used to describe any drug that has a calming or sedative effect. However, the drugs that are sometimes called "minor tranquilizers" should be called "antianxiety drugs," and the drugs that are sometimes called "major tranquilizers" should be called "antipsychotics."

Vitamins. Chemicals essential in small quantities for good health. Some vitamins are not manufactured by the body, but adequate quantities are present in a normal diet. People whose diets are inadequate or who have digestive tract or liver disorders may need to take supplementary vitamins.

Section 31.2 | Medicine's Life inside the Body

This section includes text excerpted from "A Medicine's Life inside the Body," National Institute on Aging (NIA), National Institutes of Health (NIH), October 24, 2018.

Pharmacology is the scientific field that studies how the body reacts to medicines and how medicines affect the body. Scientists funded by the National Institutes of Health (NIH) are interested in many aspects of pharmacology, including one called "pharmacokinetics," which deals with understanding the entire cycle of a medicine's life inside the body. Knowing more about each of the four main stages of pharmacokinetics collectively referred to as "absorption, distribution, metabolism, and excretion" (ADME), aids the design of medicines that are more effective and that produce fewer side effects.

ABSORPTION

The first stage of ADME is absorption. Medicines are absorbed when they travel from the site of administration into the body's circulation. A few of the most common ways to administer drugs are oral (such as swallowing an aspirin tablet), intramuscular (getting a flu shot in an arm muscle), subcutaneous (injecting insulin just under the skin), intravenous (receiving chemotherapy through a vein) or transdermal (wearing a skin patch). Medicines taken by mouth are shuttled via a special blood vessel leading from the digestive tract to the liver, where a large amount of the medicine is broken down. Other routes of drug administration bypass the liver, entering the bloodstream directly or via the skin or lungs.

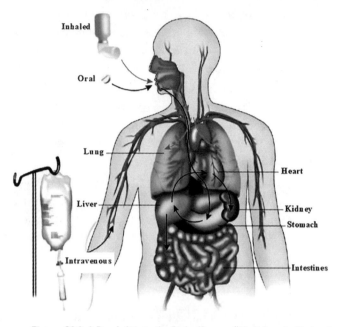

Figure 31.1. A Drug's Life in the Body *(Source: "Medicines by Design," National Institute of General Medical Sciences (NIGMS))*

DISTRIBUTION

Once a drug gets absorbed, the next stage of ADME is distribution. Most often, the bloodstream is the vehicle for carrying medicines throughout the body. During this step, side effects can occur when a drug has an effect at a site other than its target. For a pain reliever, the target organ might be a sore muscle in the leg; irritation of the stomach could be a side effect. Drugs destined for the central nervous system (CNS) face a nearly impenetrable barricade called the "blood-brain barrier" (BBB) that protects the brain from potentially dangerous substances such as poisons or viruses. Fortunately, pharmacologists have devised various ways to sneak some drugs past the BBB. Other factors that can influence distribution include protein and fat molecules in the blood that can put drug molecules out of commission by latching onto them.

METABOLISM

After a medicine has been distributed throughout the body and has done its job, the drug is broken down, or metabolized. Everything that enters the bloodstream—whether swallowed, injected, inhaled or absorbed through the skin—is carried to the body's chemical processing plant, the liver. There, substances are chemically pummeled, twisted, cut apart, stuck together, and transformed by proteins called "enzymes." Many of the products of enzymatic breakdown, or metabolites, are less chemically active than the original molecule. Genetic differences can alter how certain enzymes work, also affecting their ability to metabolize drugs. Herbal products and foods, which contain many active components, can interfere with the body's ability to metabolize drugs.

EXCRETION

The now-inactive drug undergoes excretion, the final stage of its time in the body. This removal happens via the urine or feces. By measuring the amount of a drug in urine (as well as in blood) over time, clinical pharmacologists can calculate how a person is processing a drug, perhaps resulting in a change to the prescribed dose or even the medicine. For example, if the drug is being eliminated relatively quickly, a higher dose may be needed.

Section 31.3 | The Influence of Genes on Drug Response

This section contains text excerpted from the following sources: Text in this section begins with excerpts from "What Is Pharmacogenomics?" Genetics Home Reference (GHR), National Institutes of Health (NIH), November 26, 2019; Text beginning with the heading "What Role Do Genes Play in How Medicines Work?" is excerpted from "Pharmacogenomics," National Institute of General Medical Sciences (NIGMS), March 5, 2019.

Pharmacogenomics is the study of how genes affect a person's response to drugs. This relatively new field combines pharmacology (the science of drugs) and genomics (the study of genes and their functions) to develop effective, safe medications and doses that will be tailored to a person's genetic makeup.

Many drugs that are available are "one size fits all," but they do not work the same way for everyone. It can be difficult to predict who will benefit from a medication, who will not respond at all, and who will experience negative side effects (called "adverse drug reactions"). Adverse drug reactions are a significant cause of hospitalizations and deaths in the United States. With the knowledge gained from the Human Genome Project (HGP), researchers are learning how inherited differences in genes affect the body's response to medications. These genetic differences will be used to predict whether a medication will be effective for a particular person and to help prevent adverse drug reactions. Conditions that affect a person's response to certain drugs include clopidogrel resistance, warfarin sensitivity, warfarin resistance, malignant hyperthermia, Stevens-Johnson syndrome/toxic epidermal necrolysis, and thiopurine S-methyltransferase deficiency (TPMT).

The field of pharmacogenomics is still in its infancy. Its use is currently quite limited, but new approaches are under study in clinical trials. In the future, pharmacogenomics will allow the development of tailored drugs to treat a wide range of health problems, including cardiovascular disease (CVD), Alzheimer disease (AD), cancer, human immunodeficiency virus (HIV), acquired immunodeficiency syndrome (AIDS), and asthma.

WHAT ROLE DO GENES PLAY IN HOW MEDICATIONS WORK?

Just as our genes determine our hair and eye color, they partly affect how our bodies respond to medication.

Genes are instructions, written in deoxyribonucleic acid (DNA), for building protein molecules. Different people can have different versions of the same gene. Each version has a slightly different DNA sequence. Some of these variants are common, and some are rare. And some affect health, such as those gene variants linked to certain diseases.

Scientists know that certain proteins affect how drugs work. Pharmacogenomics looks at variations in genes for these proteins. Such proteins include liver enzymes that chemically change drugs. Sometimes chemical changes can make the drugs more—or less—active in the body. Even small differences in the genes for these liver enzymes can have a big impact on a drug's safety or effectiveness.

One liver enzyme, known as "CYP2D6," acts on a quarter of all prescription drugs. For example, it converts the painkiller codeine into its active form, morphine. There are more than 160 versions of the *CYP2D6* gene. Many vary by only a single difference in their DNA sequence. Others have larger changes. Most of these variants do not affect how people respond to the drug.

Typically, people have 2 copies of each gene. However, some people have hundreds or even thousands of copies of the *CYP2D6* gene. Those with extra copies produce too much of the CYP2D6 enzyme and process the drug very fast. As a result, their bodies may convert codeine to morphine so quickly and completely that a standard dose can be an overdose. In contrast, some variants of *CYP2D6* create an enzyme that does not work. People with these variants process codeine slowly, if at all, leading to little, if any, pain relief. For them, doctors can prescribe a different drug.

HOW IS PHARMACOGENOMICS AFFECTING DRUG DESIGN, DEVELOPMENT, AND PRESCRIBING GUIDELINES?

The U.S. Food and Drug Administration (FDA) monitors drug safety in the United States. It now includes pharmacogenomic information on the labels of around 200 medications. This information can help doctors tailor drug prescriptions for individual patients by providing guidance on dose, possible side effects, or differences in effectiveness for people with certain gene variants.

Drug companies are also using pharmacogenomics to develop and market medicines for people with specific genetic profiles. By studying a drug only in people likely to benefit from it, drug companies might be able to speed up the drug's development and maximize its therapeutic benefit.

In addition, if scientists can identify genes that cause serious side effects, doctors could prescribe those drugs only to people who do not have those genes. This would allow some individuals to receive potentially lifesaving medicines that otherwise might be banned because they pose a risk for other people.

HOW IS PHARMACOGENOMICS AFFECTING MEDICAL TREATMENT?

Doctors prescribe drugs based mostly on factors such as a patient's age, weight, sex, and liver and kidney function. For a few drugs, researchers have identified gene variants that affect how people respond. In these cases, doctors can select the best medication and dose for each patient.

Additionally, learning how patients respond to medications helps to discern the different forms of their diseases.

WHAT ROLE DOES THE NATIONAL INSTITUTES OF HEALTH PLAY IN PHARMACOGENOMICS RESEARCH?

For many years, the National Institutes of Health (NIH)-funded scientists, through the Pharmacogenomics Research Network (PGRN), have studied the effect of genes on medications relevant to a wide range of conditions, including asthma, depression, cancer, and heart disease. The research findings are collected in an online resource called "PharmGKB." In addition, the Clinical Pharmacogenetics Implementation Consortium (CPIC) was started as a shared partnership between the PGRN and PharmGKB to help lower the barrier to the clinical use of pharmacogenetic tests. CPIC creates, curates, and posts freely available, peer-reviewed, evidence-based, updatable, and detailed gene/drug clinical practice guidelines. Another NIH-funded project, the Clinical Genome (ClinGen) Resource, aims to define the clinical relevance of genes and variants for use in precision medicine and research.

The NIH takes seriously the ethical and legal implications of pharmacogenomics research. It works closely with researchers, clinicians, and patient advocates to ensure research participants' privacy. And it strives to maximize the benefits of pharmacogenomics research for individuals and society. An NIH initiative where people can participate and learn more is called "All of Us."

Important goals for NIH are to further pharmacogenomics research and ensure that doctors implement the findings. This represents part of a major initiative on precision medicine that aims to tailor treatments based on each person's genes, environment, lifestyle, and other characteristics.

Section 31.4 | As You Age: You and Your Medications

This section includes text excerpted from "As You Age: You and Your Medicines," U.S. Food and Drug Administration (FDA), February 19, 2019.

As you get older you may be faced with more health conditions that you need to treat on a regular basis. It is important to be aware that more use of medicines and normal body changes caused by aging can increase the chance of unwanted or maybe even harmful drug interactions. The more you know about your medicines and the more you talk with your healthcare professionals, the easier it is to avoid problems with medicines.

As you get older, body changes can affect the way medicines are absorbed and used. For example, changes in the digestive system can affect how fast medicines enter the bloodstream. Changes in body weight can influence the amount of medicine you need to take and how long it stays in your body. The circulatory system may slow down, which can affect how fast drugs get to the liver and kidneys. The liver and kidneys also may work more slowly, affecting the way a drug breaks down and is removed from the body.

DRUG INTERACTIONS

Because of these body changes, there is also a bigger risk of drug interactions among older adults. Therefore, it is important to know about drug interactions.

- **Drug-drug interactions** happen when two or more medicines react with each other to cause unwanted effects. This kind of interaction can also cause one medicine to not work as well or even make one medicine stronger than it should be. For example, you should not take aspirin if you are taking a prescription blood thinner, such as warfarin unless your healthcare professional tells you to.
- **Drug-condition interactions** happen when a medical condition you already have makes certain drugs potentially harmful. For example, if you have high blood pressure or asthma, you could have an unwanted reaction if you take a nasal decongestant.
- **Drug-food interactions** result from drugs reacting with foods or drinks. In some cases, food in the digestive tract can affect how a drug is absorbed. Some medicines also may affect the way nutrients are absorbed or used in the body.
- **Drug-alcohol interactions** can happen when the medicine you take reacts with an alcoholic drink. For instance, mixing alcohol with some medicines may cause you to feel tired and slow your reactions.

Understanding Medications and What They Do

It is important to know that many medicines do not mix well with alcohol. As you grow older, your body may react differently to alcohol, as well as to the mix of alcohol and medicines. Keep in mind that some problems you might think are medicine-related, such as loss of coordination, memory loss, or irritability, could be the result of a mix between your medicine and alcohol.

What Side Effects Mean

Side effects are unplanned symptoms or feelings you have when taking a medicine. Most side effects are not serious and go away on their own; others can be more bothersome and even serious. To help prevent possible problems with medicines, seniors must know about the medicine they take and how it makes them feel.

Keep track of side effects to help your doctor know how your body is responding to a medicine. New symptoms or mood changes may not be a result of getting older, but could be from the medicine you are taking or another factor, such as a change in diet or routine. If you have an unwanted side effect, call your doctor right away.

TALK TO YOUR TEAM OF HEALTHCARE PROFESSIONALS

It is important to go to all your medical appointments and to talk to your team of healthcare professionals (doctors, pharmacists, nurses, or physician assistants) about your medical conditions, the medicines you take, and any health concerns you have. It may help to make a list of comments, questions, or concerns before your visit or call to a healthcare professional. Also, think about having a close friend or relative come to your appointment with you if you are unsure about talking to your healthcare professional or would prefer someone to help you understand and remember answers to your questions. Here are some other things to keep in mind:

- **All medicines count.** Tell your team of healthcare professionals about all the medicines you take, including prescription and over-the-counter (OTC) medicines, such as pain relievers, antacids, cold medicines, and laxatives. Do not forget to include eye drops, dietary supplements, vitamins, herbals, and topical medicines, such as creams and ointments.
- **Keep in touch with your doctors.** If you regularly take prescription medicine, ask your doctor to check how well it is working. Check to see whether you still need to take it and, if so, whether there is anything you can do to cut back. Do not stop taking the medicine on your own without first talking with your doctor.
- **Medical history.** Tell your healthcare professional about your medical history. The doctor will want to know whether you have any food, medicine, or other allergies. She or he also will want to know about

229

other conditions you have or had and how you are being treated or were treated for them by other doctors. It is helpful to keep a written list of your health conditions that you can easily share with your doctors. Your primary care doctor should also know about any specialist doctors you may see on a regular basis.

- **Eating habits.** Mention your eating habits. If you follow or have recently changed to a special diet (a very low-fat diet, for instance, or a high-calcium diet), talk to your doctor about this. Tell your doctor about how much coffee, tea, or alcohol you drink each day and whether you smoke. These things may make a difference in the way your medicine works.

- **Recognizing and remembering to take your medicines.** Let your healthcare professional know whether you have trouble telling your medicines apart. The doctor can help you find better ways to recognize your medicines. Also, tell your doctor if you have problems remembering when to take your medicines or how much to take. Your doctor may have some ideas to help, such as a calendar or pillbox.

- **Swallowing tablets.** If you have trouble swallowing tablets, ask your doctor, nurse, or pharmacist for ideas. Maybe there is a liquid medicine you could use or maybe you can crush your tablets. Do not break, crush, or chew tablets without first asking your healthcare professional.

- **Your lifestyle.** If you want to make your medicine schedule more simple, talk about it with your doctor. She or he may have another medicine or other ideas. For example, if taking medicine four times a day is a problem for you, maybe the doctor can give you medicine you only need to take once or twice a day.

- **Put it in writing.** Ask your healthcare professional to write out a complete medicine schedule, with directions on exactly when and how to take your medicines. Find out from your primary care doctor how your medicine schedule should be changed if you see more than one doctor.

- **Keep a record of your medicines.** List all prescription and OTC medicines, dietary supplements, vitamins, and herbals you take.

YOUR PHARMACIST CAN HELP, TOO

One of the most important services a pharmacist can offer is to talk to you about your medicines. A pharmacist can help you understand how and when to take your medicines, what side effects you might expect, or what interactions may occur. A pharmacist can answer your questions privately in the pharmacy or over the telephone.

Understanding Medications and What They Do

Here are some other ways your pharmacist can help:

- Many pharmacists keep track of medicines on their computers. If you buy your medicines at one store and tell your pharmacist all the OTC and prescription medicines or dietary supplements you take, your pharmacist can help make sure your medicines do not interact harmfully with one another.
- Ask your pharmacist to place your prescription medicines in easy-to-open containers if you have a hard time taking off child-proof caps and do not have young children living in or visiting your home. Remember to keep all medicines out of sight and reach of children.
- Your pharmacist may be able to print labels on prescription medicine containers in larger type if reading the medicine label is hard for you.
- Your pharmacist may be able to give you written information to help you learn more about your medicines. This information may be available in large type or in a language other than English.

What to Ask Your Doctor or Pharmacist

- What is the name of the medicine and what is it supposed to do? Is there a less expensive alternative?
- How and when do I take the medicine and for how long?
- Should it be taken with water, food, or with a special medicine, or at the same time as other medicines?
- What do I do if I miss or forget a dose?
- Should it be taken before, during, or after meals?
- What is the proper dose? For example, does "four times a day" means you have to take it in the middle of the night?
- What does your doctor mean by "as needed"?
- Are there any other special instructions to follow?
- What foods, drinks, other medicines, dietary supplements, or activities should I avoid while taking this medicine?
- Will any tests or monitoring be required while I am taking this medicine? Do I need to report back to the doctor?
- What are the possible side effects and what do I do if they occur?
- When should I expect the medicine to start working, and how will I know if it is working?
- Will this new prescription work safely with the other prescription and OTC medicines or dietary supplements I am taking?
- Do you have a patient profile form for me to fill out? Does it include space for my OTC drugs and any dietary supplements?

- Is there written information about my medicine? Ask the pharmacist to review the most important information with you. (Ask if it is available in large print or in a language other than English if you need it.)
- What is the most important thing I should know about this medicine? Ask the pharmacist any questions that may not have been answered by your doctor.
- Can I get a refill? If so, when?
- How and where should I store this medicine?

CUTTING MEDICINE COSTS

Medicines are an important part of treating an illness because they often allow people to remain active and independent. But, medicine can be expensive. Here are some ideas to help lower costs:

- **Tell your doctor if you are worried about the cost of your medicine.** Your doctor may not know how much your prescription costs, but may be able to tell you about another less expensive medicine, such as a generic drug or OTC product.
- **Ask for a senior citizen's discount.**
- **Shop around.** Look at prices at different stores or pharmacies. Lower medicine prices may not be a bargain if you need other services, such as home delivery, patient medication profiles, or pharmacist consultation, or if you cannot get a senior citizen discount.
- **Ask for medicine samples.** If your doctor gives you a prescription for a new medicine, ask your doctor for samples you can try before filling the prescription.
- **Buy bulk.** If you need to take medicine for a long period of time and your medicine does not expire quickly, you may be able to buy a larger amount of medicine for less money.
- **Try mail-order.** Mail-order pharmacies can provide medications at lower prices. However, it is a good idea to talk with your doctor before using such a service. Make sure to find a backup pharmacy in case there is a problem with the mail service.
- **Buy OTC medicines when they are on sale.** Check the expiration dates and use them before they expire. If you need help choosing an OTC medicine, ask the pharmacist for help.

Chapter 32 | Using Medications Safely

THE BASICS

Medications can help you feel better and get well when you are sick. But, if you do not follow the directions, medicines can hurt you.

You can lower your chances of side effects from medicines by carefully following the directions on the medicine label or from your pharmacist, doctor, or nurse.

The side effects of taking medication may be mild, such as an upset stomach. Other side effects—such as damage to your liver—can be more serious. Some side effects can even be deadly.

Take these simple steps to avoid problems with medicines.

- Follow the directions on the medicine label carefully.
- If you do not understand the directions, ask your doctor, nurse, or pharmacist to explain them to you.
- Keep a list of all medicines, vitamins, minerals, and herbs you use and share this information with your doctor at your next checkup.
- Store your medicines in a cool, dry place where children and pets cannot see or reach them.

Drug Facts Label

All over-the-counter (OTC) medicines come with a drug facts label. The information on this label can help you choose the right OTC medicine for your symptoms.

This chapter contains text excerpted from the following sources: Text beginning with the heading "The Basics" is excerpted from "Use Medicines Safely," Office of Disease Prevention and Health Promotion (ODPHP), U.S. Department of Health and Human Services (HHS), December 21, 2018; Text beginning with the heading "Managing the Benefits and Risks of Medicines" is excerpted from "Think It Through: A Guide to Managing the Benefits and Risks of Medicines," U.S. Food and Drug Administration (FDA), March 25, 2016. Reviewed December 2019; Text under the heading "Tips for Talking with Your Pharmacist to Learn How to Use Medicines Safely" is excerpted from "Stop—Learn—Go: Tips for Talking with Your Pharmacist to Learn How to Use Medicines Safely," U.S. Food and Drug Administration (FDA), October 15, 2019.

The drug facts label also gives you instructions for using the medicine safely. OTC medicines can cause side effects or harm if you use too much or do not use them correctly.

Following the directions on the drug facts label will lower your chances of side effects.

Your doctor, nurse, or pharmacist can also help you choose OTC medicines and answer any questions you may have.

TAKE ACTION
Prevent problems and mistakes with your medicines.

Follow the Directions Carefully
Be sure to read the directions carefully when taking prescription or OTC medicines. If you notice unpleasant side effects after taking medicine, such as feeling dizzy or having an upset stomach, call your doctor or nurse.

Talk to Your Doctor
Before you use any new prescription medicines, tell your doctor:
- About other medicines you use—both prescription and OTC medicines
- About any vitamins, minerals, or herbs you use (including herbal teas, creams, sprays, or gels)
- If you are allergic to any medicines
- If you have had side effects after using any medicines
- If you are pregnant or breastfeeding, because some medicines may harm your baby
- If you have any questions or concerns about the new medicine

Be sure to keep taking prescription medicines until your doctor tells you it is okay to stop—even if you are feeling better. If you are worried the medicine is making you feel worse, tell your doctor. Sometimes you can get side effects from stopping your medicine.

Ask Questions to Make Sure You Understand
To use medicine safely, you need to know:
- The name of the medicine
- Why you are using the medicine
- How to use the medicine the right way
- If there are any medicines you should not take with this one
- What the side effects could be
- How to get rid of any unused medicine safely

Using Medications Safely

Ask your doctor or nurse questions to be sure you understand how to use your medicine. Take notes to help you remember the answers. You can even ask to record the instructions on your phone.

You can also ask a pharmacist if you forget how to use a medicine or you do not understand the directions. Use these tips to talk with a pharmacist about your medicines.

Keep Track of Your Medicines

- Make a list of the medicines you use. Write down how much you use and when you use each medicine.
- Take the list with you whenever you go to a medical appointment. You may also want to make a copy to give to a family member or friend in case you have a medical emergency.
- Read and save any information that comes with your medicine.
- Keep your medicine in the box or bottle it came in so you have all of the information from the label.
- Pay attention to the color and shape of your pills. If they look different when you get a refill, ask your pharmacist to double-check that you have the right medicine.

Put Your Medicines in a Safe Place

Medicines that are stored correctly last longer and work better.
- Check for storage instructions on the medicine label—for example, some medicines need to be stored in the refrigerator.
- Store medicines that do not have special storage instructions in a cool, dry place. Medicines can break down quickly in places that are damp and warm, such as the kitchen or bathroom.
- Keep medicines away from children and pets. A locked box, cabinet, or closet is best.
- Get rid of expired (out-of-date) medicines and medicines you no longer use.

Call the Poison Control Center (800-222-1222) right away if a child or someone else accidentally uses your medicine.

MANAGING THE BENEFITS AND RISKS OF MEDICINES

Although medicines can make you feel better and help you get well, it is important to know that all medicines, both prescription and OTC, have risks as well as benefits.

The benefits of medicines are the helpful effects you get when you use them, such as lowering blood pressure, curing infection or relieving pain. The risks of medicines are the chances that something unwanted or unexpected could happen to you when you use them. Risks could be less serious things, such as an upset stomach, or more serious things, such as liver damage.

When a medicine's benefits outweigh its known risks, the U.S. Food and Drug Administration (FDA) considers it safe enough to approve. But, before using any medicine—as with many things that you do every day—you should think through the benefits and risks in order to make the best choice for you.

There are several types of risks from medicine use:

- The possibility of a harmful interaction between the medicine and food, beverage, dietary supplement (including vitamins and herbals), or another medicine. Combinations of any of these products could increase the chance that there may be interactions.
- The chance that the medicine may not work as expected.
- The possibility that the medicine may cause additional problems.

To obtain the benefits of riding in a car, you think through the risks. You consider the condition of your car and the road, for instance, before deciding to make that trip to the store.

The same is true before using any medicine. Every choice to take a medicine involves thinking through the helpful effects as well as the possible unwanted effects.

HOW DO YOU LOWER THE RISKS AND OBTAIN THE FULL BENEFITS OF MEDICINE?

In order to lower the risks and get the full benefits of the medicines you use:

- Talk to your doctor, pharmacist, or other healthcare professionals
- Know your medicines
- Read the label and follow directions
- Avoid interactions
- Monitor the medicine's effects

Weighing the Risks, Making the Choice

The benefit/risk decision is sometimes difficult to make. The best choice depends on your particular situation.

You must decide what risks you can and will accept in order to get the benefits you want. For example, if facing a life-threatening illness, you might choose to accept more risk in the hope of getting the benefits of a cure or living a longer life. On the other hand, if you are facing a minor illness, you might decide that you want to take very little risk. In many situations, the expert advice of your doctor, pharmacist, or other healthcare professionals can help you make the decision.

Using Medications Safely

Talk with Your Doctor, Pharmacist, or Other Healthcare Professionals

Keep an up-to-date, written list of all of the medicines (prescription and OTC) and dietary supplements, including vitamins and herbals, that you use—even those you only use occasionally. Share this list with all of your healthcare professionals.

Tell about any allergies or sensitivities that you may have. Inform about anything that could affect your ability to take medicines, such as difficulty swallowing or remembering to take them.

In case you are or might become pregnant, or if you are nursing a baby, do inform it to your healthcare provider.

Always ask questions about any concerns or thoughts that you may have.

Know Your Medicines—Prescription and Over-the-Counter

- The brand and generic names
- What they look like
- How to store them properly
- When, how, and how long to use them
- How and under what conditions you should stop using them
- What to do if you miss a dose
- What they are supposed to do and when to expect results
- Side effects and interactions
- Whether you need any tests or monitoring
- Always ask for written information to take with you

Read the Label and Follow Directions

Make sure you understand the directions; ask if you have questions or concerns. Always double-check that you have the right medicine. Keep medicines in their original labeled containers, whenever possible. Never combine different medicines in the same bottle.

Read and follow the directions on the label and the directions from your doctor, pharmacist, or other healthcare professional. If you stop the medicine or want to use the medicine differently than directed, consult with your healthcare professional.

Avoid Interactions

Ask if there are interactions with any other medicines or dietary supplements (including vitamins or herbal supplements), beverages, or foods.

Use the same pharmacy for all of your medicine needs, whenever possible.

Before starting any new medicine or dietary supplement (including vitamins or herbal supplements), ask again if there are possible interactions with what you are currently using.

Monitor Your Medicines' Effects—and the Effects of Other Products That You Use

Ask if there is anything you can do to minimize side effects, such as eating before you take a medicine to reduce stomach upset.

Pay attention to how you are feeling; note any changes. Write down the changes so that you can remember to tell your doctor, pharmacist, or other healthcare professional.

Know what to do if you experience side effects and when to notify your doctor. You should also know how to keep track of any improvement and when to report back.

TIPS FOR TALKING WITH YOUR PHARMACIST TO LEARN HOW TO USE MEDICINES SAFELY

Your pharmacist can help you learn how to use your prescription and nonprescription (OTC) medicines safely and effectively. You can also use these tips when talking with your other healthcare providers.

Tell Your Pharmacist

You should inform your pharmacist about:

- Every medicine you use, especially if you use multiple pharmacies, even if it is the same pharmacy chain
- Keep a record and give it to your pharmacist. List all the prescription and OTC medicines, vitamins, herbals, and other supplements you use. Tell your pharmacist exactly how you are taking the medicine.
- Do not forget to tell your pharmacist about any changes to your medicines. This includes anything you have stopped taking.
- If you have had any allergic reactions or problems with medicines, dietary supplements, food, medical devices, or other medical treatments
- What kind of reaction did you have? Did your throat swell up? Did you get a rash? Or was it a stomach ache or diarrhea?
- Any medical conditions you have or have had, including any abnormal lab results
- Anything that could affect your use of medicine, such as trouble with swallowing, reading small labels, understanding English, remembering to take your medicine, distinguishing the look of one medicine from another, paying for medicines, or transportation to the pharmacy. Your pharmacist may be able to help, so just ask!
- If you plan to start or have started something new, such as a new medicine, supplement, diet, or exercise regime. Your pharmacist can help you avoid medicines, supplements, foods, and other things that do not mix well with your medicines.

Using Medications Safely

- If you are pregnant, plan to become pregnant, breastfeeding, or plan to breastfeed
- The best phone number to reach you and your current address. This is in case the pharmacist has any questions for you or if there are any issues. If you prefer to receive text messages instead of phone calls, let your pharmacy know! Many pharmacies have the ability to text.
- If there have been any changes to your insurance plan/policy/card

Ask Your Pharmacist

There are a few questions that you should ask your pharmacist.

- What is the most important information I should know about this medicine?
- How do I pronounce the name of my medicine? Does it go by any other name(s)? What are the brand and generic (nonbrand) names?
- Are there any cheaper options? Is a generic available? Are there any copay assistance coupons?
- How does this medicine work and what is it used for?
- How and when should I use it? How much do I use? Should I take it with food or without food, before a meal or after a meal? What time of the day should I use it? How many times a day is it used? Is there a limit on how often I should use it?
- How long should I use it? Can I stop using the medicine or use less if I feel better? In what circumstances should I stop taking this medicine?
- What should I do if I …miss a dose? throw up shortly after taking a dose? use too much? lose the medicine?
- Will this take the place of anything else I am taking?
- When will the medicine start working? How should I expect to feel?
- Are there any special directions for using this?
- Should I avoid any other medicines, dietary supplements, drinks, foods, activities, or other things? Do I have to space this medicine out from any other medicines or food?
- Does this medicine contain any ingredients I am allergic to?
- Is there anything I should watch for, such as allergic reactions or side effects? What are the serious side effects? What do I do if I get any?
- Will I need any tests to check the medicine's effects (blood tests, x-rays, other)? When will I need those?
- How and where should I store this medicine? Is it stored at room temperature or refrigerated or frozen? What should I do if I left it in a hot car?
- When should I throw out this medicine? When does it expire?
- Is there a medication guide or other patient information for this medicine?

- Where and how can I get more written information?
- When should I contact my doctor about this medicine? In what situation should I call 911?

Before You Leave the Pharmacy

Before you leave the pharmacy after picking up your prescription:

- **Look to be sure you have the right medicine.** If you have bought the medicine before, make sure this medicine has the same shape, color, size, markings, and packaging. Anything different? Do not hesitate to ask your pharmacist. If it seems different when you use it, tell your pharmacist, doctor, or other healthcare professional.
- **Be sure you know the right dose for the medicine and you know how to use it.** Unsure about anything? Ask your pharmacist.
- **For liquid medicines, make sure there is a measuring spoon, cup, or syringe.** If the medicine does not come with a special measuring tool, ask your pharmacist for one. (Spoons used for eating and cooking may give the wrong dose. Do not use them.)
- **Be sure you have any information the pharmacist can give you about the medicine.** Read it and save it.
- **Get the pharmacy's phone number and hours,** so you can call back for any questions or refills.

Chapter 33 | e-Prescribing

Electronic prescribing, or "e-prescribing," is the paperless process that allows prescribers to electronically send an accurate, error-free, and understandable prescription directly to a pharmacy from the medical office, or point of care. This process decreases the likelihood of prescription errors and thus improves the quality of patient care. The inclusion of electronic prescribing in the Medicare Modernization Act (MMA) of 2003 led to a rapid transition from paper to e-prescriptions, and the July 2006 Institute of Medicine (IOM) report documenting the role e-prescribing played in reducing medication errors received widespread publicity, which helped raise awareness of the role e-prescribing plays in enhancing patient safety. Adopting standards to facilitate this improved prescription process was one of the key action items in the government's plan to expedite the adoption of electronic medical records (EMRs)—a necessary step in building a national electronic health-information infrastructure in the United States.

Although the MMA made e-prescribing optional for physicians and pharmacies, drug plans that participate in Medicare Part D are required to submit prescriptions electronically.

THE BENEFITS OF E-PRESCRIBING

E-prescribing allows healthcare providers to enter prescription information into a computer device—such as a tablet, laptop, or desktop computer—and securely transmit the prescription to pharmacies using a special software program and connectivity to a transmission network. When a pharmacy receives the e-prescription, it can begin filling the medication right away.

E-prescribing can:

- Improve healthcare quality and patient safety by reducing medication errors and automatically checking for potentially harmful drug interactions

This chapter contains text excerpted from the following sources: Text in this chapter begins with excerpts from "E-Prescribing," Centers for Medicare & Medicaid Services (CMS), August 13, 2019; Text under the heading "The Benefits of E-Prescribing" is excerpted from "What Is Electronic Prescribing?" HealthIT.gov, Office of the National Coordinator for Health Information Technology (ONC), September 10, 2019.

| Less paperwork | Easy, electronic access to your medical records | Better care coordination among health care providers | Faster, more accurate prescriptions | Fewer unnecessary tests and procedures | Greater control over your health |

Figure 33.1. How Technology Will Improve Your Health *(Source: "Electronic Health Records: How They Connect You and Your Doctors," HealthIT.gov, Office of the National Coordinator for Health Information Technology (ONC))*

- Streamlines the prescription process and makes it more convenient by allowing healthcare providers to electronically request prescription refills

In short, e-prescribing is safer, less costly, and more efficient and convenient for healthcare providers, pharmacies, and patients.

Chapter 34 | Over-the-Counter Medications

Over-the-counter (OTC) medicines are drugs you can buy without a prescription. Some OTC medicines relieve aches, pains, and itches. Some prevent or cure diseases, such as tooth decay and athlete's foot. Others help manage recurring problems, such as migraines and allergies. In the United States, the U.S. Food and Drug Administration (FDA) decides whether a medicine is safe and effective enough to sell over-the-counter. This allows you to take a more active role in your healthcare. But you also need to be careful to avoid mistakes. Make sure to follow the instructions on the drug label. If you do not understand the instructions, ask your pharmacist or healthcare provider.

ABOUT SELF-CARE: ACCESS PLUS KNOWLEDGE IS EQUAL TO POWER

American medicine cabinets contain a growing choice of nonprescription, OTC medicines to treat an expanding range of ailments. OTC medicines often do more than relieve aches, pains, and itches. Some can prevent diseases such as tooth decay, cure diseases such as athlete's foot and, with a doctor's guidance, help manage recurring conditions, such as vaginal yeast infection, migraine, and minor pain in arthritis.

The FDA determines whether medicines are prescription or nonprescription. The term "prescription" (Rx) refers to medicines that are safe and effective when used under a doctor's care. Nonprescription or OTC drugs are medicines which the FDA considers to be safe and effective for use without a doctor's prescription.

The FDA also has the authority to decide when a prescription drug is safe enough to be sold directly to consumers over the counter. This regulatory process allowing Americans to take a more active role in their healthcare is known

This chapter contains text excerpted from the following sources: Text in this chapter begins with excerpts from "Over-the-Counter Medicines," MedlinePlus, National Institutes of Health (NIH), April 21, 2016. Reviewed December 2019; Text beginning with the heading "About Self-Care: Access Plus Knowledge Is Equal to Power" is excerpted from "Over-the-Counter Medicines: What's Right for You?" U.S. Food and Drug Administration (FDA), September 3, 2013. Reviewed December 2019.

as the "Rx-to-OTC" switch. As a result of this process, more than 700 products sold over the counter nowadays use ingredients or dosage strengths available only by prescription 30 years ago.

Increased access to OTC medicines is especially important for the maturing population. Two out of three older Americans rate their health as excellent to good, but four out of five reports at least one chronic condition.

Fact is, nowadays OTC medicines offer greater opportunity to treat more of the aches and illnesses most likely to appear in later years of life. As people live longer, work longer, and take a more active role in their own healthcare, the need grows to become better informed about self-care.

The best way to become better informed—for young and old alike—is to read and understand the information on OTC labels. Next to the medicine itself, label comprehension is the most important part of self-care with OTC medicines.

With new opportunities in self-medication come new responsibilities and an increased need for knowledge. The FDA and the Consumer Healthcare Products Association (CHPA) have prepared the following information to help Americans take advantage of self-care opportunities.

Over-the-Counter Know-How: It Is on the Label

You would not ignore your doctor's instructions for using a prescription drug; so, do not ignore the label when taking an OTC medicine. Here is what to look for:

- PRODUCT NAME
- "ACTIVE INGREDIENTS": therapeutic substances in medicine
- "PURPOSE": product category (such as antihistamine, antacid, or cough suppressant)
- "USES": symptoms or diseases the product will treat or prevent
- "WARNINGS": when not to use the product, when to stop taking it, when to see a doctor, and possible side effects
- "DIRECTIONS": how much to take, how to take it, and how long to take it
- "OTHER INFORMATION": such as storage information
- "INACTIVE INGREDIENTS": substances such as binders, colors, or flavoring

You can help yourself read the label too. Always use enough light. It usually takes 3 times more light to read the same line at age 60 than at age 30. If necessary, use your glasses or contact lenses when reading labels.

Always remember to look for the statement describing the tamper-evident feature(s) before you buy the product and when you use it.

When it comes to medicines, more does not necessarily mean better. You should never misuse OTC medicines by taking them longer or in higher doses than the label recommends. Symptoms that persist are a clear signal it is time to see a doctor.

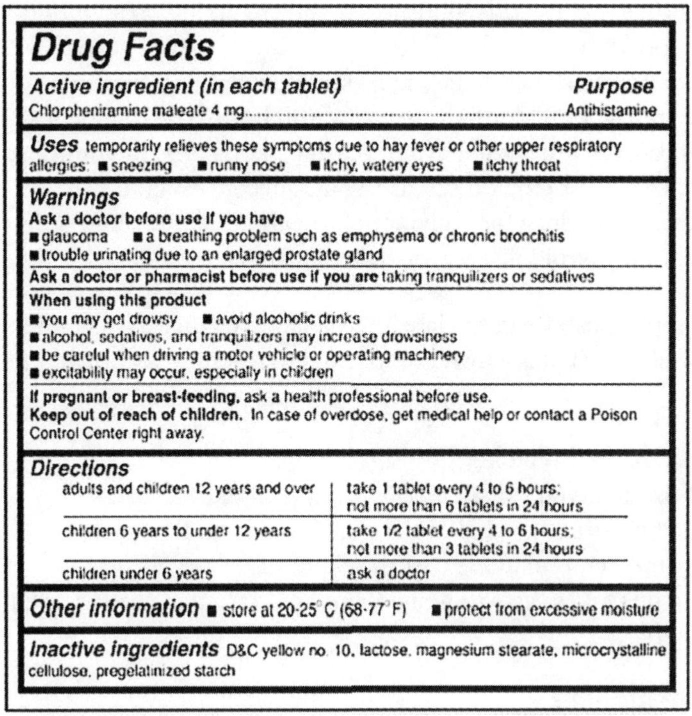

Drug Facts

Active ingredient (in each tablet)   **Purpose**
Chlorpheniramine maleate 4 mg..Antihistamine

Uses temporarily relieves these symptoms due to hay fever or other upper respiratory
allergies: ■ sneezing   ■ runny nose   ■ itchy, watery eyes   ■ itchy throat

Warnings
Ask a doctor before use if you have
■ glaucoma   ■ a breathing problem such as emphysema or chronic bronchitis
■ trouble urinating due to an enlarged prostate gland

Ask a doctor or pharmacist before use if you are taking tranquilizers or sedatives

When using this product
■ you may get drowsy   ■ avoid alcoholic drinks
■ alcohol, sedatives, and tranquilizers may increase drowsiness
■ be careful when driving a motor vehicle or operating machinery
■ excitability may occur, especially in children

If pregnant or breast-feeding, ask a health professional before use.
Keep out of reach of children. In case of overdose, get medical help or contact a Poison
Control Center right away.

Directions

adults and children 12 years and over	take 1 tablet every 4 to 6 hours; not more than 6 tablets in 24 hours
children 6 years to under 12 years	take 1/2 tablet every 4 to 6 hours; not more than 3 tablets in 24 hours
children under 6 years	ask a doctor

Other information ■ store at 20-25°C (68-77°F)   ■ protect from excessive moisture

Inactive ingredients D&C yellow no. 10, lactose, magnesium stearate, microcrystalline
cellulose, pregelatinized starch

Figure 34.1. Drug Facts Label *(Source: "Medicines in My Home," U.S. Food and Drug Administration (FDA))*

Be sure to read the label each time you purchase a product. Just because two or more products are from the same brand family does not mean they are meant to treat the same conditions or contain the same ingredients.

Remember, if you read the label and still have questions, talk to a doctor, nurse, or pharmacist.

Drug Interactions: A Word to the Wise

Although mild and relatively uncommon, interactions involving OTC drugs can produce unwanted results or make medicines less effective. It is especially important to know about drug interactions if you are taking Rx and OTC drugs at the same time.

Some drugs can also interact with foods and beverages, as well as with health conditions, such as diabetes, kidney disease, and high blood pressure.

Here are a few drug interactions cautions for some common OTC ingredients:

• Avoid alcohol if you are taking antihistamines, cough-cold products with the ingredient dextromethorphan, or drugs that treat sleeplessness.

- Do not use drugs that treat sleeplessness if you are taking prescription sedatives or tranquilizers.
- Check with your doctor before taking products containing aspirin if you are taking a prescription blood thinner or if you have diabetes or gout.
- Do not use laxatives when you have stomach pain, nausea, or vomiting.
- Unless directed by a doctor, do not use a nasal decongestant if you are taking a prescription drug for high blood pressure or depression, or if you have heart or thyroid disease, diabetes, or prostate problems.

This is not a complete list. Read the label! Drug labels change as new information becomes available. That is why it is important to read the label each time you take medicine.

Time for a Medicine Cabinet Checkup

- Be sure to look through your medicine supply at least once a year.
- Always store medicines in a cool, dry place or as stated on the label.
- Throw away any medicines that are past the expiration date.
- To make sure no one takes the wrong medicine, keep all medicines in their original containers.

Pregnancy and Breastfeeding

Drugs can pass from a pregnant woman to her unborn baby. A safe amount of medicine for the mother may be too much for the unborn baby. If you are pregnant, always talk with your doctor before taking any drugs, Rx or OTC.

Although most drugs pass into breast milk in concentrations too low to have any unwanted effects on the baby, breastfeeding mothers still need to be careful. Always ask your doctor or pharmacist before taking any medicine while breastfeeding. A doctor or pharmacist can tell you how to adjust the timing and dosing of most medicines so the baby is exposed to the lowest amount possible, or whether the drugs should be avoided altogether.

GIVING OVER-THE-COUNTER MEDICINES TO KIDS

Over-the-counter drugs rarely come in one-size-fits-all. Here are some tips about giving OTC medicines to children:

- Children are not just small adults, so do not estimate the dose based on their size.
- Read the label. Follow all directions.
- Follow any age limits on the label.
- Some OTC products come in different strengths. Be aware!
- Know the difference between a tablespoon (TBSP) and teaspoon (TSP). They are very different doses.

Over-the-Counter Medications

- Be careful about converting dose instructions. If the label says two teaspoons, it is best to use a measuring spoon or a dosing cup marked in teaspoons, not a common kitchen spoon.
- Do not play doctor. Do not double the dose just because your child seems sicker than last time.
- Before you give your child two medicines at the same time, talk to your doctor or pharmacist.
- Never let children take medicine by themselves.
- Never call medicine candy to get your kids to take it. If they come across the medicine on their own, they are likely to remember that you called it candy.

Child-Resistant Packaging

Child-resistant closures are designed for repeated use to make it difficult for children to open. Remember, if you do not relock the closure after each use, the child-resistant device cannot do its job—keeping children out!

It is best to store all medicines and dietary supplements where children can neither see nor reach them. Containers of pills should not be left on the kitchen counter as a reminder. Purses and briefcases are among the worst places to hide medicines from curious kids. And since children are natural mimics, it is a good idea not to take medicine in front of them. They may be tempted to "play house" with your medicine later on.

If you find some packages too difficult to open—and do not have young children living with you or visiting—you should know the law allows one package size for each OTC medicine to be sold without child-resistant features. If you do not see it on the store shelf, ask.

Protect Yourself against Tampering

Makers of OTC medicines seal most products in tamper-evident packaging (TEP) to help protect against criminal tampering. TEP works by providing visible evidence if the package has been disturbed. Remember, OTC packaging cannot be 100 percent tamper-proof. Here is how to help protect yourself:

- Be alert to the tamper-evident features on the package before you open it. These features are described on the label.
- Inspect the outer packaging before you buy it. When you get home, inspect the medicine inside.
- Do not buy an OTC product if the packaging is damaged.
- Do not use any medicine that looks discolored or different in any way.
- If anything looks suspicious, be suspicious. Contact the store where you bought the product. Take it back!
- Never take medicines in the dark.

Chapter 35 | What Value Do Prescription Drugs Provide to Patients?

Pharmaceutical companies are responsible for the discovery and development of medicines that help people live longer and lead healthier lives. However, the complexity of the pharmaceutical industry creates many questions for the public to consider.

PRESCRIPTION DRUGS

A substance that is intended for use in the diagnosis, cure, mitigation, treatment, or prevention of disease or illness is referred to as a "drug." Drugs are broadly classified into over-the-counter (OTC) drugs and prescription drugs. OTC drugs can be purchased directly from stores without being prescribed by a doctor.

Prescription drugs conform to the following traits:
- They are prescribed by a doctor.
- They are purchased at a pharmacy.
- They are prescribed for and intended to be used by one person.

The U.S. Food and Drug Administration (FDA) regulates prescription drugs through the New Drug Application (NDA) process. This is the official step a drug sponsor takes to ask that the FDA consider approving a new drug for marketing in the United States. An NDA incorporates all animal and human data and analyses of the data, along with information on how the drug behaves in the body and how it is produced.

Prescription drugs help people avoid death and disability caused by disease or illness and help lower the overall costs of treatment. Medical advances, along with prescription drugs, have lowered death rates for chronic diseases such as heart disease, stroke, cancer, and other deadly diseases:

- Since 1970, the death rate from heart disease has decreased by 60 percent.
- Deaths due to strokes have dropped to 7 percent since 1970.
- Cancer death rates have dropped 16 percent since 1990.
- The death rate from human immunodeficiency virus (HIV)/acquired immunodeficiency syndrome (AIDS) fell more than 75 percent from its highest point in 1995.
- The average lifespan of Americans surged from 69.7 years in 1960 to around 80 years in 2007.

The lives of more than 1 million Americans would be lost every year if not for the reduction in death rates from heart disease and stroke. Likewise, the 5-year survival rates for cancer have improved by 26 percent just since 1984. There is also a significant value in prescription samples since samples allow patients to start immediate treatment and explore treatment options before paying for a prescription. Based on these values, health economists were able to show that every $1 spent resulted in:

- Health gains of about $9.44 produced as a result of statin therapy for heart-attack survivors
- Intensive glycemic control in newly diagnosed type 2 diabetes patients, resulting in $3.77 in health gains

The treatment of asthma, which affects about 23.3 million Americans, 7 million of whom are children, has also gained consequential value from prescription drugs. Asthma is responsible for 444,000 hospitalizations, 1.7 million emergency-room visits, and around 3,600 deaths a year. As a result of the use of inhaled corticosteroids for 1 year, the risk of hospitalization was reduced by 50 percent, the number of outpatient visits by 26 percent, and monthly healthcare costs by 24 percent per patient.

Cancer is another potentially fatal disease that immensely affects Americans. During their lifetimes, 1 in 3 women and 1 in 2 men develop cancer. Since the late 1970s, the treatments and medicine researched and developed by the pharmaceutical industry has enhanced overall 5-year cancer survival rates by 36 percent. Furthermore, life expectancy for people with cancer increased by 3 years between 1980 and 2000, and 86 percent of that gain is credited to better treatment, which includes the use of prescription drugs.

VALUE-BASED PURCHASING FOR PRESCRIPTION DRUGS

Prescription drugs can be expensive and value-based purchasing is dependent on whether the price of a drug is linked to curing or improving the condition of a patient who uses it. This pricing strategy, known as "value-based purchasing" (VBP), or "value-based contracting" (VBC), is gaining attention from private insurance carriers and pharmaceutical companies.

Value-based purchasing involves contracts between insurance carriers and pharmaceutical companies that can take a variety of forms. The basic principle behind the practice is that a pharmaceutical company enters into a contract with a health-insurance carrier that includes the company's drug on its formulary (list of prescription drugs, covered by a specific healthcare plan). If patients who use the drug do not sufficiently improve or have poor reported health outcomes, then the pharmaceutical company provides discounts, rebates, or refunds to the carrier. For example, Amgen, which manufactures Repatha to treat high cholesterol levels, signed a contract with Harvard Pilgrim, an insurance carrier. Along with negotiated discounts, Amgen promised additional rebates if patients did not undergo reductions in cholesterol levels similar to clinical trial results. Or, for instance, if a Harvard Pilgrim subscriber who is prescribed Repatha, suffers a heart attack or stroke while taking the drug, Amgen will provide Harvard Pilgrim a full refund for the carrier's costs to cover the drug for that patient.

The Commonwealth Fund has published an issue brief analyzing this emerging strategy to lower drug costs while ensuring high-quality patient care. The brief's authors interviewed experts and contract professionals from nine pharmaceutical manufacturers and eight insurance carriers to determine the effect of value-based purchasing on patient outcomes and overall drug spending.

The study indicated varied results. Because sample sizes are comparatively small and pricing information for insurance formularies are often subject to strict confidentiality rules, it can be difficult to get a full picture of the effects of value-based purchasing or contracting. Nevertheless, the report authors and interviewed stakeholders found several potential benefits and drawbacks, should these practices be embraced.

Potential Benefits

- Patients may gain access to innovative and effective drugs more quickly than they might otherwise, since value-based contracting agreements can be used to encourage carriers to include new and expensive drugs in their formularies more quickly than they would without the guarantee that if the drug is ineffective in treating patients on the carriers' plans, the carrier can recover its costs for the drugs.
- Carriers can use these agreements to improve their formularies by including only the most effective drugs and removing drugs that do not offer suitable results in patient outcomes.

Potential Drawbacks

- Patients are unlikely to see any difference in out-of-pocket costs from value-based contracting programs. This is because the reimbursement rates for drugs are negotiated between insurance carriers and pharmaceutical companies. If a drug does not work for a patient who is covered by an insurance carrier's plan, then the pharmaceutical company will give the carrier a refund to cover at least a portion of the cost of the drug, but not the portion of the costs borne by the patient. Determining whether a drug was effective for a patient and issuing a refund can take years.
- There is no proven evidence that these plans make a measurable difference in prescription drug costs.

References

1. Sullivan, Thomas. "The Value of Medicine," Policy and Medicine, May 5, 2018.
2. Noble, Ashley. "Value-Based Purchasing for Prescription Drugs," National Conference of State Legislatures (NCSL), November 9, 2017.
3. "Prescription Drugs and Over-the-Counter (OTC) Drugs: Questions and Answers," U.S. Food and Drug Administration (FDA), November 13, 2017.

Chapter 36 | **Buying Prescription Drugs**

Chapter Contents

Section 36.1 | Saving Money on Prescription Drugs

This section includes text excerpted from "Saving Money on Medicines," National Institute on Aging (NIA), National Institutes of Health (NIH), May 23, 2017.

Medicines can be costly. If they are too expensive for you, the doctor may be able to suggest less expensive alternatives. If the doctor does not know the cost, ask the pharmacist before filling the prescription. You can ask your doctor if there is a generic or other less expensive choice. Your doctor may also be able to refer you to a medical assistance program that can help with drug costs.

Ask your insurance company for a copy of your drug plan "formulary"—the list of all medicines covered by your insurance company—and bring it to your doctors' appointments. Together, you and your doctor can evaluate the choice of medicines that will be most cost-effective.

You might be thinking about buying your medicines online to save some money. It is important to know which websites are safe and reliable. The U.S. Food and Drug Administration (FDA) has safety tips for buying medicines and medical products online.

Some insurance drug plans offer special prices on medicines if you order directly from them rather than filling prescriptions at a pharmacy. Contact the Centers for Medicare and Medicaid Services to learn about Medicare prescription drug plans that may help save you money, or visit www.medicare.gov/part-d. You can also contact your State Health Insurance Assistance Program (SHIP). If you are a veteran, the U.S. Department of Veterans Affairs (VA) may also be able to help with your prescriptions.

Here are some websites that can provide additional assistance:

- **Medicare Extra Help Program** (www.medicareinteractive.org/get-answers/cost-saving-programs-for-people-with-medicare/the-extra-helplow-income-subsidy-lis-program/extra-help-basics) provides information about the Social Security assistance program and application process for the Medicare Part D subsidy.
- **State Pharmaceutical Assistance Program (SPAP)** (www.medicare.gov/pharmaceutical-assistance-program/state-programs.aspx) provides information about any available state-funded assistance programs for prescription drug costs.
- **Pharmaceutical Assistance Programs (PAP)** (www.medicare.gov/pharmaceutical-assistance-program) provide information about pharmaceutical companies that offer assistance programs for the drugs they manufacture.
- **Partnership for Prescription Assistance** helps connect underinsured people with patient assistance programs for which they may be eligible.

Section 36.2 | Using Your Health-Insurance Coverage to Get Prescription Medications

This section includes text excerpted from "Getting Prescription Medications," Centers for Medicare & Medicaid Services (CMS), December 28, 2013. Reviewed December 2019.

Health plans will help pay the cost of certain prescription medications. You may be able to buy other medications, but medications on your plan's "formulary" (approved list) usually will be less expensive for you.

FAQS ON HEALTH-INSURANCE COVERAGE FOR GETTING PRESCRIPTION MEDICATIONS

Does My New Insurance Plan Cover My Prescription?

To find out which prescriptions are covered through your new plan:

- **Visit your insurer's website** to review a list of prescriptions your plan covers
- **See your Summary of Benefits and Coverage (SBC),** which you can get directly from your insurance company, or by using a link that appears in the detailed description of your plan in your Marketplace account.
- **Call your insurer directly** to find out what is covered. Have your plan information available. The number is available on your insurance card the insurer's website, or the detailed plan description in your Marketplace account.
- **Review any coverage materials** that your plan mailed to you.

What Do I Do If I Am at the Pharmacy to Pick Up My Prescription and They Say My Plan No Longer Covers It?

Some insurance companies may provide a one-time refill for your medication after you first enroll. Ask your insurance company if they offer a one-time refill until you can discuss next steps with your doctor.

If you cannot get a one-time refill, you have the right to follow your insurance company's drug exceptions process, which allows you to get a prescribed drug that is not normally covered by your health plan. Because the details of every plan's exceptions process are different, you should contact your insurance company for more information.

Generally, to get your drug covered through the exceptions process, your doctor must confirm to your health plan (orally or in writing) that the drug is appropriate for your medical condition based on one or more of the following:

- All other drugs covered by the plan have not been or would not be as effective as the drug you are asking for

Buying Prescription Drugs

- Any alternative drugs covered by your plan has caused or is likely to cause side effects that may be harmful to you
- If there is a limit on the number of doses you are allowed:
  - That the allowed dosage has not worked for your condition
  - The drug likely will not work for you based on your physical or mental makeup. For example, based on your body weight, you may need to take more doses than what is allowed by your plan.
- If you get the exception:
  - Your health plan generally will treat the drug as covered and charge you the copayment that applies to the most expensive drugs already covered on the plan (for example, a nonpreferred brand drug).
  - Any amount you pay for the drug generally will count toward your deductible and/or maximum out-of-pocket limits.

Can I Get the Noncovered Drug during the Exceptions Process?

While you are in the exceptions process, your plan may give you access to the requested drug until a decision is made.

My Insurer Denied My Request for an Exception. Now What Do I Do?

If your health insurance company will not pay for your prescription, you have the right to appeal the decision and have it reviewed by an independent third party.

Can I Go to My Regular Pharmacy to Get My Medication?

Just like different health plans cover different medications, different health plans allow you to get your medications from different pharmacies (called "in-network pharmacies"). Call your insurance company or visit their website to find out whether your regular pharmacy is in-network under your new plan and, if not, what pharmacies in your area are in-network. You can also learn if you can get your prescription delivered in the mail.

If you have additional questions, call 800-318-2596. (Toll-free TTY: 855-889-4325)

Section 36.3 | Cost May Result in Underuse of Medications

This section includes text excerpted from "Effect of Financial Stress and Positive Financial Behaviors on Cost-Related Nonadherence to Health Regimens among Adults in a Community-Based Setting," Centers for Disease Control and Prevention (CDC), April 7, 2016. Reviewed December 2019.

Little is known about the role of positive financial behaviors (behaviors that allow maintenance of financial stability with financial resources) in mitigating cost-related nonadherence (CRN) to health regimens.

One of four Americans reports financial difficulty in paying medical bills; this difficulty has significant public-health implications, especially for the 50 percent of the population that is managing chronic illness. Seven systematic reviews concluded that several factors influence adherence to treatment, but the cost to the patient is one that demonstrates a consistent negative effect. Nearly 18 percent of chronically ill Americans report underusing medications and delaying or not fulfilling therapeutic recommendations because of cost, which is referred to as "CRN" and varies by therapeutic class across chronic therapies. Nearly 56 percent of American adults with common chronic diseases self-report nonfulfillment of medication as a result of financial hardship.

Health-insurance coverage is a strong predictor of financial burden. Nearly half of Americans have literacy challenges with health insurance and pay more for healthcare out of pocket because of these challenges, despite improvements as a result of the Affordable Care Act (ACA).

Although health literacy and health insurance literacy are commonly discussed as integral for individuals to have the capacity to obtain, process, and understand basic health information or services and health insurance, financial literacy in the context of health has received little attention. Financial literacy is a set of skills and knowledge that allows individuals to make informed decisions with their financial resources, and it is associated with more frequent engagement in health-promoting behaviors. Studies show that social determinants of health that contribute to financial burden correlate with CRN. Therefore, financial burden may be experienced in the context of a growing concern for financial insecurity and may not be exclusively health-related. Given the role that cost to the patient plays in adherence to therapeutic regimens, improving financial literacy to influence positive financial behaviors (behaviors that allow individuals to maintain financial stability with their financial resources) may have implications for CRN, and may be a necessary adjunct to policy reforms.

Few interventions have aimed to mitigate CRN beyond reducing out-of-pocket costs, which have shown modest improvements in health status. Whether positive financial behavior is protective of CRN has not been explored and may have implications for behavioral interventions to promote financial literacy, especially among people who have chronic illnesses.

Researchers have examined financial stress and CRN by type of chronic condition and health insurance status in a community-dwelling sample in Michigan. They also examined the relationship between financial stress, positive financial behaviors, and CRN, testing the hypothesis that the relationship between financial stress and CRN is different between people who report lower numbers versus higher numbers of positive financial behaviors. The researchers came to the conclusion that financial literacy could be a means for promoting positive financial behavior which may in turn help reduce CRN. An intervention strategy focused on improving financial literacy may be relevant for high-risk groups who report high levels of financial stress.

Section 36.4 | How to Purchase Prescription Medicine Online Safely

This section includes text excerpted from "How to Buy Medicines Safely from an Online Pharmacy," U.S. Food and Drug Administration (FDA), January 25, 2018.

Ever been tempted to buy your medicines from an online pharmacy or another website? Protect yourself and your family by using caution when buying medicine online. There are many pharmacy websites that operate legally and offer convenience, privacy, and safeguards for purchasing medicines.

But the U.S. Food and Drug Administration (FDA) warns that there are many rogue online pharmacies that claim to sell prescription medicines at deeply discounted prices, often without requiring a valid prescription. These Internet-based pharmacies often sell unapproved or counterfeit medicines outside the safeguards followed by licensed pharmacies.

These rogue sites often prominently display a Canadian flag, but may actually be operated by criminals from the other side of the globe with no connection to Canada. Medicines bought from these websites can be dangerous and may put your health at risk.

How can you tell if an online pharmacy is operating legally? The FDA's BeSafeRx can help you identify and avoid fake online pharmacies.

SIGNS OF A ROGUE ONLINE PHARMACY

Beware of online pharmacies that:

- Allow you to buy prescription medicine without a valid prescription from your healthcare provider

- Do not have a U.S. state-licensed pharmacist available to answer your questions
- Offer very low prices that seem too good to be true
- Send spam or unsolicited e-mail offering cheap medicine
- Are located outside of the United States or ship worldwide

These pharmacies often sell medicines that can be dangerous because they may:
- Have too much or too little of the active ingredient you need to treat your disease or condition
- Not contain the right active ingredient
- Contain the wrong or other harmful ingredients

The active ingredient is what makes the medicine effective for the illness or condition it is intended to treat. If a medicine has unknown active ingredients, it could fail to have the intended effect, could have an unexpected interaction with other medicines you are taking, could cause dangerous side effects, or may cause other serious health problems, such as serious allergic reactions.

Also, these medicines may not have been stored properly, such as in a warehouse without necessary temperature controls, which may cause the medicine to be ineffective in treating the disease or condition for which you are taking it.

KNOW THE SIGNS OF A SAFE ONLINE PHARMACY

There are ways you can identify a safe online pharmacy. They:
- Require a valid prescription from a doctor or another licensed healthcare professional
- Are licensed by your state board of pharmacy, or equivalent state agency. (To verify the licensing status of a pharmacy, check your state board of pharmacy.)
- Have a U.S. state-licensed pharmacist available to answer your questions
- Are in the United States, and provide a street address

Another way to check on a website is to look for the National Association of Boards of Pharmacy's (NABP) Verified Internet Pharmacy Practice Sites™ Seal, also known as the "VIPPS® Seal." This seal means that the Internet pharmacy is safe to use because it has met state licensure requirements, as well as other NABP criteria. Visit the VIPPS website to find legitimate pharmacies that carry the VIPPS® seal.

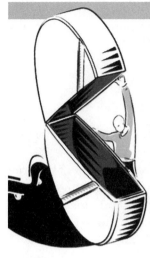

Counterfeit medicines are fake or "copycat" medicines. They may not be safe and effective, and could be dangerous to your health.

DON'T BE A VICTIM!

Buy medicines only from state-licensed pharmacies that are located in the United States. Find your state's contact information from the National Association of Boards of Pharmacy (NABP) at www.nabp.info

or

Look for this seal on Internet pharmacy Web sites. Pharmacies that carry this seal are listed at www.vipps.info.

Figure 36.1. Counterfeit Medicines *(Source: "Counterfeit Medicines: Filled with Empty Promises," U.S. Food and Drug Administration (FDA))*

Section 36.5 | Truth in Advertising: Advertisements for Prescription Drugs

This section includes text excerpted from "Prescription Drug Advertising," U.S. Food and Drug Administration (FDA), July 8, 2019.

Your healthcare provider is the best source of information about the right medicine for you. Prescription drug advertisements can provide useful information for consumers to work with their healthcare providers to make wise decisions about treatment.

PRODUCT CLAIM ADVERTISEMENTS

Product claim advertisements are the only type of advertisements that name a drug and discuss its benefits and risks. However, these advertisements must not be false or misleading in any way. The U.S. Food and Drug Administration (FDA) encourage companies to use understandable language throughout product claim ads that are directed to consumers.

All product claim advertisements, regardless of the media in which they appear, must include certain key components within the main part of the advertisements:

- The name of the drug (brand and generic)
- At least one FDA-approved use for the drug
- The most significant risks of the drug

Product claim advertisements must present the benefits and risks of a prescription drug in a balanced fashion.

Print product claim ads also must include a "brief summary" about the drug that generally includes all the risks listed in its approved prescribing information.

- Under the FDA Amendments Act of 2007, print advertisements need to include the following statement: "You are encouraged to report negative side effects of prescription drugs to the FDA. Visit MedWatch (www. fda.gov/safety/medwatch-fda-safety-information-and-adverse-event-reporting-program) or call 800-FDA-1088 (800-332-1088)."

Broadcast product claim ads (TV, radio, telephone) must include the following:

- The drug's most important risks ("major statement") presented in the audio (that is, spoken)
- Either all the risks listed in the drug's prescribing information or a variety of sources for viewers to find the prescribing information for the drug

This means that drug companies do not have to include all of a drug's risk information in a broadcast advertisement. Instead, the advertisement may tell where viewers or listeners can find more information about the drug in the FDA-approved prescribing information. This is called the "adequate provision" requirement. For broadcast advertisements, we have said that including a variety of sources of prescribing information fulfills this requirement.

Broadcast advertisements give the following sources for finding a drug's prescribing information:

- A healthcare provider (for example, a doctor)
- A toll-free telephone number
- The current issue of a magazine that contains a print advertisement
- A website address

REMINDER ADVERTISEMENTS

Reminder advertisements give the name of a drug, but not the drug's uses. These advertisements assume that the audience already knows the drug's use.

Buying Prescription Drugs

A reminder advertisement does not have to contain risk information about the drug because the advertisement does not say what the drug does or how well it works. Unlike product claim advertisements, reminder advertisements cannot suggest, in either words or pictures, anything about the drug's benefits or risks. For example, a reminder advertisement for a drug that helps treat asthma should not include a drawing of a pair of lungs, because this implies what the drug does.

Reminder advertisements are not allowed for certain prescription drugs with serious risks. Drugs with serious risks have a special warning, often called a "boxed warning," in the drug's FDA-approved prescribing information. Because of their seriousness, the risks must be included in all advertisements for these drugs.

HELP-SEEKING ADVERTISEMENTS

Help-seeking advertisements describe a disease or condition but do not recommend or suggest a specific drug treatment. Some examples of diseases or conditions discussed in help-seeking advertisements include allergies, asthma, erectile dysfunction, high cholesterol, and osteoporosis. The advertisements encourage people with these symptoms to talk to their doctor. Help-seeking advertisements may include a drug company's name and may also provide a telephone number to call for more information.

When done properly, help-seeking advertisements are not considered to be drug advertisements. Therefore, FDA do not regulate true help-seeking advertisements, but the Federal Trade Commission (FTC) does regulate them. If an advertisement recommends or suggests the use of a specific drug, however, it is considered a product claim advertisements that must comply with FDA rules.

OTHER PRODUCT CLAIM PROMOTIONAL MATERIALS

Other types of promotional materials than advertisements are used to promote the use of a drug. These are called "promotional labeling" and include brochures, materials mailed to consumers, and other types of materials given out by drug companies. If these materials mention the drug's benefit(s) they must also include the drug's prescribing information.

RISK DISCLOSURE REQUIREMENTS FOR DIFFERENT TYPES OF ADVERTISEMENTS

Different advertisements require different amounts of benefit and risk information.

Reminder advertisements do not have to include any risk information because they cannot include any claims or pictures about what a drug does or how it works. Reminder advertisements are only for drugs without certain specified serious risks.

Print product claim ads may make statements about a drug's benefit(s). They must present the drug's most important risks in the main part of the advertisement ("fair balance"). These advertisements generally must include every risk, but can present the less important risks in the detailed information known as the "brief summary."

Also, print product claim and reminder advertisements must include the following statement:

- Broadcast product claim advertisements may make statements about a drug's benefit(s). They must include the drug's most important risk information ("major statement") in a way that is clear, conspicuous, and neutral. In addition, they must include either every risk or provide enough sources for the audience to obtain the drug's prescribing information ("adequate provision").

Section 36.6 | Imported Drugs Raise Safety Concerns

This section includes text excerpted from "Imported Drugs Raise Safety Concerns," U.S. Food and Drug Administration (FDA), March 1, 2018.

Selene Seguros Rios was 18 months old in 1999 when she received 2 injections of a pain and fever drug called "Neo-Melubrina" (dipyrone) in an illegal backroom clinic in Tustin, California. That was 20 years after the U.S. Food and Drug Administration (FDA) had banned the drug in the United States because of potentially fatal side effects, including a drop in white blood cells (WBCs) that hampers the body's ability to fight off infections.

Selene died soon after the shots. Her death set off a crackdown in December 2000 on smuggling drugs from Mexico and selling them at swap meets, gift stores, clothing stores, meat markets, and other retail establishments in Southern California. "We've found drugs that were stored in tin containers and car trunks," says Daniel Hancz, Pharm.D., a pharmacist with the Health Authority Law Enforcement Task Force (HALT) in Los Angeles, an organization of police officers and other law-enforcement personnel with special training in pharmaceuticals. HALT was launched as part of the crackdown, and task force members have confiscated a variety of prescription drugs being sold illegally. Experts say the problem mirrors what goes on in nearby Mexico, where easy access to prescription drugs is common. Marv Shepherd, Ph.D., director of the Pharmacoeconomic Center at the University of Texas at Austin, places drugs available in Mexico into two categories. "Plenty of drugs that require a prescription in the United States. HALT was launched as part of the crackdown, such as antibiotics, cardiac drugs, and birth control pills (BCPs)—are available OTC in Mexico," he says. "Then there are controlled substances like Valium, which you do need a prescription for in Mexico."

The FDA's Office of Criminal Investigations (OCI) in Los Angeles has teamed with HALT to uncover major black-market pharmacy rings selling Spanish-labeled pharmaceuticals. Ring members have been arrested and accused of violating the Federal Food, Drug, and Cosmetic Act (FD&C Act). Local lawmakers have stiffened penalties, and many illegal pharmacies have been shut down. Other drug sellers have taken their businesses underground, moving from storefronts to private homes in an attempt to hide.

As in Selene's case, some criminals have falsely claimed to have a medical background and not only illegally sold drugs, but administered injections. Hancz says that HALT has seized prescription drugs found mostly in Latinx, Asian, and Russian immigrant communities, where some undocumented immigrants, fearing that their immigration status may be discovered, have sought healthcare in back rooms. The U.S. Attorney's Office for the Central District of California has indicated that legitimate or state-licensed clinics exist where immigrants can be treated safely regardless of immigration status.

The list of safety risks is long, but the principal problems involve the use of prescription drugs without a physician's supervision and the danger of buying drugs of unknown origin and quality. "I've seen eye medications that look like they're 20 years old," Hancz says. "The drugs could be old, contaminated, or counterfeit. And if you experience some kind of allergic reaction or other side effect, it's hard to trace the problem and treat it."

Whether you are searching for a cheaper price or dodging the doctor's office, the FDA warns against using unapproved drugs. And just because a drug is approved in a foreign country, that does not mean it is approved in the United States. Drug standards and regulations vary from country to country, and the FDA is responsible only for those marketed and sold inside the United States.

Joe McCallion, a consumer safety officer in the FDA's Office of Regulatory Affairs (ORA), sums it up this way: "If you buy drugs that come from outside the U.S., the FDA doesn't know what you're getting, which means safety can't be assured."

BENEFITS OF A CLOSED SYSTEM

Under the FD&C Act, the interstate shipment of any prescription drug that lacks required FDA approval is illegal. Interstate shipment includes importation—bringing drugs from a foreign country into the United States.

Drugs sold in the United States also must have proper labeling that conforms with the FDA's requirements, and must be made in accordance with good manufacturing practices. As part of the FDA's high standards, drugs can be manufactured only at plants registered with the agency, whether those facilities are domestic or foreign. If a foreign firm is listed as a manufacturer or supplier of a drug's ingredients on a new drug application, the FDA generally travels to that site to inspect it.

After the FDA approves a drug, manufacturers still are subject to FDA inspections and must continue to comply with good manufacturing practices. "With an unapproved drug, you can't be sure that it has been shipped, handled, and stored under conditions that meet U.S. requirements," McCallion says.

Along with legal requirements on manufacturing, U.S. pharmacists and wholesalers must be licensed or authorized in the states where they operate, and limits on how drugs can be distributed lessen the likelihood that counterfeit or poor-quality drugs will turn up. It is because of such safeguards that the process of getting drugs onto U.S. pharmacy shelves is commonly referred to as a "closed" distribution system.

Counterfeit drugs—phony replicas of pharmaceuticals—can surface anywhere. Historically, they have been more common in foreign countries than in the United States. And while the Internet has given customers the convenience of buying drugs from the privacy of their own homes, it is also opened up windows for crooks to crawl through.

In an investigation that ended in the indictment of seven people and five companies in the spring of 2002, undercover agents in the Manhattan District Attorney's Office in New York bought more than 25,000 counterfeit Viagra pills. They pretended to sell the impotence pills and uncovered four supply streams from China and India.

Some of the little blue pills arrived in the mail stuffed inside a teddy bear and stereo speakers. The exporters used a machine to punch the pills with Pfizer's logo, and intermediaries sold the pills over the Internet to brokers and consumers.

In this case, all the counterfeit pills tested had some of Viagra's active ingredient (sildenafil citrate) with varying potency, according to Barbara Thompson, a spokeswoman for the Manhattan District Attorney's Office. With fake drugs, "You could be getting some of an active ingredient or you could be getting nothing at all," she says.

That is what happened with a batch of Viagra worth $150,000 that HALT seized from Los Angeles gift shops. "It looked perfect," says Hancz. "But there was nothing there—just lactose, dye, and other filling agents."

LIMITS ON REIMPORTATION

The FD&C Act also states that prescription drugs made in the United States and exported to a foreign country can only be reimported by the drug's original manufacturer. Even when original manufacturers reimport drugs, the drugs must be real, properly handled, and relabeled for sale in the United States if necessary.

Buying Prescription Drugs

The Medicine Equity and Drug Safety Act (MEDS), enacted in 2000, would have allowed prescription drugs manufactured in the United States and exported to certain foreign countries to be reimported from those countries for sale to American consumers. Supporters of the bill hoped that lower drug pricing in other countries would be passed along to consumers. But, former U.S. Department of Health and Human Services (HHS) secretary Tommy G. Thompson responded by saying that, while he believed strongly in access to affordable drugs, he could not implement the act because it would sacrifice public safety by opening up the closed distribution system in the United States.

Though the law was enacted in 2000, before the bill can take effect, one provision requires that the HHS secretary determine whether adequate safety could be maintained and whether costs could be reduced significantly. Both Thompson and his predecessor, Donna Shalala, concluded that these conditions could not be guaranteed.

"Once an FDA-approved prescription drug is exported for sale in another country, it is no longer subject to U.S. requirements and it can no longer be monitored by U.S. regulators," Thompson wrote in a letter to Sen. James Jeffords, Ind-Vt., one of the bill's sponsors. "In addition, it may not have the U.S.-approved labeling. Instead, it may have labeling for the country to which it is exported."

GUIDANCE ON PERSONAL USE

Although importing unapproved prescription drugs is illegal, the FDA's guidance on importing prescription drugs for personal use recognizes that there may be circumstances in which the FDA can exercise discretion to not take action against the illegal importation.

The personal use guidance was first adopted in 1954, and it was modified in 1988 in response to concerns that certain acquired immunodeficiency syndrome (AIDS) treatments were not available in the United States. The guidance allows individuals with serious conditions, such as a rare form of cancer, to get treatments that are legally available in foreign countries but are not approved in the United States.

The current policy is not a law or a regulation, but serves as guidance for FDA personnel. The importation of certain unapproved prescription medications for personal use may be allowed in some circumstances if all of these factors apply:

- If the intended use is for a serious condition for which effective treatment may not be available domestically
- If the product is not considered to represent an unreasonable risk
- If the individual seeking to import the drug affirms in writing that it is for the patient's own use and provides the name and address of the U.S.-licensed doctor responsible for her or his treatment with the drug

or provides evidence that the drug is for continuation of a treatment begun in a foreign country

- If the product is for personal use and is a three-month supply or less and not for resale, since larger amounts would lend themselves to commercialization
- If there is no known commercialization or promotion to U.S. residents by those involved in distribution of the product

That means if you buy your high blood pressure or other medication from a foreign country because it Is cheaper—even though a drug with the same name is approved for sale in the United States—generally the drug will be considered unapproved and the FDA's personal use guidance will not apply. The U.S. Drug Enforcement Administration (DEA) has additional requirements for controlled drugs.

THE SAME GOES FOR CANADA

Neena Quirion, director of the Maine Council of Senior Citizens in Augusta, has organized bus trips to Canada for her members and estimates that 25 seniors collectively saved about $19,000 on an overnight trip. "Paying for drugs is a real hardship for so many people," she says. "One lady takes about 15 different medications."

Quirion says they have obtained prescriptions from a doctor who is licensed to practice medicine in both Maine and Canada and who performs a physical examination on each person before writing prescriptions. "Our feeling is that the quality of the drugs is the same," she says. "Everything's very regulated in Canada."

Greg Thompson, Pharm.D., a pharmacy professor at the University of Southern California, agrees. "Getting drugs from Canada under the doctor's orders is different than getting drugs from Mexico on your own," he says. "Regulations in Mexico aren't as strict."

But even if you obtain drugs from a place or in a manner that you consider to be safe, according to the FDA, you are almost always obtaining unapproved drugs. "The law applies evenly to all countries outside of FDA's jurisdiction," says Thomas McGinnis, Pharm.D., director of pharmacy affairs in the FDA's Office of Policy and Planning (OPP).

So, what about the belief often mentioned in the media that drugs sold in Canada are exactly the same as drugs sold in the United States—made in the exact same manufacturing plants? Some may be, and some may not. For example, drugs sold and distributed in Canada by Eli Lilly Canada come from the company's manufacturing facilities throughout the world—the United States, Europe, Asia, and South America.

Buying Prescription Drugs

Manufacturing facilities that make drugs for Canadians have been approved and registered by Health Canada's Health Products and Food Branch, the federal agency responsible for regulating drugs sold in Canada. This agency is responsible for approving the product labeling, which must be made available in Canada's two official languages, English and French.

But the FDA does not have authority to approve drugs sold in Canada. And if a Canadian company is selling drugs only for export to the United States, and not to Canadian citizens, Health Canada may not regulate the drugs or the company at all. Drugs coming to the United States from Canada may be coming from some other country and simply passing through Canada. The drugs could also be counterfeit, contaminated, or subpotent, among other things,

Experts at the FDA say it would be hard for you to know whether drugs sold outside of the United States meet FDA standards and have been manufactured in a plant listed on an FDA-approved new drug application. "Even if you did know," McCallion says, "existing law requires you to prove it. The burden is on the importer to prove that the drug meets legal requirements—that includes having an FDA-approved label in English." The fact also remains that a drug made in this country can only be reimported back into this country by the original manufacturer, he adds.

Barbara Wells, executive director of the National Association of Pharmacy Regulatory Authorities (NAPRA) in Ontario, Canada, says that the practice of U.S. residents filling prescriptions in Canada is an issue that her organization is concerned about. "Our members do not feel that Canadian pharmacists should be breaking laws of jurisdictions in which their patients reside," she says.

INTERNET CHALLENGES

When it comes to buying prescription drugs online, Canada is dealing with some of the same regulatory challenges that occur in the United States.

The NAPRA has signed an agreement with the National Association of Boards of Pharmacy (NABP) in the United States and has developed a program in Canada modeled after the NABP's Verified Internet Pharmacy Practice Sites (VIPPS), a voluntary certification program.

A VIPPS® seal of approval indicates that an online pharmacy complies with state licensing and inspection requirements, along with other VIPPS criteria dealing with such areas as patient rights to privacy and authentication of orders.

The NABP developed the service in 1999 after consumers complained to state pharmacy boards about rogue sites posing as legitimate pharmacies. Sites can pop up overnight and disappear just as quickly, and there is little the U.S. government can do if you get swindled. The FDA suggests you steer clear of foreign websites. If you buy medicine from a domestic site, remember that the legitimate ones require a valid prescription.

The FDA sends warning letters over the Internet to suspicious sites. About 30 percent of Internet sites that receive the FDA's letters stop their illegal activity. The FDA also sends copies of the letters to the home governments of the websites when the locations can be identified.

"We seek out the cooperation of foreign governments because we have limited reach in a foreign land," says David Horowitz, director of the Office of Compliance (OC) for the FDA's Center for Drug Evaluation and Research (CDER). "That is one of the major challenges of Internet enforcement."

HOW THE FDA WORKS WITH U.S. CUSTOMS AND BORDER PROTECTION

The exact amount of imported drugs that come into the United States is hard to track, and the high volume makes it impossible to examine them all. In one pilot program, the FDA and the CBP examined 1,908 packages of drug products from 19 countries that came through a mail facility in Carson, Calif., during a 5-week period.

The FDA estimates that a total of 16,500 packages could have been set aside if there were enough resources to handle them. Of the 1,908 packages, 721 were detained, and the addressees were notified that the products appeared to violate the FD&C Act.

The FDA's enforcement efforts focus on drugs for commercial use, fraudulent drugs, and products that pose an unreasonable health risk.

If a bag or package arouses suspicion, customs will set it aside and contact the nearest office of the FDA or the DEA for advice on whether to release or detain the drug product. Even though your bag may not be checked, it is against the law not to properly declare imported medications to customs. Failure to declare products could result in penalties. Possession of certain medications without a prescription from a licensed physician may violate federal, state, and local laws.

Prescription drugs should be stored in their original containers, and you should have a copy of your doctor's prescription or letter of instruction. If a drug is detained, the FDA is required by law to send you a written notice asking whether you can show that the product meets legal requirements. If you cannot, the drug could be destroyed or returned to the sender.

POTENTIAL HEALTH RISKS WITH IMPORTED DRUGS
Quality Assurance Concerns

Medications that have not been approved for sale in the United States may not have been manufactured under quality assurance procedures designed to produce a safe and effective product.

Counterfeit Potential

Some imported medications—even those that bear the name of a United States—approved product—may, in fact, be counterfeit versions that are unsafe or even completely ineffective.

Buying Prescription Drugs

Presence of Untested Substances

Imported medications and their ingredients, although legal in foreign countries, may not have been evaluated for safety and effectiveness in the United States. These products may be addictive or contain other dangerous substances.

Risks of Unsupervised Use

Some medications, whether imported or not, are unsafe when taken without adequate medical supervision. You may need a medical evaluation to ensure that the medication is appropriate for you and your condition. Or, you may require medical checkups to make sure that you are taking the drug properly, it is working for you, and that you are not having unexpected or life-threatening side effects.

Labeling and Language Issues

The medication's label, including instructions for use and possible side effects, may be in a language you do not understand or may make medical claims and suggest specific uses that have not been adequately evaluated for safety and effectiveness.

Lack of Information

An imported medication may lack information that would permit you to be promptly and correctly treated for a dangerous side effect caused by the drug.

Chapter 37 | Generic Drugs

Chapter Contents

Section 37.1 | Facts about Generic Drugs

This section includes text excerpted from "Generic Drug Facts," U.S. Food and Drug Administration (FDA), June 1, 2018.

A generic drug is a medication created to be the same as an existing approved brand-name drug in dosage form, safety, strength, route of administration, quality, and performance characteristics.

GENERIC MEDICINES WORK THE SAME AS BRAND-NAME MEDICINES

A generic medicine works in the same way and provides the same clinical benefit as its brand-name version. This standard applies to all U.S. Food and Drug Administration (FDA)-approved generic medicines. A generic medicine is the same as a brand-name medicine in dosage, safety, effectiveness, strength, stability, and quality, as well as in the way it is taken and should be used.

The FDA's Generic Drugs Program conducts a rigorous review to make sure generic medicines meet these requirements. In addition, FDA conducts 3,500 inspections of manufacturing plants a year, ensuring compliance with the agency's regulations on good manufacturing practices.

The staff at the FDA also continually monitor drug products to make certain medicines at all levels of the supply chain, from active pharmaceutical ingredients (API) to products being sold to consumers, are safe, effective, and high quality. In the event of reports of negative patient side effects or other reactions, the FDA investigates and, when appropriate, may require changes in how a medicine (both brand-name and generic versions) is used or manufactured.

GENERIC DRUGS MUST MEET HIGH STANDARDS TO RECEIVE FDA'S APPROVAL

The FDA requires drug companies to demonstrate that the generic medicine can be effectively substituted and provide the same clinical benefit as the brand-name medicine that it copies. The abbreviated new drug application (ANDA) submitted by drug companies must show the generic medicine is the same as the brand-name version in the following ways:

- The active ingredient in the generic medicine is the same as in the brand-name drug/innovator drug.
- The generic medicine has the same strength, use indications, form (such as a tablet or an injectable), and route of administration (such as oral or topical).
- The inactive ingredients of the generic medicine are acceptable.
- The generic medicine is manufactured under the same strict standards as the brand-name medicine.

- The container in which the medicine will be shipped and sold is appropriate, and the label is the same as the brand-name medicine's label.

APPROVED GENERIC MEDICINES ARE GENERALLY ONLY SOLD AFTER PATENTS AND EXCLUSIVITIES PROTECTING THE BRAND-NAME VERSION END

Patents and exclusivities are forms of protection for drug makers that may affect how and when a generic drug is approved and can be sold. New brand-name drugs are usually protected by patents (issued by the U.S. Patent and Trademark Office (USPTO)) that prohibit others from selling generic versions of the same drug. Periods of marketing exclusivity for brand-name drugs can also impact the approval of generic drugs.

GENERIC MEDICINES COST LESS THAN BRAND-NAME MEDICINES

Generic medicines tend to cost less than their brand-name counterparts because they do not have to repeat animal and clinical (human) studies that were required of the brand-name medicines to demonstrate safety and effectiveness. In addition, multiple applications for generic drugs are often approved to market a single product; this creates competition in the marketplace, typically resulting in lower prices.

The reduction in upfront research costs means that, although generic medicines have the same therapeutic effect as their branded counterparts, they are typically sold at substantially lower costs. When multiple generic companies market a single approved product, market competition typically results in prices about 85 percent less than the brand-name. According to the Intercontinental Medical Statistics (IMS) Health Institute, generic drugs saved the U.S. healthcare system $1.67 trillion from 2007 to 2016.

Section 37.2 | FAQs about Generic Drugs

This section includes text excerpted from "Generic Drugs: Questions and Answers," U.S. Food and Drug Administration (FDA), June 1, 2018.

WHAT ARE GENERIC DRUGS?

A generic drug is a medication created to be the same as an already marketed brand-name drug in dosage form, safety, strength, route of administration, quality, performance characteristics, and intended use. These similarities help to demonstrate bioequivalence, which means that a generic medicine works in the same way and provides the same clinical benefit as its brand-name version. In other words, you can take a generic medicine as an equal substitute for its brand-name counterpart.

DO GENERIC MEDICINES WORK THE SAME AS BRAND-NAME MEDICINES?

Yes. Any generic medicine modeled after a brand-name medicine must perform the same in the body as the brand-name medicine. This standard applies to all generic medicines. A generic medicine is the same as a brand-name medicine in dosage, safety, effectiveness, strength, stability, and quality, as well as in the way it is taken and the way it should be used. Generic medicines use the same active ingredients as brand-name medicines and work the same way, so they have the same risks and benefits as the brand-name medicines. The U.S. Food and Drug Administration's (FDA) Generic Drugs Program conducts a rigorous review to make certain generic medicines meet these standards, in addition to conducting 3,500 inspections of manufacturing plants a year and monitoring drug safety after the generic medicine has been approved and brought to market.

It is important to note that there will always be a slight, but not medically important, level of natural variability—just as there is for one batch of brand-name medicine compared with the next batch of brand-name products. This variability can and does occur during manufacturing, for both brand-name and generic medicines. When a medicine, generic or brand-name, is mass produced, very small variations in purity, size, strength, and other parameters are permitted. FDA limits how much variability is acceptable.

For example, in a very large research study comparing generics with brand-name medicines, it was found that there were very small differences (approximately 3.5%) in absorption into the body between the generic and the brand-name medicines. Some generics were absorbed slightly more, some slightly less. This amount of difference is expected and acceptable, whether for one batch of brand-name medicine tested against another batch of the same brand, or for a generic tested against a brand-name medicine. As a rule, the difference for the generic-to-brand comparison was about the same as the brand-to-brand comparison.

WHY DO BRAND-NAME DRUGS LOOK DIFFERENT FROM THEIR GENERIC VERSIONS?

Trademark laws in the United States do not allow a generic drug or medicine to look exactly similar other drugs already on the market. Generic medicines and brand-name medicines share the same active ingredient, but other characteristics, such as colors and flavorings, that do not affect the performance, safety, or effectiveness of the generic medicine, may be different.

WHY DO GENERIC MEDICINES COST LESS THAN BRAND-NAME MEDICINES?

Generic drugs or medicines become available only after a rigorous review by the FDA and after a set period of time that the brand-name version has been on the market exclusively. This is because new drugs, similar to other new products, are usually protected by patents that prohibit others from making and selling copies of the same drug. The patent protects the company's investment in the drug's development by giving the company the sole right to sell the drug while the patent is in effect. Because it takes such a long time to bring a new drug to market, this period of exclusivity allows drug companies to recoup the costs associated with bringing a new drug to market. The FDA also grants certain periods of marketing exclusivity to brand-name drugs that can prohibit the approval of generic drugs. Once these patents and marketing exclusivities expire (or if the patents are success-fully challenged by the generic drug company), the generic drug can be approved.

Generic drugs also tend to cost less than their brand-name counterparts because generic drug applicants do not have to repeat animal and clinical (human) studies that were required of the brand-name medicines to demon-strate safety and effectiveness. This is why the application is called an "abbrevi-ated new drug application" (ANDA). This, together with competition between the brand-name drug and multiple generic drugs, is a large part of the reason generic medicines cost much less.

In fact, multiple generic companies are often approved to market a single product; this creates competition in the marketplace, typically resulting in lower prices.

The reduction in upfront research costs means that, although generic medi-cines have the same therapeutic effect as their branded counterparts, they are typ-ically sold at substantial discounts, an estimated 80 to 85 percent less, compared with the price of the brand-name medicine. According to the Intercontinental Medical Statistics (IMS) Health Institute, generic drugs saved the U.S. healthcare system $1.67 trillion from 2007 to 2016.

WHAT STANDARDS MUST GENERIC MEDICINES MEET TO RECEIVE U.S. FOOD AND DRUG ADMINISTRATION APPROVAL?

Drug companies can submit an abbreviated new drug application (ANDA) for approval to market a generic drug that is the same as (or bioequivalent to) the brand-name version. The FDA's Office of Generic Drugs (OGD) reviews the application to make certain drug companies have demonstrated that the generic medicine can be substituted for the brand-name medicine that it copies.

An ANDA must show the generic medicine is equivalent to the brand in the following ways:

- The active ingredient is the same as that of the brand-name drug/ innovator drug.

- An active ingredient in a medicine is the component that makes it pharmaceutically active—effective against the illness or condition it is treating.
- Generic drug companies must provide evidence that shows that their active ingredient is the same as that of the brand-name medicine they copy, and the FDA must review that evidence.
- The generic medicine is the same strength.
- The medicine is the same type of product (such as a tablet or an injectable).
- The medicine has the same route of administration (such as oral or topical).
- It has the same use indications.
- The inactive ingredients of the medicine are acceptable.
  - Some differences, which must be shown to have no effect on how the medicine functions, are allowed between the generic and the brand-name version.
  - Generic drug companies must submit evidence that all the ingredients used in their products are acceptable, and the FDA must review that evidence.
- It lasts for at least the same amount of time.
  - Most medicines break down, or deteriorate over time.
  - Generic drug companies must do months-long "stability tests" to show that their versions last for at least the same amount of time as the brand-name.
- It is manufactured under the same strict standards as the brand-name medicine.
  - It meets the same batch requirements for identity, strength, purity, and quality.
  - The manufacturer is capable of making the medicine correctly and consistently.
  - Generic drug manufacturers must explain how they intend to manufacture the medicine and must provide evidence that each step of the manufacturing process will produce the same result each time. FDA scientists review those procedures, and FDA inspectors go to the generic drug manufacturer's facility to verify that the manufacturer is capable of making the medicine consistently and to check that the information the manufacturer has submitted to the FDA is accurate.
  - Often, different companies are involved (such as one company manufacturing the active ingredient and another company manufacturing the finished medicine). Generic drug manufacturers

must produce batches of the medicine they want to market and provide information about the manufacturing of those batches for the FDA to review.

- The container in which the medicine will be shipped and sold is appropriate.
- The label is the same as the brand-name medicine's label.
  - The drug information label for the generic medicine should be the same as the brand-name label. One exception is if the brand-name drug is approved for more than one use and that use is protected by patents or exclusivities. A generic medicine can omit the protected use from its labeling and only be approved for a use that is not protected by patents or exclusivities, so long as that removal does not take away information needed for safe use. Labels for generic medicines can also contain certain changes when the drug is manufactured by a different company, such as a different lot number or company name.
- Relevant patents or exclusivities are addressed.
  - As an incentive to develop new medicines, drug companies are awarded patents and exclusivities that may delay FDA approval of applications for generic medicines. The FDA must comply with the delays in approval that the patents and exclusivities impose.

The ANDA process does not, however, require the drug applicant to repeat costly animal and clinical research on ingredients or dosage forms already approved for safety and effectiveness. This allows generic medicines to be brought to market more quickly and at lower cost, allowing for increased access to medications by the public.

IS A GENERIC VERSION OF YOUR BRAND-NAME MEDICINE AVAILABLE?

In addition to asking your local pharmacist for assistance, there are three ways to find out if there is a generic version of your brand-name medicine available:

- Use Drugs@FDA, a catalog of FDA-approved drug products, including their drug labeling.
- Search for generic equivalents by using the online version of the "Orange Book."
  - First, search by proprietary or "brand" name.
  - Second, search again by the active ingredient name.
  - If other manufacturers are listed besides the brand-name manufacturer in result for searches by the "active ingredient," they are the generic product manufacturers.
- For very recent approvals, consult the First Generics List.

Generic Drugs

If you are unable to locate a generic version of your brand-name medicine, it may be that the brand-name medicine is still within the period of time when it has exclusive rights to the marketplace, to allow drug companies to recoup their costs for the initial research and marketing of the brand-name or innovator drug. It is only after both patent and other periods of exclusivity are resolved that the FDA can approve generic versions of the medicine.

DOES THE FDA MONITOR SIDE EFFECTS OR SAFETY ISSUES WITH GENERIC MEDICINES?

Yes. After the FDA approves any medicine, including generics, it continues to examine the medicine's safety. The FDA takes several actions to ensure the safety and quality before and after a new or generic medicine is marketed.

The staff at the FDA continually monitors drug products to make certain medicines at all levels of the supply chain, from active pharmaceutical ingredients (APIs) to products being sold to consumers, are safe, effective, and high quality.

The FDA also monitors and investigates reports of negative patient side effects or other reactions. The investigations may lead to changes in how a product (brand-name and generic counterparts) is used or manufactured.

Due to limited resources, the FDA is unable to perform independent clinical studies, and the agency lacks the regulatory authority to require the generic industry to conduct such studies. The FDA will, however, continue to investigate these reports to ensure that it has all the facts about these possible treatment failures and will make recommendations to healthcare professionals and the public if the need arises. Currently, to better understand what may cause problems with certain formulations if, in fact, they are linked to specific generic products, the FDA is encouraging the generic industry to investigate whether, and under what circumstances, such problems occur.

WHERE CAN YOU FIND MORE INFORMATION ABOUT GENERIC MEDICINES?

Contact your doctor, pharmacist, or other healthcare provider for information on generic medicines. For more information, you can also:
- Visit the FDA's Generic Drugs Program (www.fda.gov/drugs/buying-using-medicine-safely/generic-drugs)
- Call toll-free: 888-INFO-FDA (888-463-6332)

Chapter 38 | Other Types of Drugs

Chapter Contents

Section 38.1 | Biosimilars

This section includes text excerpted from "Biosimilars: More Treatment Choices and Innovation," U.S. Food and Drug Administration (FDA), October 23, 2017.

Biosimilar products provide more treatment options to patients, potentially lowering treatment costs and increasing access to lifesaving medications.

The U.S. Food and Drug Administration (FDA) has approved biosimilar products to treat conditions such as cancer, Crohn disease and colitis, irritable bowel syndrome (IBS), rheumatoid arthritis (RA), psoriasis, and more.

But, what are biosimilars? To answer this question, it helps to first know what biological products (biologics) are.

BIOSIMILARS: MEDICATIONS FROM LIVING ORGANISMS

Biologics are medicines that generally come from living organisms, which can include humans, animals and microorganisms, such as yeast and bacteria.

That makes biologics different from conventional medications, which are generally made from chemicals, or are chemically synthesized. Generally, it is relatively easy to define the structure of a conventional medicine.

Unlike conventional medications, biologics cannot be made by following a chemical "recipe." Because biologics come from living organisms, they are variable in nature and their structures are generally more complex and not as easy to define and characterize. In turn, developing biologics generally is a far more difficult process than manufacturing conventional drugs.

A biosimilar is a biologic that is highly similar to another biologic that is already approved by the FDA (known as the "reference product"). A biosimilar is not similar to a generic drug. It is not an exact duplicate of the reference product. Biosimilars have allowable differences. Any differences between the proposed biosimilar product and reference product are carefully evaluated by the FDA to ensure the biosimilar meets the FDA's high approval standards.

BIOSIMILARS ARE SAFE AND EFFECTIVE

The FDA rigorously and thoroughly evaluates a biologic's safety and effectiveness before granting it approval.

Because the structure of a biologic and the process used to make it are typically complex, developing a biosimilar generally is not as easy as producing a generic drug, which is a copy of a brand name, conventional drug.

Before approving a biosimilar, FDA experts must conclude, among other things, that there are no clinically meaningful differences between the biosimilar and its reference product—the already approved biologic—in terms of safety, purity, and potency. This thorough evaluation helps to ensure that all biosimilar products are safe and effective and meet the agency's high standards for approval.

A biosimilar must have the same strength, dosage form, and route of administration (injection in the arm, for example) as the reference product. It also must be manufactured following Current Good Manufacturing Practices, which covers manufacturing, facilities, and controls for the manufacturing, processing, packaging, or holding of a drug product. This helps to prevent manufacturing mistakes or unacceptable impurities and ensures product quality.

Patients can rest assured that they will be able to rely upon the safety and effectiveness of an FDA-approved biosimilar, just as they can rely on the safety and effectiveness of the reference product that the biosimilar was compared to.

As in the case of other biologics, biosimilars generally must be prescribed by a doctor.

Biologics are among the fastest growing segments of the prescription product market. The FDA approval of additional biosimilars will help stimulate competition. Patients will have more treatment options and potentially less expensive alternatives to approved products.

Section 38.2 | Homeopathic Products

This section includes text excerpted from "Homeopathic Products," U.S. Food and Drug Administration (FDA), October 24, 2019.

WHAT IS HOMEOPATHY?

Homeopathy is an alternative medical practice that was developed in the late 1700s. Homeopathy is generally based on two main principles:
- That a substance that causes symptoms in a healthy person can be used in diluted form to treat symptoms and illnesses, a principle known as "like-cures-like"
- The more diluted the substance, the more potent it is, which is known as the "law of infinitesimals"

Historically, homeopathic products have been identified through "provings," in which substances are administered to healthy volunteers in concentrations that cause symptoms. Symptoms experienced by volunteers are recorded to indicate possible therapeutic uses for the substances. In other words, if a substance causes a particular symptom, individuals experiencing that symptom would be treated with a diluted solution made from that substance.

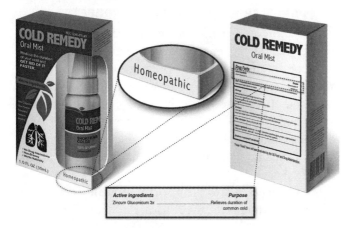

Figure 38.1. Homeopathic Products

WHAT ARE HOMEOPATHIC PRODUCTS AND HOW CAN YOU TELL YOU ARE TAKING ONE?

There are no U.S. Food and Drug Administration (FDA)-approved products labeled as homeopathic; this means that any product labeled as homeopathic is being marketed in the U.S. without FDA evaluation for safety or effectiveness. These products are often marketed as natural, safe, and effective alternatives to approved prescription and nonprescription products, and are sold online and in major retail stores.

Products labeled as homeopathic can contain a wide range of substances, including ingredients derived from plants, healthy or diseased animal or human sources, minerals, and chemicals.

Products labeled as homeopathic generally include:

- The word "Homeopathic"
- The ingredients listed in terms of dilution, e.g., 1X, 6X, 2C

IS THE FDA CONCERNED ABOUT THE SAFETY OF HOMEOPATHIC PRODUCTS?

While products labeled as homeopathic are generally labeled as highly diluted, some of these products have been found to contain measurable amounts of active ingredients, and therefore, could cause significant patient harm. Additionally, the FDA has tested products that were improperly manufactured, which can cause incorrect dilutions and increase the potential for contamination. Further, some products labeled as homeopathic are marketed to treat serious diseases or conditions. The FDA alerts consumers and pet owners not to use products manufactured by King Bio, including Dr. King's homeopathic-labeled drug and pet products.

WHAT SHOULD CONSUMERS KNOW ABOUT HOMEOPATHIC PRODUCTS?

Products labeled as homeopathic and marketed in the U.S. have not been reviewed by the FDA for safety and effectiveness to diagnose, treat, cure, prevent or mitigate any diseases or conditions. The FDA's evidence-based drug reviews play an essential role in ensuring that drugs are made with quality manufacturing processes, and are safe and effective for their intended uses. Products that have not been evaluated for safety and effectiveness may harm consumers who choose to treat serious diseases or conditions with such products, and consumers may be foregoing treatment with a medical product that has been scientifically proven to be safe and effective.

The FDA recommends consumers talk to their doctor or healthcare professional about safe and effective treatments for their disease or condition.

HOW ARE HOMEOPATHIC PRODUCTS REGULATED?

Under the Federal Food, Drug, and Cosmetic Act (FFDCA), homeopathic products are subject to the same requirements related to approval, adulteration and misbranding as other drug products. There are currently no homeopathic products approved by the FDA.

In 1988, the FDA issued a Compliance Policy Guide (CPG) 400.400, entitled "Conditions Under Which Homeopathic Drugs May be Marketed," which described the agency's enforcement policy. On October 24, 2019, the FDA withdrew CPG 400.400 because it is inconsistent with their risk-based approach to regulatory and enforcement action. The FDA also issued a revised draft guidance: *Drug Products Labeled as Homeopathic,* for public comment. Since homeopathic drug products have not been approved by the FDA for any use, they may not meet modern standards for safety, effectiveness, and quality. This revised draft guidance proposes a comprehensive, risk-based enforcement approach to homeopathic products marketed without FDA approval.

The FDA's proposed approach prioritizes regulatory and enforcement actions involving unapproved homeopathic products that pose the greatest risk to patients. Many homeopathic products will likely fall outside the risk-based categories described in the revised draft guidance.

IS THE FDA GOING TO REMOVE HOMEOPATHIC PRODUCTS FROM THE MARKET?

The FDA's top concern is patient safety. When the draft guidance is finalized, it will specify the categories of products the agency intends to prioritize for enforcement. In the interim, before the draft guidance is finalized, the FDA intends to apply its general approach to prioritizing risk-based regulatory and enforcement action.

Section 38.3 | Orphan Products

This section includes text excerpted from "Orphan Products: Hope for People with Rare Diseases," U.S. Food and Drug Administration (FDA), March 1, 2018.

Jumping Frenchmen of Maine sounds similar to an uproarious, modern-day stage show or even a new-wave rock group. But, it is neither. It is the name of an unusual disorder that causes an extreme startle reaction to unexpected noises or sights. Though little is known about Jumping Frenchmen of Maine, the disorder and more than 6,000 other rare or "orphan" diseases are receiving increasing attention from the government, patient groups, and the pharmaceutical industry.

An orphan disease is defined as "a condition that affects fewer than 200,000 people nationwide." This includes diseases as familiar as cystic fibrosis (CF), Lou Gehrig disease, and Tourette syndrome (TS), and as unfamiliar as Hamburger disease, Job syndrome, and acromegaly, or "gigantism." Some diseases have patient populations of fewer than a 100. Collectively, however, they affect as many as 25 million Americans, according to the National Institutes of Health (NIH), and that makes the diseases and—finding treatments for them—a serious public-health concern.

MOST INHERIT ORPHAN DISEASES

New rare diseases are discovered every year. Most are inherited and caused by alterations or defects in genes (mutations). Others can be acquired as a result of environmental and toxic conditions. Genes are pieces of deoxyribonucleic acid (DNA), part of the code that determines the traits and individual characteristics of all living things. Each human cell contains around 30,000 genes. Besides influencing features such as eye and hair color, genes also can play a role in the development of diseases and in their transmission from parent to child.

As disparate as rare diseases are, patients share many common frustrations. For example, for one-third of people with a rare disease, getting an accurate diagnosis can take one to five years. And people often are so isolated that they may never know anyone else with the same disease. Patients often must travel long distances to visit the few doctors knowledgeable about their illnesses, and the costs involved with diagnosis, treatment, and other related expenses can be exorbitant.

MANAGING RARE DISEASES

Many rare diseases or conditions can be difficult to diagnose and manage because in their early stages, symptoms may be absent or masked, misunderstood, or confused with other diseases.

For example, adrenomyeloneuropathy (AMN), one of a group of genetically determined progressive disorders known as "leukodystrophies" that affect the brain, spinal cord, and peripheral nerves, is often misdiagnosed as multiple sclerosis (MS), according to the United Leukodystrophy Foundation. Since diagnosis of neurological conditions relies on subtle and circumstantial evidence, even the most experienced clinicians may have difficulty distinguishing between the two. For rare-disease patients, there may be no cures, but treatments of the symptoms can help. Participating in a clinical trial may be a way to receive the most advanced care for some diseases. People who experience unexplained symptoms, recurrent infections, and pain that have gone undiagnosed for a long period of time might want to visit a referral center that is experienced in diagnosing patients with rare diseases. Some rare diseases do not have clearly defined treatment guidelines and require the specific skills of an expert physician. Be sure to go to a hospital that is familiar with treating people with multiple problems.

ADOPTING THE "ORPHANS"

Before the passage of rare-disease laws in the United States, patients diagnosed with a rare disease were denied access to effective medicines because prescription drug manufacturers rarely could make a profit from marketing drugs to such small groups. Consequently, the prescription-drug industry did not adequately fund research for orphan product development. Other potential sources, such as research hospitals and universities, also lacked the capital and business expertise to develop treatments for small patient groups. Despite the urgent health need for these medicines, they came to be known as "orphans" because companies were not interested in adopting them.

This changed in 1983 when Congress passed the Orphan Drug Act (ODA). The ODA created financial incentives for drug and biologics manufacturers, including tax credits for costs of clinical research, government grant funding, assistance for clinical research, and a seven-year period of exclusive marketing given to the first sponsor of an orphan-designated product who obtains market approval from the U.S. Food and Drug Administration (FDA) for the same indication. At the same time, federal programs at the FDA and the NIH began encouraging product development, as well as clinical research for products targeting rare diseases.

Since 1983, the ODA has resulted in the development of more than 250 orphan drugs, which are now available to treat a potential patient population of more than 13 million Americans. In contrast, the decade before 1983 saw fewer than 10 such products developed without government assistance. As a result of the ODA, treatments are available to people with rare diseases who once had no hope for survival.

Other Types of Drugs

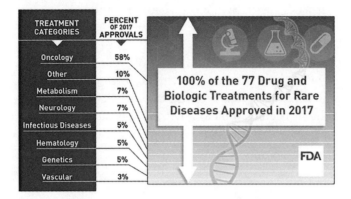

Figure 38.2. Drug and Biologic Treatment for Rare Diseases: Approval Status *(Source: "Taking New Steps to Meet the Challenges of Rare Diseases—FDA Marks the 11th Rare Disease Day," U.S. Food and Drug Administration (FDA))*

"A lot of people are affected," says Marlene E. Haffner, M.D., M.P.H., director of the FDA's Office of Orphan Products Development (OOPD). "That makes it a major public-health impact, and in time, we are going to see even more rare diseases requiring treatment."

Despite the success of the ODA, however, rare-disease advocacy groups argue that the plight of people with orphan diseases deserves even more attention.

PATIENT SUPPORT GROUPS

Rare diseases affect so few people that information about them may be difficult to find, making the situation more traumatic and stressful. Before Congress enacted the ODA, families coping with a rare disease usually struggled alone. Support could only be found through telephone calls to other families suffering with similar diseases, and only if the names were provided by doctors.

Support groups such as the National Organization for Rare Disorders (NORD) have worked aggressively for over two decades now to draw attention to people with rare diseases, and especially to the lack of treatment options. Paramount in NORD's ongoing cause are efforts to promote legislation, such as ODA, that encourages further research and continuing development of products that are necessary—and often life-saving—and to provide easier access to such treatments.

The role of the support group is evolving. Recent trends at the FDA and the NIH in encouraging scientists to become involved with patient support groups has brought research even farther along.

New web-based support groups continue to proliferate. Not only are people receiving comfort from others with the same conditions, but they are learning from each other's experiences as well. By the late 1990s, most nonprofit organizations had websites where people could ask questions and get immediate responses.

Nevertheless, people diagnosed with a rare disease often are vulnerable to misguided assistance. While Stephen C. Groft, Pharm.D., director of the NIH's Office of Rare Diseases, encourages people to use the Internet to find information, he also warns that it is dangerous to rely solely on the computer for medical advice.

Section 38.4 | Precision Medicine

This section contains text excerpted from the following sources: Text in this section begins with excerpts from "Precision Medicine," U.S. Food and Drug Administration (FDA), September 27, 2018; Text under the heading "Some Potential Benefits of Precision Medicine" is excerpted from "What Are Some Potential Benefits of Precision Medicine and the Precision Medicine Initiative?" Genetics Home Reference (GHR), National Institutes of Health (NIH), November 26, 2019.

Most medical treatments are designed for the "average patient" as a one-size-fits-all-approach, which may be successful for some patients, but not for others. Precision medicine, sometimes known as "personalized medicine" is an innovative approach to tailoring disease prevention and treatment that takes into account differences in people's genes, environments, and lifestyles. The goal of precision medicine is to target the right treatments to the right patients at the right time.

Advances in precision medicine have already led to powerful new discoveries and the U.S. Food and Drug Administration (FDA)-approved treatments that are tailored to specific characteristics of individuals, such as a person's genetic makeup, or the genetic profile of an individual's tumor. Patients with a variety of cancers routinely undergo molecular testing as part of patient care, enabling physicians to select treatments that improve chances of survival and reduce exposure to adverse effects.

NEXT GENERATION SEQUENCING TESTS

Precision care will only be as good as the tests that guide diagnosis and treatment. Next Generation Sequencing (NGS) tests are capable of rapidly identifying or 'sequencing' large sections of a person's genome and are important advances in the clinical applications of precision medicine. Patients, physicians and researchers can use these tests to find genetic variants that help them diagnose, treat, and understand more about human disease.

SOME POTENTIAL BENEFITS OF PRECISION MEDICINE

Precision medicine holds promise for improving many aspects of health and healthcare. Some of these benefits will be apparent soon, as the All of Us Research Program continues and new tools and approaches for managing data are developed. Other benefits will result from long-term research in precision medicine and may not be realized for years.

Potential benefits of the Precision Medicine Initiative include:

- New approaches for protecting research participants, particularly patients' privacy and the confidentiality of their data
- Design of new tools for building, analyzing, and sharing large sets of medical data
- Improvement of FDA oversight of tests, drugs, and other technologies to support innovation while ensuring that these products are safe and effective
- New partnerships of scientists in a wide range of specialties, as well as people from the patient advocacy community, universities, pharmaceutical companies, and others
- Opportunity for a million people to contribute to the advancement of scientific research

Potential long-term benefits of research in precision medicine include:

- Wider ability of doctors to use patients' genetic and other molecular information as part of routine medical care
- Improved ability to predict which treatments will work best for specific patients
- Better understanding of the underlying mechanisms by which various diseases occur
- Improved approaches to preventing, diagnosing, and treating a wide range of diseases
- Better integration of electronic health records (EHRs) in patient care, which will allow doctors and researchers to access medical data more easily

Chapter 39 | Taking Medications

Chapter Contents

Section 39.1 | Tips for Taking Medications

This section includes text excerpted from "Why You Need to Take Your Medications as Prescribed or Instructed," U.S. Food and Drug Administration (FDA), February 16, 2016. Reviewed December 2019.

TIPS TO HELP YOU TAKE YOUR MEDICINE

Taking your medicine as prescribed or medication adherence is important for controlling chronic conditions, treating temporary conditions, and overall long-term health and well-being. A personal connection with your healthcare provider or pharmacist is an important part of medication adherence. "Because your pharmacist is an expert in medications, they can help suggest how best to take your medications," says Kimberly DeFronzo, R.Ph., M.S., M.B.A., a Consumer Safety Officer in U.S. Food and Drug Administration's (FDA) Center for Drug Evaluation and Research (CDER). However, you play the most important part by taking all of your medications as directed.

Here are tips that may help:

- Take your medication at the same time every day.
- Tie taking your medications with a daily routine such as brushing your teeth or getting ready for bed. Before choosing mealtime for your routine, check if your medication should be taken on a full or empty stomach.
- Keep a "medicine calendar" with your pill bottles and note each time you take a dose.
- Use a pill container. Some types have sections for multiple doses at different times, such as morning, lunch, evening, and night.
- When using a pill container, refill it at the same time each week. For example, every Sunday morning after breakfast.
- Purchase timer caps for your pill bottles and set them to go off when your next dose is due. Some pillboxes also have timer functions.
- When traveling, be certain to bring enough of your medication, plus a few days extra, in case your return is delayed.
- If you are flying, keep your medications in your carry-on bag to avoid lost luggage. Temperatures inside the cargo hold could damage your medication.

Section 39.2 | **Know When Antibiotics Work**

This section includes text excerpted from "Be Antibiotics Aware: Smart Use, Best Care," Centers for Disease Control and Prevention (CDC), November 18, 2019.

Antibiotic resistance is one of the most urgent threats to the public's health. Antibiotic resistance occurs when bacteria develop the ability to defeat the drugs designed to kill them. Each year in the United States, at least 2 million people get infected with antibiotic-resistant bacteria, and at least 23,000 people die as a result.

Antibiotics save lives, but any time antibiotics are used, they can cause side effects and lead to antibiotic resistance. About 30 percent of antibiotics, or 47 million prescriptions, are prescribed unnecessarily in doctors' offices and emergency departments in the United States, which makes improving antibiotic prescribing and use a national priority.

Helping healthcare professionals improve the way they prescribe antibiotics, and improving the way we take antibiotics, helps keep us healthy now, helps fight antibiotic resistance, and ensures that these life-saving drugs will be available for future generations.

WHEN ANTIBIOTICS ARE NEEDED

Antibiotics are only needed for treating certain infections caused by bacteria. People rely on antibiotics to treat serious infections, such as pneumonia, and life-threatening conditions including sepsis, the body's extreme response to an infection. Effective antibiotics are also needed for people who are at high risk of developing infections. Some of those at high risk for infections include patients undergoing surgery, patients with end-stage kidney disease, or patients receiving cancer therapy (chemotherapy).

WHEN ANTIBIOTICS ARE NOT NEEDED

Antibiotics do not work on viruses, such as those that cause colds, flu, bronchitis, or runny noses, even if the mucus is thick, yellow, or green.

Antibiotics are only needed for treating infections caused by bacteria, but even some bacterial infections get better without antibiotics. Antibiotics are not needed for many sinus infections and some ear infections. Antibiotics save lives, and when a patient needs antibiotics, the benefits usually outweigh the risk of side effects and antibiotic resistance. When antibiotics are not needed, they will not help you, and the side effects could still cause harm. Common side effects of antibiotics can include:
- Rash
- Dizziness

Taking Medications

- Nausea
- Diarrhea
- Yeast infections

More serious side effects include *Clostridioides difficile* infection (also called "*C. difficile*" or "*C. diff*"), which causes severe diarrhea that can lead to severe colon damage and death. People can also have severe and life-threatening allergic reactions.

WHAT YOU CAN DO TO FEEL BETTER

Talk with your healthcare professional about the best treatment for you or your loved one's illness. If you need antibiotics, take them exactly as prescribed. Talk with your healthcare professional if you have any questions about your antibiotics, or if you develop any side effects—especially, severe diarrhea, since that could be a *C. difficile* infection, which needs to be treated immediately.

Respiratory viruses usually go away in a week or two without treatment. Ask your healthcare professional about the best way to feel better and get relief from symptoms while your body fights off the virus. To stay healthy and keep others healthy:

- Clean your hands
- Cover coughs
- Stay home when sick
- Get recommended vaccines, such as the flu vaccine

Section 39.3 | Kids Are Not Just Small Adults: Advice on Giving Medicine to Your Child

This section includes text excerpted from "Kids Aren't Just Small Adults—Medicines, Children, and the Care Every Child Deserves," U.S. Food and Drug Administration (FDA), December 20, 2017.

CARING WHILE GIVING ANY MEDICINE TO AN INFANT OR A CHILD

Use care when giving any medicine to an infant or a child. Even over-the-counter (OTC) medicines that you buy are serious medicines. The following is advice for giving OTC medicine to your child, from the U.S. Food and Drug Administration (FDA) and the makers of OTC medicines:

- **Always read and follow the Drug Facts label on your OTC medicine.** This is important for choosing and safely using all OTC medicines. Read the label every time, before you give the medicine. Be sure you clearly understand how much medicine to give and when the medicine can be taken again.

- **Know the "active ingredient" in your child's medicine.** This is what makes the medicine work and is always listed at the top of the Drug Facts label. Sometimes an active ingredient can treat more than one medical condition. For that reason, the same active ingredient can be found in many different medicines that are used to treat different symptoms. For example, a medicine for a cold and a medicine for a headache could each contain the same active ingredient. So, if you are treating a cold and a headache with two medicines and both have the same active ingredient, you could be giving two times the normal dose. If you are confused about your child's medicines, check with a doctor, nurse, or pharmacist.

- **Give the right medicine, in the right amount, to your child.** Not all medicines are right for an infant or a child. Medicines with the same brand name can be sold in many different strengths, such as infants, children, and adult formulas. The amount and directions are also different for children of different ages or weights. Always use the right medicine and follow the directions exactly. Never use more medicine than directed, even if your child seems sicker than the last time.

- **Talk to your doctor, pharmacist, or nurse to find out what mixes well and what does not.** Medicines, vitamins, supplements, foods, and beverages do not always mix well with each other. Your healthcare professional can help.

- **Use the dosing tool that comes with the medicine, such as a dropper or a dosing cup.** A different dosing tool, or a kitchen spoon, could hold the wrong amount of medicine.

- **Know the difference between a tablespoon (tbsp.) and a teaspoon (tsp.).** Do not confuse them! A tablespoon holds three times as much medicine as a teaspoon. On measuring tools, a teaspoon (tsp.) is equal to "5 cc" or "5 mL."

- **Know your child's weight.** Directions on some OTC medicines are based on weight. Never guess the amount of medicine to give to your child or try to figure it out from the adult dose instructions. If a dose is not listed for your child's age or weight, call your doctor or other members of your healthcare team.

- **Prevent a poison emergency by always using a child-resistant cap.** Relock the cap after each use. Be especially careful with any products that contain iron; they are the leading cause of poisoning deaths in young children.

Taking Medications

- **Store all medicines in a safe place.** Medicines are tasty, colorful, and many can be chewed. Kids may think that these products are candy. To prevent an overdose or poisoning emergency, store all medicines and vitamins in a safe place out of your child's (and even your pet's) sight and reach. If your child takes too much, call the Poison Center Hotline at 800-222-1222 (open 24 hours every day, 7 days a week) or call 911.
- **Check the medicine three times.** First, check the outside packaging for such things as cuts, slices, or tears. Second, once you are at home, check the label on the inside package to be sure you have the right medicine. Make sure the lid and seal are not broken. Third, check the color, shape, size, and smell of medicine. If you notice anything different or unusual, talk to a pharmacist or another healthcare professional.

Chapter 40 | **Adverse Drug Reactions**

FROM MINOR TO LIFE-THREATENING
Unwanted or Unexpected Drug Reactions

Drugs approved by the U.S. Food and Drug Administration (FDA) for sale in the United States must be safe—which means that the benefits of the drug appear to be greater than the known risks—and effective. However, both prescription and over-the-counter (OTC) drugs have side effects. Side effects, also known as "adverse events," are unwanted or unexpected events or reactions to a drug. Side effects can vary from minor problems such as a runny nose to life-threatening events, such as an increased risk of a heart attack.

Several things can affect who does and does not have a side effect when taking a drug—age, gender, allergies, how the body absorbs the drug, other drugs, vitamins and dietary supplements that you may be taking. Common side effects include upset stomach, dry mouth, and drowsiness. A side effect is considered serious if the result is: death; life-threatening; hospitalization; disability or permanent damage; or exposure prior to conception or during pregnancy caused birth defects.

Side effects can happen when you:
- Start taking a new drug, dietary supplement, or vitamin/mineral
- Stop taking a drug that you have been on for a while
- When you increase or decrease the amount of a drug that you take

Reducing Your Risk

There are several ways to learn about side effects for your drugs and to reduce your risk of experiencing a side effect.
- Ask your healthcare professional about any possible side effects and what, if any steps should be taken to reduce the risk when you are

This chapter includes text excerpted from "Finding and Learning about Side Effects (Adverse Reactions)," U.S. Food and Drug Administration (FDA), July 19, 2018.

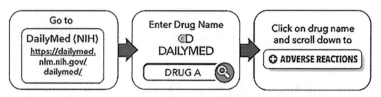

Figure 40.1. How to Find Out about Drug Side Effects

prescribed a drug. For example, she or he may recommend taking the drug with food to lower the chance of getting nausea.

- Ask your pharmacist for the patient prescribing information when you receive your prescription. This document will include possible common and serious side effects.
- Read the pharmacy label and any stickers that may be attached to the prescription bottle. The label and stickers have information on how to take the drug and possible side effects.

When a Side Effect Occurs

Should you experience a side effect, you may be able to lessen or eliminate the effects. Work with your healthcare professional to see if adjusting the dosage or switching to a different medication will ease or eliminate the side effect. Sometimes simply switching from two separate medications to a combination product, if available, will make a difference. Other options, such as a lifestyle or dietary change, may be suggested by your healthcare professional.

Reporting Side Effects

When side effects do occur, you are encouraged to report them to the FDA's MedWatch, a program for reporting serious problems with human medical products, including drugs.

MedWatch has a consumer reporting form, FDA 3500B. Written in plain language and designed to be consumer friendly, the form starts off with a page of some commonly asked questions and answers to help guide the user in submitting the form, and then asks simple questions about the problem. In addition to formal reports, MedWatch has a toll-free line (800-332-1088) to answer questions.

BE AN ACTIVE MEMBER OF YOUR HEALTHCARE TEAM

By taking time to learn about the possible side effects of a drug and working with your healthcare provider and pharmacist, you will be better prepared to reduce your chance of experiencing a side effect or coping with any side effects that you may experience.

Adverse Drug Reactions

WHERE CAN YOU FIND DETAILED SIDE EFFECT INFORMATION FOR A DRUG?

DailyMed, from the National Institutes of Health (NIH), contains detailed information about FDA-approved drugs. Please use these instructions to find information about a particular drug.

Chapter 41 | Drug Interactions: What You Should Know

Do you take two or more prescription drugs or a prescription drug and over-the-counter (OTC) drug together? If you do, this can cause more harm than good if you are not careful.

RECOGNIZING DRUG INTERACTIONS

Drug-drug interactions occur when two or more drugs—prescription and/or OTC—react with each other. Some drug interactions can make the drug you take less effective. And some combinations of drugs can be dangerous. For example, mixing a drug you take to help you sleep (a sedative) and a drug you take for allergies (an antihistamine) can slow your reactions and make driving a car or operating machinery dangerous.

Not all drugs work in the same way in all people. You could be harmed and not helped by a drug designed to treat cold symptoms. For example, if you have high blood pressure, cold medications containing a decongestant may actually raise your blood pressure.

FOOD AND DRUG INTERACTIONS

There are also times that a drug should not be taken with certain foods or beverages. For example, some drug instructions will say not to drink a citrus juice, such as grapefruit, when taking the medicine and others will instruct you not to drink alcohol.

This chapter contains text excerpted from the following sources: Text in this chapter begins with excerpts from "Drug Interactions: Understanding the Risk," U.S. Food and Drug Administration (FDA), July 27, 2016. Reviewed December 2019; Text under the heading "Tips to Avoid Problems" is excerpted from "Avoiding Drug Interactions," U.S. Food and Drug Administration (FDA), November 10, 2008. Reviewed December 2019.

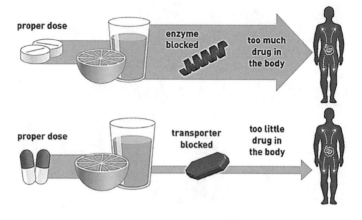

Figure 41.1. How Fruit Juice Affects Some Drugs *(Source: "Grapefruit Juice and Some Drugs Don't Mix," U.S. Food and Drug Administration (FDA))*

UNDERSTAND YOUR DRUG AND POSSIBLE SIDE EFFECTS

You can reduce the risk of harmful drug interactions and side effects by understanding the drugs that you take. Every time you use a drug, take the time to learn about possible drug interactions and read the drug label.

Talk to your healthcare providers and pharmacist about all the drugs that you take. Discuss all OTC and prescription drugs, dietary supplements, vitamins, botanicals, minerals and herbals you take, as well as the foods you eat. Also, read the package insert for each prescription drug you take. The package insert provides more information about potential OTC and prescription drug interactions. Before taking a drug, ask your doctor or pharmacist the following questions:

- Can I take it with other drugs?
- What are the possible side effects and what to do if I experience them?
- Should I avoid certain foods, beverages or other products?

TIPS TO AVOID PROBLEMS

There are lots of things you can do to take prescription or OTC medications in a safe and responsible manner.

- Always read drug labels carefully.
- Learn about the warnings for all the drugs you take.
- Keep medications in their original containers so that you can easily identify them.
- Ask your doctor what you need to avoid when you are prescribed a new medication. Ask about food, beverages, dietary supplements, and other drugs.
- Check with your doctor or pharmacist before taking an OTC drug if you are taking any prescription medications.

Drug Interactions: What You Should Know

- Use one pharmacy for all of your drug needs.
- Keep all of your healthcare professionals informed about everything that you take.
- Keep a record of all prescription drugs, OTC drugs, and dietary supplements (including herbs) that you take. Try to keep this list with you at all times, but especially when you go on any medical appointment.

Chapter 42 | **Preventing Medication Errors**

A medication error is defined as "any preventable event that may cause or lead to inappropriate medication use or patient harm while the medication is in the control of the healthcare professional, patient, or consumer," according to the National Coordinating Council for Medication Error Reporting and Prevention (NCC MERP).

Medication errors can occur throughout the medication-use system. Such as, when prescribing a drug, upon entering information into a computer system, when the drug is being prepared or dispensed, or when the drug is given to or taken by a patient.

The U.S. Food and Drug Administration (FDA) receives more than 100,000 U.S. reports each year associated with a suspected medication error. The FDA reviews the reports and classifies them to determine the cause and type of error. The reports come from drug manufacturers, healthcare professionals, and consumers through MedWatch, the agency's safety information and adverse event reporting program. Serious harmful results of a medication error may include:

- Death
- Life-threatening situation
- Hospitalization
- Disability
- Birth defect

LOOKING FOR WAYS TO REDUCE MEDICATION ERRORS

The FDA looks for ways to prevent medication errors. Before drugs are approved for marketing, the FDA reviews the drug name, labeling, packaging, and product design to identify and revise information that may contribute to medication errors. For example, the FDA reviews:

This chapter includes text excerpted from "Working to Reduce Medication Errors," U.S. Food and Drug Administration (FDA), August 23, 2019.

- **Proposed proprietary (brand) names** to minimize confusion among drug names. With the help of simulated prescriptions and computerized models, the FDA determines the acceptability of proposed proprietary names to minimize medication errors associated with product name confusion.
- **Container labels** to help healthcare providers and consumers select the right drug product. If a drug is made in multiple strengths—e.g., 5 mg, 10 mg, and 25 mg,—the labels of those three containers should be easy to differentiate. The label design may use different colors or identify the strength in large bold numbers and letters.
- **Prescribing and patient information** to ensure the directions for prescribing, preparing, and use are clear and easy to read.

After drugs are approved for marketing in the United States, the FDA monitors and evaluates medication error reports. The FDA may require a manufacturer to revise the labels, labeling, packaging, product design or proprietary name to prevent medication errors. The FDA may also issue communications alerting the public about a medication error safety issue, by way of drug safety communications, drug safety alerts, medication guides, and drug safety podcasts.

Getting the Right Drug to the Right Patient

The FDA also put into place rules requiring barcodes on certain drug and biological product labels. Barcodes allow healthcare professionals to use barcode scanning equipment to verify that the right drug—in the right dose and right route of administration—is being given to the right patient at the right time. This system is intended to help reduce the number of medication errors that occur in hospitals and other healthcare settings.

The FDA has published several guidances to help manufacturers design their drug labels, labeling, packaging, and select drug names in a way to minimize or eliminate hazards that can contribute to medication errors. For example, in 2016, the FDA issued a final guidance titled, *Safety Considerations for Product Design to Minimize Medication Errors*. To avoid errors and encourage safe use of drugs, the guidance recommendations include:

- **Tablets and other oral dosage forms** should have distinct and legible imprint codes so healthcare providers and consumers can verify the drug product and strength.
- **Oral syringes and other dosing devices** copackaged with a liquid oral dosage form should be appropriate for the doses to be measured. Dosing errors have been reported when an oral syringe is labeled in milligrams but the dose is prescribed in milliliters.
- **The package design** should protect the consumer against incorrect use. Medications applied to the skin (topical) should not be packaged

in containers that look similar to the containers usually associated with eye, ear, nasal, or oral products. Similar looking containers have resulted in people putting a topical product in the eye, ear, nose, and mouth.

OVER-THE-COUNTER AND PRESCRIPTION DRUG LABELING

According to a Harris Interactive Market Research Poll conducted for the National Council on Patient Information and Education (NCPIE) and released in January 2002, consumers tend to overlook important label information on over-the-counter (OTC) drugs. In response to that report, the FDA now requires a standardized "Drug Facts" label on more than 100,000 OTC drug products. Modeled after the Nutrition Facts label on foods, Drug Facts helps consumers compare and select OTC medicines, and follow the instructions. The label clearly lists active ingredients, inactive ingredients, uses, warnings, dosage, directions, and other information, such as how to store the medicine.

In 2006, the FDA revised its rules for the content and format of prescribing information for prescription drug and biological products. The revised look helps healthcare professionals find the information they need more easily and quickly. The FDA also makes updated prescribing information available on the Web at Drugs@FDA.

CONSUMERS PLAY AN IMPORTANT ROLE

Consumers can also play an important role in reducing medication errors. Here are some drug safety tips:

- **Know the various risks and causes for medication errors.**
- **Find out what drug you are taking and what it is for.** Rather than simply letting the doctor write you a prescription and send you on your way, be sure to ask the name of the drug and the purpose of the drug.
- **Find out how to take the drug and make sure you understand the directions.** Ask if the medicine needs to be kept in the refrigerator.
- **Check the container's label every time you take a drug.** This is especially important if you are taking several drugs because it will lower your risk of accidentally taking the wrong medicine.
- **Keep drugs stored in their original containers.** Many pills look alike, so keeping them in their original containers will help know the name of the drug and how to take them. If you are having trouble keeping multiple medications straight, ask your doctor or pharmacist about helpful aids.
- **Keep an updated list of all medications taken for health reasons,** including OTC drugs, supplements, medicinal herbs, and other substances. Give a copy of this list to your healthcare provider.

- Be aware of the risk of drug/drug or drug/food interactions.
- If in doubt or you have questions about your medication, ask your pharmacist or other healthcare provider.
- **Report suspected medication errors** to MedWatch.

Chapter 43 | Unapproved, Counterfeit, and Misused Drugs

Chapter Contents

Section 43.1 | Unapproved and Counterfeit Drugs

This section contains text excerpted from the following sources: Text under the heading "Unapproved Drugs" is excerpted from "Unapproved Drugs," U.S. Food and Drug Administration (FDA), October 17, 2019; Text under the heading "Counterfeit Drugs" is excerpted from "Counterfeit Medicine," U.S. Food and Drug Administration (FDA), September 13, 2019.

UNAPPROVED DRUGS

Unapproved prescription drugs pose significant risks to patients because they have not been reviewed by the U.S. Food and Drug Administration (FDA) for safety, effectiveness or quality. Without FDA's review, there is no way to know if these drugs are safe and effective for their intended use, whether they are manufactured in a way that ensures consistent drug quality or whether their label is complete and accurate. Unapproved drugs have resulted in patient harm, and the agency works to protect patients from the risks posed by these drugs.

Preserving Patient Access to Medically Necessary Drugs

The agency balances its goal to eliminate unapproved prescription drugs from the market with patient access to medically necessary drugs. The FDA carefully considers the possible effects on patient access, including whether any action would likely lead to a disruption in the drug supply, before initiating an action against an unapproved drug.

The agency permits some unapproved drugs to be marketed if they are relied on by healthcare professionals to treat serious medical conditions when there is no FDA-approved drug to treat the condition or there is insufficient supply of FDA-approved drugs.

The FDA's Approval Is Required by Law

The federal law requires all new prescription drugs in the United States be shown to be safe and effective for their intended use prior to marketing. However, some drugs are available in the United States even though they have never received the required FDA approval. Many healthcare professionals and patients are unaware that some of the drugs prescribed are not FDA approved.

The FDA permits some unapproved prescription drugs to be marketed if:
- The drug is subject to an open drug efficacy study implementation (DESI) program proceeding
- Healthcare professionals rely on the drug to treat serious medical conditions when there is no FDA-approved drug to treat the condition
- There is insufficient supply of an FDA-approved drug

The law allows some unapproved prescription drugs to be lawfully marketed if they meet the criteria of generally recognized as safe and effective (GRASE) or grandfathered. However, the agency is not aware of any human prescription drug that is lawfully marketed as grandfathered.

Unapproved Drugs Program

The agency's Unapproved Drugs Program has a two-prong approach to help assure patient safety. First, the agency encourages manufacturers of unapproved drugs to obtain approval to be legally marketed in the U.S. Second, the FDA has worked to remove unapproved drugs from the market. Many potentially unsafe drugs have been removed from the market since 2006, including several drugs with significant safety concerns. The agency uses a risk-based approach, giving enforcement priority to drugs that pose the highest risk to public health, without imposing undue burden on patients or unnecessarily disrupting the availability of drugs on the market.

In 2011, the FDA issued a final guidance, *Guidance for FDA Staff and Industry, Marketed Unapproved Drugs—Compliance Policy Guide, Section 440.100: Marketed New Drugs without Approved by New Drug Application (NDA) or Abbreviated New Drug Application (ANDA)*, which describes the FDA's enforcement priorities.

Search Marketed Drugs Listed with the FDA, Including Unapproved Drugs

Drugs marketed in the United States, with or without FDA approval, can be identified in the following databases:
- National Drug Code (NDC) Directory publishes data derived from information submitted to the agency as part of drug listing requirements, including information on unapproved drugs. NDC numbers are provided for all listed drugs, regardless of approval status. Information in the directory does not indicate that the FDA has verified the information provided.
- Drugs@FDA lists information on FDA-approved drugs since 1998, including patient information, labels and approval letters.
- Orange Book identifies FDA-approved drugs.

Unapproved Drugs and Drug Prices

There are many factors that contribute to drug pricing. When there is a sole source of an FDA-approved drug, market dynamics may enable the company that sought approval to set a higher price than when the drug faces competition. Patients and healthcare professionals can, however, have confidence that the FDA-approved version has been shown to be safe and effective for its intended use and that it is manufactured according to federal quality standards.

Unapproved, Counterfeit, and Misused Drugs

While the FDA does not have the authority to regulate drug prices, it is keenly aware of price fluctuations that can occur on the heels of its regulatory actions and takes steps within its authority to minimize the duration, if not the extent, of those price hikes. Although following the FDA approval process may result in cost increases for a drug over the short term, the risks to the individual patient are substantially reduced and the benefits are assured for the long term.

COUNTERFEIT DRUGS

Counterfeit medicine is fake medicine. It may be contaminated or contain the wrong or no active ingredient. They could have the right active ingredient but at the wrong dose. Counterfeit drugs are illegal and may be harmful to your health.

The FDA takes all reports of suspect counterfeits seriously and, in order to combat counterfeit medicines, is working with other agencies and the private sector to help protect the nation's drug supply from the threat of counterfeits.

Tips for Reducing Your Chances of Buying Counterfeit Medicines*

Counterfeiting happens all over the world, but it is most common in countries where there are few or no rules about making drugs. An estimated 10 to 30 percent of medicines sold in developing countries are counterfeit. In the industrialized world (countries such as the United States, Australia, Japan, Canada, New Zealand, and those in the European Union), estimates suggest that less than 1 percent of medicines sold are counterfeit.

The only way to know if a drug is counterfeit is through chemical analysis done in a laboratory. Counterfeit drugs may look strange or be in poor-quality packaging, but they often seem identical to the real thing. The only way to make sure you have the real thing is to bring all the drugs you will need during your trip with you from the United States, rather than buying them while you are traveling.

If an emergency occurs and you must buy drugs during your trip, you can reduce your chances of buying drugs that are counterfeit.

- Buy medicines only from licensed pharmacies and get a receipt. Do not buy medicines from open markets.
- Ask the pharmacist whether the drug has the same active ingredient as the one that you were taking.
- Make sure that the medicine is in its original packaging.
- Look closely at the packaging. Sometimes poor-quality printing or otherwise strange-looking packaging will indicate a counterfeit product.

Text excerpted from "Counterfeit Medicines," Centers for Disease Control and Prevention (CDC), October 23, 2017

What You Should Do If You Have Received or Taken Counterfeit Medicine*

First, talk to the pharmacist where you bought the medicine or contact your healthcare professional for medical advice.

After your safety is assured, the FDA needs your help in protecting the safety of others! In order to ensure that only safe and effective drug products are available on the market, the FDA relies on the voluntary reporting of suspect counterfeit drugs from consumers, healthcare professionals, and other drug supply chain partners.

If you are aware of suspicious activity that may be associated with counterfeit prescription drugs, please contact the FDA's Office of Criminal Investigations (OCI).

If you find a website you think is illegally selling human drugs, animal drugs, medical devices, biological products, foods, dietary supplements or cosmetics over the Internet, please report it to the FDA. If your report:

- Involves a life-threatening situation due to an FDA-regulated product you purchased from a Website, call 866-300-4374 or 301-796-8240 immediately. (Also contact your health professional for medical advice.)
- Involves a serious reaction or problem with an FDA-regulated product, fill out the FDA's MedWatch reporting form. (Also contact your health professional for medical advice.)

To report e-mails promoting medical products that you think might be illegal, forward the e-mail to webcomplaints@ora.fda.gov.

Text excerpted from "What Should I Do If I Believe I Have Received or Taken Counterfeit Medicine? Information for Consumers and Health Providers," U.S. Food and Drug Administration (FDA), February 19, 2016

Section 43.2 | Misuse of Prescription Pain Relievers

This section includes text excerpted from "Misuse of Prescription Pain Relievers: The Buzz Takes Your Breath Away Permanently," U.S. Food and Drug Administration (FDA), January 10, 2018.

IF YOU THINK YOU HAVE HEARD IT BEFORE, YOU ARE DEAD WRONG

How many times has someone told you a "party" drug could lead to more serious problems—such as addiction, brain damage, or even death? You have probably heard it so many times, it is getting hard to believe. Especially when kids around you are smoking, drinking, and rolling. But all drugs have real potential for harm—even prescription pain relievers. When abused alone, or taken with other drugs, prescription pain medications can kill you. And the death toll from misuse and abuse is rising steadily.

THINK TWICE—BECAUSE YOU ONLY DIE ONCE

Prescription pain relievers, when used correctly and under a doctor's supervision, are safe and effective. But abuse them, or mix them with illegal drugs or alcohol, and you could wind up in the morgue. Even using prescription pain relievers with other prescription drugs (such as antidepressants) or over-the-counter (OTC) medications (such as cough syrups and antihistamines), can lead to life-threatening respiratory failure. That is why people just like you are dropping pills at parties, and dropping dead. They are not downing handfuls of pills, either. With some prescription pain relievers, all it takes is one pill.

DRUGS TO WATCH OUT FOR

The most dangerous prescription pain relievers are those containing drugs known as "opioids," such as morphine and codeine. Some common drugs containing these substances include Darvon, Demerol, Dilaudid, OxyContin, Tylenol with Codeine, and Vicodin. Your friends probably call these drugs by their street names: ac/dc, coties, demmies, dillies, hillbilly heroin, OC, oxy, oxycotton, percs, and vics to name a few. Whatever you call them, remember one thing—they can be killers.

SYMPTOMS OF OVERDOSE

If you, or any of your friends, have taken prescription pain relievers, here are the danger signs to watch for:

- Slow breathing (less than ten breaths a minute is really serious trouble)
- Small, pinpoint pupils
- Confusion
- Being tired, nodding off, or passing out
- Dizziness
- Weakness
- Apathy (they do not care about anything)
- Cold and clammy skin
- Nausea
- Vomiting
- Seizures

A lot of these symptoms can make people think your friend is drunk. And you may be tempted to let them sleep it off, or tell their parents they had too much to drink. But do not. Your friend could go to sleep and never wake up.

WHAT YOU CAN DO IF A FRIEND IS OVERDOSING

Make an anonymous call to 911 or your friend's parents if you are too scared to identify yourself. Try to get your friend to respond to you by calling out her/his name. Make your friend wake up and talk to you. Shake her/his if you have to. Otherwise, your friend could suffer brain damage, fall into a coma, or die.

ADDICTION CAN BE A LIVING DEATH

If you abuse prescription pain relievers and are lucky enough to cheat death, you are still in big trouble. Prescription pain relievers can be addictive. The longer you take them, the more your body needs them. Try to stop, and you could experience withdrawal symptoms.

Addiction to prescription pain relievers is similar to that of being hooked on heroin and the withdrawal is not much different: bone and muscle pain, diarrhea, vomiting, cold flashes, and insomnia.

If you, or someone you know is abusing or is addicted, get professional help. You can also ask for help from parents, doctors, relatives, teachers, or school guidance counselors. Substance abuse ruins lives. Do not let it happen to your friends—or you.

Chapter 44 | Where and How to Dispose of Unused Medicines

Section 44.1 | Drug Take-Back Locations

This section includes text excerpted from "Drug Disposal: Drug Take Back Locations," U.S. Food and Drug Administration (FDA), December 18, 2018.

Medicine take-back options are the best way to safely dispose of most types of unneeded or expired prescription and over-the-counter (OTC) medicines.

Note that there are a few, select medicines with specific instructions to immediately flush down the toilet only if a drug take-back option is not readily available.

Before disposing of prescription medicines using a drug take-back option, be sure to remove all personal information on the label of pill bottles or medicine packaging. Do note that all medicines dropped off at these locations will be destroyed and discarded.

There are generally two kinds of take-back options; permanent collection locations and periodic events.

PERMANENT COLLECTION LOCATIONS

Some facilities and businesses are registered with the U.S. Drug Enforcement Administration (DEA) to collect old, unused, unneeded, or expired medicines. These authorized drug-collection locations safely and securely gather and dispose of pharmaceuticals containing controlled substances, as well as other medicines.

In your community, such authorized collection locations may be in retail pharmacies, hospital or clinic pharmacies, and law enforcement agencies/facilities. Some authorized collectors may also offer mail-back programs or collection receptacles (drop-off boxes) to assist you in safely disposing of your unused medicines.

Finally, you can go to Google Maps and type in "drug disposal near me" or "medication disposal near me" to find your nearest drug disposal site.

Find an authorized drug-collection site near you or call the DEA's Diversion Control Division Registration Call Center at 800-882-9539 for more information.

PERIODIC EVENTS

The DEA periodically hosts National Prescription Drug Take Back events. During these Drug Take Back Days, temporary drug-collection sites are set up in communities nationwide for safe disposal of prescription drugs.

Local law enforcement agencies may also sponsor medicine take back events in your community. You can also contact your local waste-management authorities to learn about events in your area.

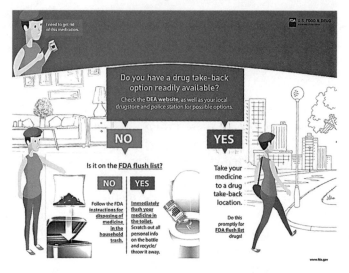

Figure 44.1. Drug Disposal Options *(Source: "Disposal of Unused Medicines: What You Should Know," U.S. Food and Drug Administration (FDA))*

Section 44.2 | Disposing of Medicines at Home

This section includes text excerpted from "Where and How to Dispose of Unused Medicines," U.S. Food and Drug Administration (FDA), May 1, 2019.

Is your medicine cabinet full of expired drugs or medications you no longer use? Your medicine is for you. What is safe for you might be harmful for someone else. You can dispose of your expired, unwanted, or unused medicines through a drug take-back program—or you can do it at home.

HOW TO DISPOSE OF MEDICINES AT HOME

When a take-back option is not readily available, there are two ways to dispose of prescription and over-the-counter (OTC) medicine, depending on the drug.

Flushing Medicines

Because some medicines could be especially harmful to others, they have specific directions to immediately flush them down the sink or toilet when they are no longer needed, and a take-back option is not readily available.

How will you know? Check the label or the patient information leaflet with your medicine. Or consult the U.S. Food and Drug Administration's (FDA) list of medicines recommended for disposal by flushing when a take-back option is not readily available.

Disposing Medicines in Household Trash

Almost all medicines, except those on the FDA flush list, can be thrown into your household trash. These include prescription and over-the-counter (OTC) drugs in pills, liquids, drops, patches, creams, and inhalers.

Follow these steps:

- Remove the drugs from their original containers and mix them with something undesirable, such as used coffee grounds, dirt, or cat litter. This makes the medicine less appealing to children and pets and unrecognizable to someone who might intentionally go through the trash looking for drugs.
- Put the mixture in something you can close (a resealable zipper storage bag, empty can, or other container) to prevent the drug from leaking or spilling out.
- Throw the container in the garbage.
- Scratch out all your personal information on the empty medicine packaging to protect your identity and privacy. Throw the packaging away.

If you have a question about your medicine, ask your healthcare provider or pharmacist.

DISPOSING OF FENTANYL PATCHES

Some prescription drugs—such as powerful narcotic pain medicines and other controlled substances—have instructions for flushing to reduce the danger of overdose from unintentional or illegal use. One example is the fentanyl patch. This adhesive patch delivers a strong pain medicine through the skin. Even after a patch is used, a lot of the medicine remains. That is why the drug comes with instructions to flush used or leftover patches.

DISPOSING OF INHALER PRODUCTS

One environmental concern involves inhalers used by people who have asthma or other breathing problems, such as chronic obstructive pulmonary disease (COPD). Read handling instructions on the labeling of inhalers and aerosol products. These products could be dangerous if punctured or thrown into a fire or incinerator. To properly dispose of these products and follow local regulations and laws, contact your trash and recycling facility.

FLUSHING DRUGS AND THE WATER SUPPLY

Some people wonder if it is okay to flush certain medicines when a take-back option is not readily available. There are concerns about the small levels of drugs

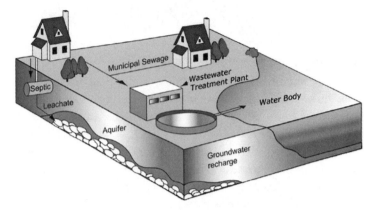

Figure 44.2. How Improper Disposal of Medicines May End Up in Our Drinking Water Sources *(Source: "How to Dispose of Medicines Properly," U.S. Environmental Protection Agency (EPA))*

In homes that use septic tanks, prescription and over-the-counter (OTC) drugs flushed down the toilet can leach into the ground and seep into groundwater. In cities and towns where residences are connected to wastewater treatment plants, prescription and OTC drugs poured down the sink or flushed down the toilet can pass through the treatment system and enter rivers and lakes. They may flow downstream to serve as sources for community drinking water supplies. Water treatment plants are generally not equipped to routinely remove medicines.

that may be found in surface water, such as rivers and lakes, and in drinking-water supplies.

"The main way drug residues enter water systems is by people taking medicines and then naturally passing them through their bodies," says Raanan Bloom, Ph.D., an environmental assessment expert at the FDA. "Many drugs are not completely absorbed or metabolized by the body and can enter the environment after passing through wastewater treatment plants."

The FDA and the U.S. Environmental Protection Agency (EPA) take the concerns of flushing certain medicines in the environment seriously. Still, there has been no sign of environmental effects caused by flushing recommended drugs. In fact, the FDA published a paper to assess this concern, finding negligible risk of environmental effects caused by flushing recommended drugs.

Part 5 | Managing Chronic Disease

Chapter 45 | Self-Management of Chronic Illness

Chapter Contents

Section 45.1 | Take Charge of Your Health

This section contains text excerpted from the following sources: Text beginning with the heading "The Basics" is excerpted from "Take Charge of Your Healthcare," Office of Disease Prevention and Health Promotion (ODPHP), U.S. Department of Health and Human Services (HHS), August 9, 2019; Text under the heading "Get Moving to Take Charge of Your Health" is excerpted from "Get Moving to Take Charge of Your Health," National Institute of Diabetes and Digestive and Kidney Diseases (NIDDK), September 2011. Reviewed December 2019.

THE BASICS

When you play an active role in your healthcare, you can improve the quality of the care that you and your family get. Start by speaking up and asking questions at the doctor's office.

Healthcare is a team effort, and you are the most important member of the team! Your team also includes doctors, nurses, pharmacists, and insurance providers.

To take charge of your healthcare you should:
- Keep track of important health information
- Know your family's health history
- See a doctor regularly for checkups
- Be prepared for medical appointments
- Ask your doctor, nurse, or pharmacist questions
- Follow up after your appointment

TAKE ACTION!

Follow these steps to play an active role in your healthcare.

Keep Track of Important Health Information

Keeping all your health information in one place will make it easier to manage your healthcare. Take this information with you to every medical appointment.

To start your own personal health record, write down:
- Your name and birth date
- The name and phone number of a friend or relative to call if there is an emergency
- Telephone numbers and addresses of all the places where you get medical care, including your pharmacy
- Your blood type
- Dates and results of checkups and screening tests
- All the shots (vaccinations) you have had—and the dates that you got them
- Medicines you take, how much you take, and why you take them
- Any health conditions you have, including allergies
- Any important health conditions that run in your family

If you are not sure about some of this information, check with your doctor's office.

Know Your Family Health History

Your family's health history is an important part of your personal health record. Use this family health history tool to keep track of health conditions that run in your family.

See a Doctor Regularly for Checkups

Getting regular checkups with your doctor or nurse can help you stay healthy. If you do not have a doctor or nurse, check out these tips for choosing a doctor you can trust.

Regular checkups can help find problems early, when they may be easier to treat.

- Use the myhealthfinder tool (healthfinder.gov/myhealthfinder/default. aspx) to get personalized health recommendations based on your age and sex.
- Get information about shots to help you stay healthy.
- Protect your health by getting recommended screenings.

If you need help finding healthcare, use these tools to help you choose a doctor, hospital, or nursing home.

What about Cost

Under the Affordable Care Act (ACA), insurance plans must cover many preventive services such as screenings and shots. Plans must also cover well-child visits through age 21 and well-woman visits.

Depending on your insurance plan, you may be able to get preventive services at no cost to you. Check with your insurance company for more information.

- Find out which services are covered under the ACA.
- Find out which services are covered by Medicare.

If you do not have insurance, check out these resources to help you get healthcare.

- Visit HealthCare.gov to find insurance options for your family.
- For low-cost or free services, find a health center near you (www. findahealthcenter.hrsa.gov/) and make an appointment.

Write Down Your Questions Ahead of Time

Write down any questions you have about your health. Take the list with you to your doctor, nurse, or pharmacist. Use the question builder tool (www.ahrq. gov/patients-consumers/question-builder.html) to build your list of questions.

Make the Most of Doctor Visits

Take your list of questions and personal health record with you to the appointment. You may also want to ask a family member or friend to go with you to help take notes.

Be sure to talk about any changes since your last visit, such as:

- New medicines you are taking, including over-the-counter (OTC) medicines
- Herbs, home remedies, and vitamins you are taking
- Recent illnesses or surgeries
- Important changes in your life, such as becoming unemployed or a death in the family
- Health concerns or issues
- Health information you have found online or heard from others

Follow Up after Your Appointment

It can take time and hard work to make the healthy changes you talked about with your doctor or nurse. Remember to:

- Call if you have any questions—or if you experience side effects from a medicine
- Schedule follow-up appointments for tests or lab work if you need to
- Contact the doctor to get test results if you need to

GET MOVING TO TAKE CHARGE OF YOUR HEALTH

You do not have to do boring exercise routines to be active. Fun activities can be good for you, too!

Be Active to Look and Feel Better!

Do not do it because you are "supposed to." Be active to:

- Get better control of your weight, a more toned look, and stronger muscles
- Have more energy for other fun times, such as hanging out with your friends
- Make friends who share your interests in dance, sports, or other activities
- Improve your mood and ability to focus for sports and school

Get Up and Move!

- Be active for 60 minutes a day. (You do not have to do it all at once.)
- Enjoy the outdoors with these activities: jumping rope, playing frisbee or flag-football, and skateboarding.
- Join a school sports or dance team. Jump into a neighborhood pick-up game of basketball or softball.

- Pitch in to help keep your area's sidewalks, sports fields, parks, and athletic centers clean and usable.

Here is how your activity can add up:
- 10 minutes of walking/biking to a friend's house
- 30 minutes of shooting hoops
- +20 minutes of dancing

Stay Active Indoors Too!
- Play indoor sports when it is cold or wet outside.
- Sit less. Watching TV, gaming, and surfing the web are fun but inactive, so spend less time in front of the screen.
- Dance to your favorite music by yourself, or have a dance party with friends.
- If you have a gaming system, choose active dance and sports games that track your movement.

Have Fun with Your Friends!
- Be active with your friends to support each other and make moving fun.
- Mix it up. Choose different kinds of group activity:
- Sports
- Active games
- Actions that get you moving, such as walking around the mall
- Take the President's Challenge (www.fitness.gov) or sign up with your friends for other fun, lively challenges

Section 45.2 | Adopt a Healthy Eating Plan

This section contains text excerpted from the following sources: Text beginning with the heading "The Importance of Good Nutrition" is excerpted from "Importance of Good Nutrition," U.S. Department of Health and Human Services (HHS), January 26, 2017; Text under the heading "What a Healthy Eating Plan Comprises Of" is excerpted from "Healthy Eating for a Healthy Weight," Centers for Disease Management and Prevention (CDC), April 12, 2019.

THE IMPORTANCE OF GOOD NUTRITION

Your food choices each day affect your health—how you feel today, tomorrow, and in the future.

Good nutrition is an important part of leading a healthy lifestyle. Combined with physical activity, your diet can help you to reach and maintain a healthy weight, reduce your risk of chronic diseases (such as heart disease and cancer), and promote your overall health.

THE IMPACT OF NUTRITION ON YOUR HEALTH

Unhealthy eating habits have contributed to the obesity epidemic in the United States: about one-third of U.S. adults (33.8%) are obese and approximately 17 percent (or 12.5 million) of children and adolescents aged 2 to 19 years are obese. Even for people at a healthy weight, a poor diet is associated with major health risks that can cause illness and even death. These include heart disease, hypertension (high blood pressure), type 2 diabetes, osteoporosis, and certain types of cancer. By making smart food choices, you can help protect yourself from these health problems.

The risk factors for adult chronic diseases, such as hypertension and type 2 diabetes, are increasingly seen in younger ages, often a result of unhealthy eating habits and increased weight gain. Dietary habits established in childhood often carry into adulthood, so teaching children how to eat healthy at a young age will help them stay healthy throughout their life.

The link between good nutrition and healthy weight, reduced chronic disease risk, and overall health is too important to ignore. By taking steps to eat healthy, you will be on your way to getting the nutrients your body needs to stay healthy, active, and strong. As with physical activity, making small changes in your diet can go a long way, and it is easier than you think!

Eat Healthy

Now that you know the benefits, it is time to start eating healthy.

WHAT A HEALTHY EATING PLAN COMPRISES OF

A healthy lifestyle involves many choices. Among them, choosing a balanced diet or healthy eating plan. So how do you choose a healthy eating plan? According to the *Dietary Guidelines for Americans 2015–2020*, a healthy eating plan:

- Emphasizes fruits, vegetables, whole grains, and fat-free or low-fat milk and milk products
- Includes lean meats, poultry, fish, beans, eggs, and nuts
- Is low in saturated fats, trans fats, cholesterol, salt (sodium), and added sugars
- Stays within your daily calorie needs

If "healthy eating" makes you think about the foods you cannot have, try refocusing on all the new foods you can eat.

Section 45.3 | **Stress and Your Health**

This section includes text excerpted from "Manage Stress," Office of Disease Prevention and Health Promotion (ODPHP), U.S. Department of Health and Human Services (HHS), August 20, 2019.

THE BASICS ABOUT STRESS

Not all stress is bad. But long-term stress can lead to health problems. Preventing and managing long-term stress can lower your risk for other conditions such as heart disease, obesity, high blood pressure, and depression.

You can prevent or reduce stress by:

- Planning ahead
- Deciding which tasks need to be done first
- Preparing for stressful events

Some stress is hard to avoid. You can find ways to manage stress by:

- Noticing when you feel stressed
- Taking time to relax
- Getting active and eating healthy
- Talking to friends and family

What Are the Benefits of Managing Stress?

Over time, long-term stress can lead to health problems. Managing stress can help you:

- Sleep better
- Control your weight
- Get sick less often
- Feel better faster when you do get sick
- Less muscle tensions
- Be in a better mood
- Get along better with family and friends

TAKE ACTION TO MANAGE STRESS

You cannot always avoid stress, but you can take steps to deal with stress in a positive way. Follow these tips for preventing and managing stress. Being prepared and feeling in control of your situation might help lower your stress.

Plan Your Time

Think ahead about how you are going to use your time. Write a to-do list and figure out what is most important—then do that thing first. Be realistic about how long each task will take.

Prepare Yourself

Prepare ahead for stressful events such as a hard conversation with a loved one. You can:

- Picture what the room will look like and what you will say
- Think about different ways the conversation could go—and how you could respond
- Have a plan for ending the conversation early if you need time to think

Relax with Deep Breathing or Meditation

Deep breathing and meditation can help relax your muscles and clear your mind.

- Learn how to use deep breathing to relax
- Try meditating for a few minutes a day

Relax Your Muscles

Stress causes tension in your muscles. Try stretching or taking a hot shower to help you relax.

Get Active

Regular physical activity can help prevent and manage stress. It can also help relax your muscles and improve your mood.

- Aim for 2 hours and 30 minutes a week of moderate-intensity physical activity. Try going for a bike ride or taking a walk.
- Do strengthening activities—such as push-ups or lifting weights—at least 2 days a week.
- Remember that any amount of physical activity is better than none.

Eat Healthy

Give your body plenty of energy by eating healthy—including vegetables, fruits, and lean sources of protein.

Drink Alcohol Only in Moderation

Avoid using alcohol or other drugs to manage stress. If you choose to drink, drink only in moderation. This means no more than one drink a day for women and no more than two drinks a day for men.

Talk to Friends and Family

Tell your friends and family if you are feeling stressed. They may be able to help.

Get Help If You Need It

Stress is a normal part of life. But, if your stress does not go away or keeps getting worse, you may need help.

Over time, stress can lead to serious problems such as depression or anxiety.

- If you are feeling down or hopeless, talk with your doctor about depression.
- If you are feeling anxious, find out how to get help for anxiety.
- If you have lived through a traumatic event (such as a tragedy, crime, or natural disaster).

A mental-health professional (such as a psychologist or social worker) can help treat these conditions with talk therapy (called "psychotherapy") or medicine.

Finally, keep in mind that lots of people need help dealing with stress—it is nothing to be ashamed of.

Section 45.4 | Exercise Can Improve Some Chronic Disease Conditions

This section contains text excerpted from the following sources: Text in this section begins with excerpts from "Physical Activity Prevents Chronic Disease," Centers for Disease Control and Prevention (CDC), April 30, 2019; Text under the heading "Physical Activity Has Many Health Benefits" is excerpted from "Physical Activity Has Many Health Benefits," Office of Disease Prevention and Health Promotion (ODPHP), U.S. Department of Health and Human Services (HHS), November 6, 2019.

Regular physical activity helps improve your overall health, fitness, and quality of life (QOL). It also helps reduce your risk of chronic conditions such as, type

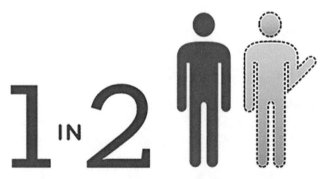

About 1 in 2 adults live with a chronic disease. About half of this group have two or more.

Figure 45.1. Chronic Diseases among Adults *(Source: "Physical Activity—Why It Matters," Centers for Disease Control and Prevention (CDC))*

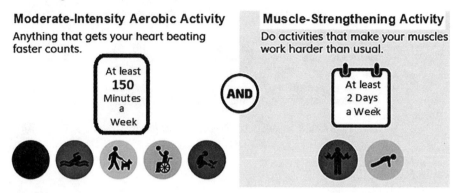

Figure 45.2. How Much Activity Do Adults Need? *(Source: "What's Your Move," Office of Disease Prevention and Health Promotion (ODPHP), U.S. Department of Health and Human Services (HHS))*

2 diabetes, heart disease, many types of cancer, depression and anxiety, and dementia.

WHAT IS PHYSICAL ACTIVITY?
Cardio or Aerobic Activity
- Moderate or vigorous intensity, every minute counts
- Gets you breathing harder and your heart beating faster
- Examples: Brisk walking, biking, dancing, and yard work

Muscle Strengthening
- Works best when you work all your body's major muscle groups
- Includes legs, hips, back, chest, abs, shoulders, and arms
- Examples: Free weights, crunches, elastic bands, and squats

Everyone can benefit from physical activity—no matter your age, sex, race or ethnicity, health condition, shape or size.

How Much Physical Activity Do You Need?
Preschool-aged children. Children who are 3 to 5 years, should be physically active throughout the day. They should be provided with plenty of opportunities for active play.

Kids. Kids who are 6 to 17 years, should spend 1 hour or more of physical activity each day

Adults. Adults should spend at least 150 minutes of moderate-intensity aerobic activity every week, plus muscle-strengthening activities at least 2 days a week.

Fitting regular physical activity into your schedule may seem hard at first, but you can reach your goals through different types and amounts of physical activity each week.

Physical Activity Prevents

1 in 8 cases of breast cancer	1 in 8 cases of colorectal cancer	1 in 12 cases of diabetes	1 in 15 cases of heart disease

Figure 45.3. Importance of Physical Activity *(Source: "Physical Activity—Why It Matters," Centers for Disease Control and Prevention (CDC))*

Tips to Get and Stay Active

- Talk to your doctor if you have a chronic condition such as type 2 diabetes or heart disease.
- Get the support of your friends and family—and invite them to get active with you!
- Start slowly and add time, frequency, or intensity every week.
- Schedule physical activity for times in the day or week when you are most energetic.
- Plan ahead. Make physical activity part of your daily or weekly schedule.
- Walk instead of drive to nearby destinations or park the car farther away and fit in a walk to your destination.
- Support improvements in your neighborhood that make it easier to walk or bike to where you want to go.

PHYSICAL ACTIVITY HAS MANY HEALTH BENEFITS

All Americans should be regularly physically active to improve overall health and fitness and to prevent many adverse health outcomes. The benefits of physical activity occur in generally healthy people, in people at risk of developing chronic diseases, and in people with current chronic conditions or disabilities.

Physical activity affects many health conditions, and the specific amounts and types of activity that benefit each condition vary. In developing public-health guidelines, the challenge is to integrate scientific information across all health benefits and identify a critical range of physical activity that appears to have an effect across the health benefits. One consistent finding from research studies is that once the health benefits from physical activity begin to accrue, additional amounts of activity provide additional benefits.

Although some health benefits seem to begin with as little as 60 minutes (1 hour) a week, research shows that a total amount of 150 minutes (2 hours and 30 minutes) a week of moderate-intensity aerobic activity, such as brisk walking, consistently reduces the risk of many chronic diseases and other adverse health outcomes.

Examining the Relationship between Physical Activity and Health

In many studies covering a wide range of issues, researchers have focused on exercise, as well as on the more broadly defined concept of physical activity. Exercise is a form of physical activity that is planned, structured, repetitive, and performed with the goal of improving health or fitness. So, although all exercise is physical activity, not all physical activity is exercise.

Studies have examined the role of physical activity in many groups—men and women, children, teens, adults, older adults, people with disabilities, and women during pregnancy and the postpartum period. These studies have focused on the role that physical activity plays in many health outcomes, including:

- Premature (early) death
- Diseases, such as coronary heart disease (CHD), stroke, some cancers, type 2 diabetes, osteoporosis, and depression
- Risk factors for disease, such as high blood pressure and high blood cholesterol
- Physical fitness, such as aerobic capacity, and muscle strength and endurance
- Functional capacity (the ability to engage in activities needed for daily living)
- Mental health, such as depression and cognitive function
- Injuries or sudden heart attacks

These studies have also prompted questions as to what type and how much physical activity is needed for various health benefits. To answer this question, investigators have studied three main kinds of physical activity: aerobic, muscle-strengthening, and bone strengthening. Investigators have also studied balance and flexibility activities.

Major Research Findings

- Regular physical activity reduces the risk of many adverse health outcomes.
- Some physical activity is better than none.
- For most health outcomes, additional benefits occur as the amount of physical activity increases through higher intensity, greater frequency, and/ or longer duration.
- Most health benefits occur with at least 150 minutes a week of moderate-intensity physical activity, such as brisk walking. Additional benefits occur with more physical activity.

- Both aerobic (endurance) and muscle-strengthening (resistance) physical activity are beneficial.
- Health benefits occur for children and adolescents, young and middle-aged adults, older adults, and those in every studied racial and ethnic group.
- The health benefits of physical activity occur for people with disabilities.
- The benefits of physical activity far outweigh the possibility of adverse outcomes.

Health Benefits Associated with Regular Physical Activity
Children and Adolescents
- Improved cardiorespiratory and muscular fitness
- Improved bone health
- Improved cardiovascular and metabolic health biomarkers
- Favorable body composition
- Reduced symptoms of depression

Adults and Older Adults
- Lower risk of early death
- Lower risk of coronary heart disease
- Lower risk of stroke
- Lower risk of high blood pressure
- Lower risk of adverse blood lipid profile
- Lower risk of type 2 diabetes
- Lower risk of metabolic syndrome
- Lower risk of colon cancer
- Lower risk of breast cancer
- Prevention of weight gain
- Weight loss, particularly when combined with reduced calorie intake
- Improved cardiorespiratory and muscular fitness
- Prevention of falls
- Reduced depression
- Better cognitive function (for older adults)
- Better functional health (for older adults)
- Reduced abdominal obesity
- Lower risk of hip fracture
- Lower risk of lung cancer
- Lower risk of endometrial cancer
- Weight maintenance after weight loss
- Increased bone density
- Improved sleep quality

Self-Management of Chronic Illness

Note: The Advisory Committee rated the evidence of health benefits of physical activity as strong, moderate, or weak. To do so, the Committee considered the type, number, and quality of studies available, as well as the consistency of findings across studies that addressed each outcome. The Committee also considered evidence for causality and dose-response in assigning the strength-of-evidence rating.

Section 45.5 | Tips for Dealing with Pain

This section contains text excerpted from the following sources: Text in this section begins with excerpts from "Managing Pain," *NIH News in Health,* National Institutes of Health (NIH), October 2018; Text under the heading "Nondrug Pain Management" is excerpted from "Nondrug Pain Management," MedlinePlus, National Institutes of Health (NIH), August 27, 2018.

Most people experience some kind of pain during their lives. Pain serves an important purpose: it warns the body when it is in danger. Think of when your hand touches a hot stove. But ongoing pain causes distress and affects the quality of life (QOL). Pain is the number one reason people see a doctor.

OPIOIDS NOT ALWAYS NEEDED

Opioids are often prescribed for acute pain. Acute pain is short-term pain, the kind experienced after an accident or an operation. But other drugs may be just as effective for acute pain, even after surgery, explains Dr. Dena Fischer, a dental-health expert at the National Institutes of Health (NIH). Some of these drugs, such as acetaminophen or ibuprofen, do not require a prescription.

People may think that prescription drugs work better for acute pain. But that is often not the case, Fischer says. Using something other than an opioid first can be especially important to manage acute pain in fields such as dentistry, she adds.

Many people receiving opioid prescriptions from dentists are teens or young adults who have never been prescribed an opioid before.

"Research is starting to tell us that people who receive an opioid prescription as a teenager have a tendency to continue to take opioids for nonmedical purposes in the long term," Fischer says.

Healthcare providers who decide their patient needs an opioid are now being encouraged to give only a few pills at a time. People who receive shorter prescriptions are less likely to misuse their pills by taking more than prescribed or taking them after the pain is gone. This also cuts down the chance that the pills could be taken by others.

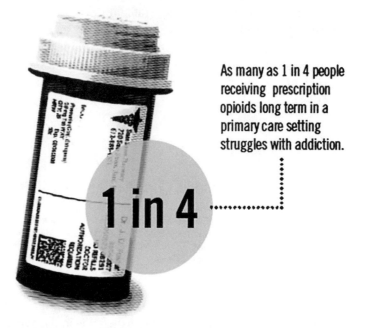

As many as 1 in 4 people receiving prescription opioids long term in a primary care setting struggles with addiction.

1 in 4

Figure 45.4. Opioids and Risk of Addiction *(Source: "Promoting Safer and More Effective Pain Management," Centers for Disease Control and Prevention (CDC))*

WHEN PAIN IS CHRONIC

Managing chronic pain is more complicated than treating acute pain. More than 25 million people in the United States alone live with chronic pain, which is pain that lasts more than 3 months.

Many things can cause chronic pain. For example, Dr. Michael Oshinsky, NIH pain expert says, a muscle that was damaged in an accident may heal relatively quickly. But if a nerve was also hurt, it can continue to send pain signals long after the body has repaired the muscle.

Other types of chronic pain are driven by brain changes, explains Dr. David Williams, an NIH-funded pain researcher at the University of Michigan. When these changes happen, the brain continues to perceive pain even though the injury has healed. For people with this type of chronic pain, sometimes called "central pain," opioids and some other kinds of pain medications can actually make the pain worse.

Research has shown that talk therapies, such as cognitive-behavioral therapy (CBT), can help many people with chronic central pain. These types of therapies "emphasize behaving in different ways or thinking in different ways that alter the perception of pain," Williams explains. "Pain is a combination of a sensory and an emotional experience."

Self-Management of Chronic Illness

Cognitive-behavioral therapy can also help people with chronic pain management-related health problems, such as problems sleeping, feeling tired, or trouble concentrating. This can increase QOL for people with chronic pain. It can also have overlapping effects.

"Pain processing and sleep and thinking and mood all share the same neurotransmitters in the brain," Williams says. "So, by improving something like sleep, you're also improving pain."

Nonopioid drugs can help some people with chronic pain too, Oshinsky says. Many of these drugs were first developed to treat different health conditions, such as seizures, depression, or anxiety. But, they can also change the way the brain processes pain.

Some people benefit from devices that stimulate the nerves directly to block pain signals from reaching the brain, Oshinsky adds. Different devices can work on different parts of the nervous system, from the nerves in the skin to the spinal cord.

People with certain types of pain have also been shown to benefit from exercise, acupuncture, massage therapy, or yoga.

EXPANDING THE OPTIONS

The alternatives to opioids available in the market do not work for everyone's pain. More nonopioid, nonaddictive treatment options could help reduce the number of opioids prescribed each year. The NIH launched the Helping to End Addiction Long-Term (HEAL) Initiative to address the shortage of effective medications for chronic pain and other issues contributing to the opioid crisis. Some of the research funded by HEAL will focus on understanding how chronic pain develops. A better understanding of how acute pain becomes chronic could reveal new treatment targets.

Researchers funded by HEAL also hope to learn how to predict who will develop chronic pain from acute pain. This information could be used to guide early pain management, Oshinsky explains. HEAL will fund research into new treatments for opioid misuse and addiction as well.

More options for pain management could help doctors better personalize pain treatment. "It could be a little more like precision medicine, where you try to identify what flavour of pain the patient has, and then match the treatments we have available to the needs of that patient," Williams explains.

Dealing Safely with Pain

You can do the following if you are prescribed an opioid:

- Ask if there are ways besides opioids to relieve your pain.
- Make sure your healthcare provider knows about all other medications you are taking.

- Let your healthcare provider know if you or others in your family have had any problems with addiction, such as with alcohol, prescription medications, or illicit drugs.
- Ask about the risks of taking an opioid.
- Ask how to take the opioid and how long you should take it.
- Never use alcohol when taking an opioid.
- Store opioids in a safe place out of sight and out of reach of children, preferably in a locked cabinet.
- Dispose of leftover prescription medicine quickly and properly.

NONDRUG PAIN MANAGEMENT

There are many nondrug treatments that can help with pain. It is important to check with your healthcare provider before trying any of them:

- **Acupuncture** involves stimulating acupuncture points. These are specific points on your body. There are different acupuncture methods. The most common one involves inserting thin needles through the skin. Others include using pressure, electrical stimulation, and heat. Acupuncture is based on the belief that qi (vital energy) flows through the body along paths, called "meridians." Practitioners believe that stimulating the acupuncture points can rebalance the qi. Research suggests that acupuncture can help manage certain pain conditions.
- **Biofeedback techniques** use electronic devices to measure body functions such as breathing and heart rate. This teaches you to be more aware of your body functions so you can learn to control them. For example, a biofeedback device may show you measurements of your muscle tension. By watching how these measurements change, you can become more aware of when your muscles are tense and learn to relax them. Biofeedback may help to control pain, including chronic headaches and back pain.
- **Electrical stimulation** involves using a device to send a gentle electric current to your nerves or muscles. This can help treat pain by interrupting or blocking the pain signals. Types include:
  - Transcutaneous electrical stimulation (TENS)
  - Implanted electric nerve stimulation
  - Deep brain or spinal cord stimulation
- **Massage therapy** is a treatment in which the soft tissues of the body are kneaded, rubbed, tapped, and stroked. Among other benefits, it may help people relax, and relieve stress and pain.
- **Meditation** is a mind-body practice in which you focus your attention on something, such as an object, word, phrase, or breathing. This helps you to minimize distracting or stressful thoughts or feelings.

- **Physical therapy** uses techniques such as heat, cold, exercise, massage, and manipulation. It can help to control pain, as well as condition muscles and restore strength.
- **Psychotherapy (talk therapy)** uses methods such as discussion, listening, and counseling to treat mental and behavioral disorders. It can also help people who have pain, especially chronic pain, by:
    - Teaching them coping skills, to be able to better deal with the stress that pain can cause
    - Addressing negative thoughts and emotions that can make pain worse
    - Providing them with support
- **Relaxation therapy** can help reduce muscle tension and stress, lower blood pressure, and control pain. It may involve tensing and relaxing muscles throughout the body. It may be used with guided imagery (focusing the mind on positive images) and meditation.
- **Surgery** can sometimes be necessary to treat severe pain, especially when it is caused by back problems or serious musculoskeletal injuries. There are always risks to getting surgery, and it does not always work to treat pain. So, it is important to go through all of the risks and benefits with your healthcare provider.

Section 45.6 | Relaxation Techniques for Health

This section includes text excerpted from "Relaxation Techniques for Health," National Center for Complementary and Integrative Health (NCCIH), May 2016. Reviewed December 2019.

WHAT ARE RELAXATION TECHNIQUES?

Relaxation techniques include a number of practices, such as progressive relaxation, guided imagery, biofeedback, self-hypnosis, and deep breathing exercises. The goal is similar in all: to produce the body's natural relaxation response, characterized by slower breathing, lower blood pressure, and a feeling of increased well-being.

Meditation and practices that include meditation with movement, such as yoga and tai chi, can also promote relaxation.

Stress management programs commonly include relaxation techniques. Relaxation techniques have also been studied to see whether they might be of value in managing various health problems.

The Importance of Practice

Relaxation techniques are skills, and as of other skills, they need practice. People who use relaxation techniques frequently are more likely to benefit from them. Regular, frequent practice is particularly important if you are using relaxation techniques to help manage a chronic health problem. Continuing use of relaxation techniques is more effective than short-term use.

Various relaxation techniques are described below.

Autogenic Training

In autogenic training, you learn to concentrate on the physical sensations of warmth, heaviness, and relaxation in different parts of your body.

Biofeedback-Assisted Relaxation

Biofeedback techniques measure body functions and give you information about them so that you can learn to control them. Biofeedback-assisted relaxation uses electronic devices to teach you to produce changes in your body that are associated with relaxation, such as reduced muscle tension.

Deep Breathing or Breathing Exercises

This technique involves focusing on taking slow, deep, even breaths.

Guided Imagery

For this technique, people are taught to focus on pleasant images to replace negative or stressful feelings. Guided imagery may be self-directed or led by a practitioner or a recording.

Progressive Relaxation

This technique, also called "Jacobson relaxation" or "progressive muscle relaxation," involves tightening and relaxing various muscle groups. Progressive relaxation is often combined with guided imagery and breathing exercises.

Self-Hypnosis

In self-hypnosis programs, people are taught to produce the relaxation response when prompted by a phrase or nonverbal cue (called a "suggestion").

WHAT THE SCIENCE SAYS ABOUT THE EFFECTIVENESS OF RELAXATION TECHNIQUES

Researchers have evaluated relaxation techniques to see whether they could play a role in managing a variety of health conditions, including the following.

Anxiety. Studies have shown that relaxation techniques may reduce anxiety in people with ongoing health problems, such as heart disease or inflammatory bowel disease (IBD), and in those who are having medical procedures, such as breast biopsies or dental treatment. Relaxation techniques have also been shown to be useful for older adults with anxiety. On the other hand, relaxation techniques may not be the best way to help people with generalized anxiety disorder (GAD). GAD is a mental-health condition, lasting for months or longer, in which a person is often worried or anxious about many things and finds it hard to control the anxiety. Studies indicate that long-term results are better in people with GAD who receive a type of psychotherapy called "cognitive-behavioral therapy" (CBT) than in those who are taught relaxation techniques.

Asthma. There has not been enough research to show whether relaxation techniques can relieve asthma symptoms in either adults or children.

Childbirth. Relaxation techniques, such as guided imagery, progressive muscle relaxation, and breathing techniques may be useful in managing labor pain. Studies have shown that women who were taught self-hypnosis have a decreased need for pain medicine during labor. Biofeedback has not been shown to relieve labor pain.

Depression. An evaluation of 15 studies concluded that relaxation techniques are better than no treatment in reducing symptoms of depression but are not as beneficial as psychological therapies, such as CBT.

Epilepsy. There is no reliable evidence that relaxation techniques are useful in managing epilepsy.

Fibromyalgia. Studies of guided imagery for fibromyalgia have had inconsistent results. A 2013 evaluation of the research concluded that electromyographic (EMG) biofeedback, in which people are taught to control and reduce muscle tension, helped to reduce fibromyalgia pain, at least for short periods of time. However, EMG biofeedback did not affect sleep problems, depression, fatigue, or health-related quality of life (QOL) in people with fibromyalgia, and its long-term effects have not been established.

Headache. Biofeedback has been studied for both tension headaches and migraines. An evaluation of high-quality studies concluded that there is conflicting evidence about whether biofeedback can relieve tension headaches. Studies have shown decreases in the frequency of migraines in people who were using biofeedback. However, it is unclear whether biofeedback is better than a placebo. Relaxation techniques other than biofeedback have been studied for tension headaches. An evaluation of high-quality studies found conflicting evidence on whether relaxation techniques are better than no treatment or a placebo. Some studies suggest that other relaxation techniques are less effective than biofeedback.

Heart disease. In people with heart disease, studies have shown relaxation techniques can reduce stress and anxiety and may also have beneficial effects on physical measures, such as heart rate.

High blood pressure. Stress can lead to a short-term increase in blood pressure, and the relaxation response has been shown to reduce blood pressure on a short-term basis, allowing people to reduce their need for blood pressure medication. However, it is uncertain whether relaxation techniques can have long-term effects on high blood pressure.

Insomnia. There is evidence that relaxation techniques can be helpful in managing chronic insomnia. Relaxation techniques can be combined with other strategies for getting a good night's sleep, such as maintaining a consistent sleep schedule; avoiding caffeine, alcohol, heavy meals, and strenuous exercise too close to bedtime; and sleeping in a quiet, cool, dark room.

Irritable bowel syndrome (IBS). An evaluation of research results by the American College of Gastroenterology (ACG) concluded that relaxation techniques have not been shown to help IBS. However, other psychological therapies, including CBT and hypnotherapy, are associated with overall symptom improvement in people with IBS.

Menopause symptoms. Relaxation techniques have been studied for hot flashes and other symptoms associated with menopause, but the quality of the research is not high enough to allow definite conclusions to be reached.

Menstrual cramps. Some research suggests that relaxation techniques may be beneficial for menstrual cramps, but definite conclusions cannot be reached because of the small number of participants in the studies and the poor quality of some of the research.

Nausea. An evaluation of the research evidence concluded that some relaxation techniques, including guided imagery and progressive muscle relaxation, are likely to be effective in relieving nausea caused by cancer chemotherapy when used in combination with antinausea drugs.

Nightmares. Some studies have indicated that relaxation exercises may be an effective approach for nightmares of unknown cause and those associated with posttraumatic stress disorder (PTSD). However, an assessment of many studies concluded that relaxation is less helpful than more extensive forms of treatment (psychotherapy or medication).

Pain. Evaluations of the research evidence have found promising but not conclusive evidence that guided imagery may help relieve some musculoskeletal pain (pain involving the bones or muscles) and other types of pain. An analysis of data on hospitalized cancer patients showed that those who received integrative medicine therapies, such as guided imagery and relaxation response training, during their hospitalization had reductions in both pain and anxiety.

Pain in children and adolescents. A 2014 evaluation of the scientific evidence found that psychological therapies, which may include relaxation techniques as well as other approaches, such as CBT, can reduce pain in children and adolescents with chronic headaches or other types of chronic pain. The evidence is particularly promising for headaches: the effect on pain may last for several months after treatment, and the therapies also help to reduce anxiety.

Posttraumatic stress disorder. Studies of biofeedback and other relaxation techniques for PTSD have had inconsistent results.

Rheumatoid arthritis (RA). There is limited evidence that biofeedback or other relaxation techniques might be valuable additions to treatment programs for RA.

Ringing in the ears (Tinnitus). Only a few studies have evaluated relaxation techniques for ringing in the ears. The limited evidence from these studies suggests that relaxation techniques might be useful, especially in reducing the intrusiveness of the problem.

Smoking cessation. Limited evidence suggests that guided imagery may be a valuable tool for people who are working to quit smoking. In a study that compared the two techniques, autogenic training was found to be less effective than CBT as a quit-smoking aid. However, this study involved patients in an alcohol detoxification program, so its results may not be applicable to other people. Preliminary research suggests that a guided relaxation routine might help reduce cigarette cravings.

Temporomandibular joint (TMJ) dysfunction. Problems with the TMJ (the joint that connects the jaw to the side of the head) can cause pain and difficulty moving the jaw. A few studies have shown that programs that include relaxation techniques may help relieve symptoms of TMJ dysfunction.

WHAT THE SCIENCE SAYS ABOUT THE SAFETY AND SIDE EFFECTS OF RELAXATION TECHNIQUES

Relaxation techniques are generally considered safe for healthy people. However, occasionally, people report negative experiences, such as increased anxiety, intrusive thoughts, or fear of losing control.

There have been rare reports that certain relaxation techniques might cause or worsen symptoms in people with epilepsy or certain psychiatric conditions, or with a history of abuse or trauma. People with heart disease should talk to their healthcare provider before doing progressive muscle relaxation.

WHO TEACHES RELAXATION TECHNIQUES?

A variety of professionals, including physicians, psychologists, social workers, nurses, and complementary-health practitioners, may teach relaxation techniques. Also, people sometimes learn the simpler relaxation techniques on their own.

MORE TO CONSIDER

If you have severe or long-lasting symptoms of any kind, see your healthcare provider. You might have a condition that needs to be treated promptly. For example, if depression or anxiety persists, it is important to seek help from a qualified healthcare professional.

Tell all your healthcare providers about any complementary or integrative health approaches you use. Give them a full picture of what you do to manage your health. This will help ensure coordinated and safe care.

Section 45.7 | The Health Benefits of Having Pets

This section includes text excerpted from "The Power of Pets," *NIH News in Health,* National Institutes of Health (NIH), February 2018.

Nothing compares to the joy of coming home to a loyal companion. The unconditional love of a pet can do more than keep you company. Pets may also decrease stress, improve heart health, and even help children with their emotional and social skills.

An estimated 68 percent of U.S. households have a pet. But, who benefits from an animal? And which type of pet brings health benefits?

Over the past 10 years, the National Institutes of Health (NIH) has partnered with the Mars Corporation's Waltham Centre for Pet Nutrition to answer questions such as these by funding research studies. Scientists are looking at what the potential physical- and mental-health benefits are for different animals—from fish to guinea pigs to dogs and cats.

POSSIBLE HEALTH EFFECTS

Research on human–animal interactions is still relatively new. Some studies have shown positive health effects, but the results have been mixed.

Interacting with animals has been shown to decrease levels of cortisol (a stress-related hormone) and lower blood pressure. Other studies have found that animals can reduce loneliness, increase feelings of social support, and boost your mood.

Self-Management of Chronic Illness

The NIH/Mars Partnership is funding a range of studies focused on the relationship humans have with animals. For example, researchers are looking into how animals might influence child development. They are studying animal interactions with kids who have autism, attention deficit hyperactivity disorder (ADHD), and other conditions.

"There's not one answer about how a pet can help somebody with a specific condition," explains Dr. Layla Esposito, who oversees NIH's Human–Animal Interaction Research Program. "Is your goal to increase physical activity? Then you might benefit from owning a dog. You have to walk a dog several times a day and you're going to increase physical activity. If your goal is reducing stress, sometimes watching fish swim can result in a feeling of calmness. So there's no one type fits all."

The NIH is funding large-scale surveys to find out the range of pets people live with and how their relationships with their pets relate to health.

"We're trying to tap into the subjective quality of the relationship with the animal—that part of the bond that people feel with animals—and how that translates into some of the health benefits," explains Dr. James Griffin, a child-development expert at the NIH.

ANIMALS HELPING PEOPLE

Animals can serve as a source of comfort and support. Therapy dogs are especially good at this. They are sometimes brought into hospitals or nursing homes to help reduce patients' stress and anxiety.

"Dogs are very present. If someone is struggling with something, they know how to sit there and be loving," says Dr. Ann Berger, a physician and researcher at the NIH Clinical Center (CC) in Bethesda, Maryland. "Their attention is focused on the person all the time."

Berger works with people who have cancer and terminal illnesses. She teaches them about mindfulness to help decrease stress and manage pain.

"The foundations of mindfulness include attention, intention, compassion, and awareness," Berger says. "All of those things are things that animals bring to the table. People kind of have to learn it. Animals do this innately."

Researchers are studying the safety of bringing animals into hospital settings because animals may expose people to more germs. A study is looking at the safety of bringing dogs to visit children with cancer, Esposito says. Scientists will be testing the children's hands to see if there are dangerous levels of germs transferred from the dog after the visit.

Dogs may also aid in the classroom. A study found that dogs can help children with ADHD focus their attention. Researchers enrolled 2 groups of children diagnosed with ADHD into 12-week group-therapy sessions. The first group of kids read to a therapy dog once a week for 30 minutes. The second group read to puppets that resembled dogs.

Kids who read to the real animals showed better social skills and more sharing, cooperation, and volunteering. They also had fewer behavioral problems.

Another study found that children with autism spectrum disorder (ASD) were calmer while playing with guinea pigs in the classroom. When the children spent 10 minutes in a supervised group playtime with guinea pigs, their anxiety levels dropped. The children also had better social interactions and were more engaged with their peers. The researchers suggest that the animals offered unconditional acceptance, making them a calm comfort to the children.

"Animals can become a way of building a bridge for those social interactions," Griffin says. He adds that researchers are trying to better understand these effects and who they might help.

Animals may help you in other unexpected ways. A study showed that caring for fish helped teens with diabetes better manage their disease. Researchers had a group of teens with type 1 diabetes care for a pet fish twice a day by feeding and checking water levels. The caretaking routine also included changing the tank water each week. This was paired with the children reviewing their blood glucose (blood sugar) logs with parents.

Researchers tracked how consistently these teens checked their blood glucose. Compared with teens who were not given a fish to care for, fish-keeping teens were more disciplined about checking their own blood glucose levels, which is essential for maintaining their health.

While pets may bring a wide range of health benefits, an animal may not work for everyone. Studies suggest that early exposure to pets may help protect young children from developing allergies and asthma. But for people who are allergic to certain animals, having pets in the home can do more harm than good.

HELPING EACH OTHER

Pets also bring new responsibilities. Knowing how to care for and feed an animal is part of owning a pet. The NIH/Mars Partnership funds studies looking into the effects of human–animal interactions for both the pet and the person.

Remember that animals can feel stressed and fatigued, too. It is important for kids to be able to recognize signs of stress in their pet and know when not to approach. Animal bites can cause serious harm.

"Dog bite prevention is certainly an issue parents need to consider, especially for young children who don't always know the boundaries of what's appropriate to do with a dog," Esposito explains.

Researchers will continue to explore the many health effects of having a pet. "We're trying to find out what's working, what's not working, and what's safe—for both the humans and the animals," Esposito says.

Chapter 46 | **Preventing Infection at Home and Work**

Germs are a part of everyday life and are found in our air, soil, water, and in and on our bodies. Some germs are helpful, others are harmful. Many germs live in and on our bodies without causing harm and some even help us to stay healthy. Only a small portion of germs are known to cause infection.

HOW DO INFECTIONS OCCUR?

An infection occurs when germs enter the body, increase in number, and cause a reaction of the body. Three things are necessary for an infection to occur: source, susceptible person, and transmission.

Source

A source is an infectious agent or germ and refers to a virus, bacteria, or other microbes.

In healthcare settings, germs are found in many places. People who may be a potential source of germs include:

- Patients
- Healthcare workers
- Visitors and household members

People can be sick with symptoms of an infection or colonized with germs (not have symptoms of an infection but able to pass the germs to others).

Germs are also found in the healthcare environment. Examples of environmental sources of germs include:

- Dry surfaces in patient care areas (e.g., bed rails, medical equipment, countertops, and tables)

This chapter contains text excerpted from the following sources: Text in this chapter begins with excerpts from "How Infections Spread," Centers for Disease Control and Prevention (CDC), January 7, 2016. Reviewed December 2019; Text under the heading "How to Prevent Infections" is excerpted from "Infection Control," MedlinePlus, National Institutes of Health (NIH), June 3, 2019; Text beginning with the heading "Wash Your Hands Often to Stay Healthy" is excerpted from "When and How to Wash Your Hands," Centers for Disease Control and Prevention (CDC), October 3, 2019.

- Wet surfaces, moist environments, and biofilms (e.g., cooling towers, faucets and sinks, and equipment such as ventilators)
- Indwelling medical devices (e.g., catheters and intravenous (IV) lines)
- Dust or decaying debris (e.g., construction dust or wet materials from water leaks)

Susceptible Person

A susceptible person is someone who is not vaccinated or otherwise immune, or a person with a weakened immune system who has a way for germs to enter the body. For an infection to occur, germs must enter a susceptible person's body and invade tissues, multiply, and cause a reaction.

Devices such as IV catheters and surgical incisions can provide an entryway, whereas a healthy immune system helps fight infection.

When patients are sick and receive medical treatment in healthcare facilities, the following factors can increase their susceptibility to infection.

- Patients in healthcare who have underlying medical conditions, such as diabetes, cancer, and organ transplantation are at increased risk for infection because often these illnesses decrease the immune system's ability to fight infection.
- Certain medications used to treat medical conditions, such as antibiotics, steroids, and certain cancer-fighting medications increase the risk of some types of infections.
- Lifesaving medical treatments and procedures used in healthcare, such as urinary catheters, tubes, and surgery increase the risk of infection by providing additional ways that germs can enter the body.

Recognizing the factors that increase patients' susceptibility to infection allows providers to recognize risks and perform basic infection prevention measures to prevent infection from occurring.

Transmission

"Transmission" refers to the way germs are moved to the susceptible person.

Germs do not move themselves. Germs depend on people, the environment, and/or medical equipment to move in healthcare settings.

There are a few general ways that germs travel in healthcare settings—through contact (i.e., touching), sprays and splashes, inhalation, and sharps injuries (i.e., when someone is accidentally stuck with a used needle or sharp instrument).

- Contact moves germs by touch (example: multiresistant *Staphylococcus aureus* (MRSA) or vancomycin-resistant enterococci (VRE)). For example, healthcare provider hands become contaminated by touching germs present on medical equipment or high touch surfaces and then carry the germs on their hands and spread to a susceptible person when proper hand hygiene is not performed before touching the susceptible person.

- Sprays and splashes occur when an infected person coughs or sneezes, creating droplets which carry germs short distances (within approximately 6 feet). These germs can land on a susceptible person's eyes, nose, or mouth and can cause infection (example: pertussis or meningitis).
    - Close range inhalation occurs when a droplet containing germs is small enough to breathe in but not durable over distance.
- Inhalation occurs when germs are aerosolized in tiny particles that survive on air currents over great distances and time and reach a susceptible person. Airborne transmission can occur when infected patients cough, talk, or sneeze germs into the air (example: tuberculosis (TB) or measles), or when germs are aerosolized by medical equipment or by dust from a construction zone (example: Nontuberculous mycobacteria or *aspergillus*).
- Sharps injuries can lead to infections (example: human immunodeficiency virus (HIV), hepatitis B virus (HBV), hepatitis C virus (HCV)) when bloodborne pathogens enter a person through a skin puncture by a used needle or sharp instrument.

HOW TO PREVENT INFECTIONS

Proper hand washing is the most effective way to prevent the spread of infections. If you are a patient, do not be afraid to remind friends, family, and healthcare providers to wash their hands before getting close to you.

Other steps that you can take include:

- Covering coughs and sneezes
- Staying up-to-date with immunizations
- Using gloves, masks, and protective clothing
- Making tissues and hand cleaners available
- Following hospital guidelines when dealing with blood or contaminated items

WASH YOUR HANDS OFTEN TO STAY HEALTHY

Handwashing is one of the best ways to protect yourself and your family from getting sick. Learn when and how you should wash your hands to stay healthy.

You can help yourself and your loved ones stay healthy by washing your hands often, especially during these key times when you are likely to get and spread germs:

- Before, during, and after preparing food

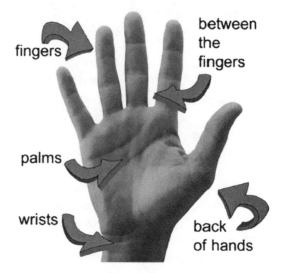

Figure 46.1. Wash Your Hands Thoroughly *(Source: "Where to Wash," U.S. Department of Veterans Affairs (VA))*

- Before eating food
- Before and after caring for someone at home who is sick with vomiting or diarrhea
- Before and after treating a cut or wound
- After using the toilet
- After changing diapers or cleaning up a child who has used the toilet
- After blowing your nose, coughing, or sneezing
- After touching an animal, animal feed, or animal waste
- After handling pet food or pet treats
- After touching garbage

FOLLOW FIVE STEPS TO WASH YOUR HANDS THE RIGHT WAY

Washing your hands is easy, and it is one of the most effective ways to prevent the spread of germs. Clean hands can stop germs from spreading from one person to another and throughout an entire community—from your home and workplace to child care facilities and hospitals.

Follow these five steps every time.

- **Wet** your hands with clean, running water (warm or cold), turn off the tap, and apply soap.
- **Lather** your hands by rubbing them together with the soap. Lather the backs of your hands, between your fingers, and under your nails.
- **Scrub** your hands for at least 20 seconds. Need a timer? Hum the "Happy Birthday" song from beginning to end twice.

Preventing Infection at Home and Work

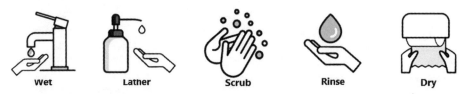

Figure 46.2. Five Steps to Wash Your Hands the Right Way *(Source: "Stop Germs! Wash Your Hands," Centers for Disease Control and Prevention (CDC))*

- **Rinse** your hands well under clean, running water.
- **Dry** your hands using a clean towel or air dry them.

How to Use Hand Sanitizer

- Apply the gel product to the palm of one hand (read the label to learn the correct amount).
- Rub your hands together.
- Rub the gel over all the surfaces of your hands and fingers until your hands are dry. This should take around 20 seconds.

Caution

Swallowing alcohol-based hand sanitizers can cause alcohol poisoning if more than a couple of mouthfuls are swallowed. Keep it out of reach of young children and supervise their use.

Chapter 47 | **Chronic Illness and Depression**

It is common to feel sad or discouraged after a heart attack, cancer diagnosis, or if you are trying to manage a chronic condition such as pain. You may be facing new limits on what you can do and feel anxious about treatment outcomes and the future. It may be hard to adapt to a new reality and to cope with the changes and ongoing treatment that come with the diagnosis. Your favorite activities, such as hiking or gardening, may be harder to do.

Temporary feelings of sadness are expected, but if these and other symptoms last longer than a couple of weeks, you may have depression. Depression affects your ability to carry on with daily life and to enjoy work, leisure, friends, and family. The health effects of depression go beyond mood—depression is a serious medical illness with many symptoms, including physical ones. Some symptoms of depression are:

- Feeling sad, irritable, or anxious
- Feeling empty, hopeless, guilty, or worthless
- Loss of pleasure in usually enjoyed hobbies or activities, including sex
- Fatigue and decreased energy, and feeling listless
- Trouble concentrating, remembering details, and making decisions
- Not being able to sleep, or sleeping too much. Waking up too early.
- Eating too much or not wanting to eat at all, possibly with unplanned weight gain or loss
- Thoughts of death, suicide, or suicide attempts
- Aches or pains, headaches, cramps, or digestive problems without a clear physical cause and/or that do not ease even with treatment

This chapter includes text excerpted from "Chronic Illness and Mental Health: Recognizing and Treating Depression," National Institute of Mental Health (NIMH), December 18, 2015. Reviewed December 2019.

PEOPLE WITH OTHER CHRONIC MEDICAL CONDITIONS HAVE A HIGHER RISK OF DEPRESSION

The same factors that increase the risk of depression in otherwise healthy people also raise the risk in people with other medical illnesses. These risk factors include a personal or family history of depression, or loss of family members to suicide.

However, there are some risk factors directly related to having another illness. For example, conditions such as Parkinson disease (PD) and stroke cause changes in the brain. In some cases, these changes may have a direct role in depression. Illness-related anxiety and stress can also trigger symptoms of depression.

Depression is common among people who have chronic illnesses such as:

- Cancer
- Coronary heart disease (CHD)
- Diabetes
- Epilepsy
- Multiple sclerosis (MS)
- Stroke
- Alzheimer disease (AD)
- Human immunodeficiency virus (HIV)/acquired immunodeficiency syndrome (AIDS)
- Parkinson disease (PD)
- Systemic lupus erythematosus (SLE)
- Rheumatoid arthritis (RA)

Sometimes symptoms of depression may follow a medical diagnosis but lift as you adjust or as the other condition is treated. In other cases, certain medications used to treat an illness may trigger depression. Depression may persist, even as physical health improves.

Research suggests that people who have depression and another medical illness tend to have more severe symptoms of both illnesses. They may have more difficulty adapting to their co-occurring illness and more medical costs than those who also do not have depression.

It is not yet clear whether the treatment of depression when another illness is present can improve physical health. However, it is still important to seek treatment. It can make a difference in day-to-day life if you are coping with a chronic or long-term illness.

PEOPLE WITH DEPRESSION ARE AT HIGHER RISK FOR OTHER MEDICAL CONDITIONS

It may have come as no surprise that people with a medical illness or condition are more likely to suffer from depression. The reverse is also true: the risk of developing some physical illnesses is higher in people with depression.

Chronic Illness and Depression

People with depression have an increased risk of cardiovascular disease, diabetes, stroke, and AD, for example. Research also suggests that people with depression are at higher risk for osteoporosis relative to others. The reasons are not yet clear. One factor with some of these illnesses is that many people with depression may have less access to good medical care. They may have a harder time caring for their health, for example, seeking care, taking prescribed medication, eating well, and exercising.

Ongoing research is also exploring whether physiological changes seen in depression may play a role in increasing the risk of physical illness. In people with depression, scientists have found changes in the way several different systems in the body function, all of which can have an impact on physical health:

- Signs of increased inflammation
- Changes in the control of heart rate and blood circulation
- Abnormalities in stress hormones
- Metabolic changes typical of those seen in people at risk for diabetes

It is not yet clear whether these changes, seen in depression, raise the risk of other medical illness. However, the negative impact of depression on mental health and everyday life is clear.

DEPRESSION IS TREATABLE EVEN WHEN OTHER ILLNESS IS PRESENT

Do not dismiss depression as a normal part of having a chronic illness. Effective treatment for depression is available and can help even if you have another medical illness or condition. If you or a loved one think you have depression, it is important to tell your healthcare provider and explore treatment options.

You should also inform your healthcare provider about all the treatments or medications you are already receiving, including treatment for depression (prescribed medications and dietary supplements). Sharing information can help avoid problems with multiple medications interfering with each other. It also helps the provider stay informed about your overall health and treatment issues.

Recovery from depression takes time, but treatment can improve the quality of life (QOL) even if you have a medical illness. Treatments for depression include:

- **Cognitive-behavioral therapy (CBT), or talk therapy**, that helps people change negative thinking styles and behaviors that may contribute to their depression. Interpersonal and other types of time-limited psychotherapy have also been proven effective, in some cases combined with antidepressant medications.
- **Antidepressant medications,** including, but not limited to, selective serotonin reuptake inhibitors (SSRIs), and serotonin and norepinephrine reuptake inhibitors (SNRIs).

- **While electroconvulsive therapy (ECT)** is generally reserved for the most severe cases of depression, newer brain stimulation approaches, including transcranial magnetic stimulation (TMS), can help some people with depression without the need for general anesthesia and with few side effects.

Chapter 48 | Use of Technologies in Managing Diseases and Improving Health

Chapter Contents

Section 48.1 | Rehabilitative and Assistive Technology

This section includes text excerpted from "About Rehabilitative and Assistive Technology," *Eunice Kennedy Shriver* National Institute of Child Health and Human Development (NICHD), October 24, 2018.

Rehabilitative and assistive technologies are tools, equipment, or products that can help people with disabilities function successfully at school, home, work, and in the community.

Assistive technology can be as simple as a magnifying glass or as complex as a digital communication system. An assistive device can be as large as a power wheelchair lift for a van or as small as a handheld hook that assists with buttoning a shirt.

Tools to help people recover or improve their functioning after injury or illness are sometimes called "rehabilitative technology." But, the term is often used interchangeably with the term "assistive technology."

Rehabilitative engineers use scientific principles to study how people with disabilities function in society. They study barriers to optimal function and design solutions so that people with disabilities can interact successfully in their environments.

The *Eunice Kennedy Shriver* National Institute of Child Health and Human Development (NICHD) supports research on developing and evaluating technologies, devices, instruments, and other aids to help people with disabilities achieve their full potential.

WHAT ARE SOME TYPES OF ASSISTIVE DEVICES AND HOW ARE THEY USED?

Some examples of assistive technologies are:

- **Mobility aids**, such as wheelchairs, scooters, walkers, canes, crutches, prosthetic devices, and orthotic devices.
- **Hearing aids** to help people hear or hear more clearly.
- **Cognitive aids**, including computer or electrical assistive devices, to help people with memory, attention, or other challenges in their thinking skills.
- **Computer software and hardware**, such as voice recognition programs, screen readers, and screen enlargement applications, to help people with mobility and sensory impairments use computers and mobile devices.
- **Tools**, such as automatic page turners, book holders, and adapted pencil grips to help learners with disabilities participate in educational activities.
- **Closed captioning** to allow people with hearing problems to watch movies, television programs, and other digital media.

- **Physical modifications** in the built environment, including ramps, grab bars, and wider doorways to enable access to buildings, businesses, and workplaces.
- **Lightweight, high-performance mobility devices** that enable persons with disabilities to play sports and be physically active.
- **Adaptive switches and utensils** to allow those with limited motor skills to eat, play games, and accomplish other activities.
- **Devices and features of devices** to help perform tasks, such as cooking, dressing, and grooming; specialized handles and grips, devices that extend reach, and lights on telephones and doorbells are a few examples.

WHAT ARE SOME TYPES OF REHABILITATIVE TECHNOLOGIES?

Rehabilitative technologies and techniques help people recover or improve function after injury or illness. Examples include the following:

- **Robotics.** Specialized robots help people regain and improve function in arms or legs after a stroke.
- **Virtual reality.** People who are recovering from injury can restrain themselves to perform motions within a virtual environment.
- **Musculoskeletal modeling and simulations.** These computer simulations of the human body can pinpoint underlying mechanical problems in a person with a movement-related disability. This technique can help improve assistive aids or physical therapies.
- **Transcranial magnetic stimulation (TMS).** TMS sends magnetic impulses through the skull to stimulate the brain. This system can help people who have had a stroke recover movement and brain function.
- **Transcranial direct current stimulation (tDCS).** In tDCS, a mild electrical current travels through the skull and stimulates the brain. This can help recover movement in patients recovering from stroke or other conditions.
- **Motion analysis.** Motion analysis captures video of human motion with specialized computer software that analyzes the motion in detail. The technique gives healthcare providers a detailed picture of a person's specific movement challenges to guide proper therapy.

HOW DOES REHABILITATIVE TECHNOLOGY BENEFIT PEOPLE WITH DISABILITIES?

Rehabilitative technology can help restore or improve function in people who have developed a disability due to disease, injury, or aging. Appropriate assistive technology often helps people with disabilities compensate, at least in part, for a limitation.

Use of Technologies in Managing Diseases and Improving Health

For example, assistive technology enables students with disabilities to compensate for certain impairments. This specialized technology promotes independence and decreases the need for other support.

Rehabilitative and assistive technology can enable individuals to:

- Care for themselves and their families
- Work
- Learn in typical school environments and other educational institutions
- Access information through computers and reading
- Enjoy music, sports, travel, and the arts
- Participate fully in community life

Assistive technology also benefits employers, teachers, family members, and everyone who interacts with people who use the technology.

As assistive technologies become more commonplace, people without disabilities are benefiting from them. For example, people for whom English is a second language are taking advantage of screen readers. Older individuals are using screen enlargers and magnifiers.

The person with a disability, along with her or his caregivers and a team of professionals and consultants, usually decide which type of rehabilitative or assistive technology would be most helpful. The team is trained to match particular technologies to specific needs to help the person function better or more independently. The team may include family doctors, regular and special education teachers, speech-language pathologists, rehabilitation engineers, occupational therapists, and other specialists, including representatives from companies that manufacture assistive technology.

What Conditions May Benefit from Assistive Devices?

Some disabilities are quite visible, while others are "hidden." Most disabilities can be grouped into the following categories:

- **Cognitive disability:** intellectual and learning disabilities/disorders, distractibility, reading disorders, and inability to remember or focus on large amounts of information
- **Hearing disability:** hearing loss or impaired hearing
- **Physical disability:** paralysis, difficulties with walking or other movement, inability to use a computer mouse, slow response time, and difficulty controlling movement
- **Visual disability:** blindness, low vision, and color blindness
- **Mental conditions:** posttraumatic stress disorder (PTSD), anxiety disorders, mood disorders, eating disorders, and psychosis

Hidden disabilities are those that might not be immediately apparent when you look at someone. They can include visual impairments, movement problems, hearing impairments, and mental-health conditions.

Some medical conditions may also contribute to disabilities or may be categorized as hidden disabilities under the Americans with Disabilities Act (ADA). For example, epilepsy; diabetes; sickle cell conditions; human immunodeficiency virus (HIV)/acquired immunodeficiency syndrome (AIDS); cystic fibrosis (CF); cancer; and heart, liver, or kidney problems may lead to problems with mobility or daily function, and may be viewed as disabilities under the law. The conditions may be short term or long term; stable or progressive; constant or unpredictable; and changing, treatable, or untreatable. Many people with hidden disabilities can benefit from assistive technologies for certain activities or during certain stages of their diseases or conditions.

People who have spinal cord injuries (SCIs), traumatic brain injury (TBI), cerebral palsy (CP), muscular dystrophy (MD), spina bifida, osteogenesis imperfecta (OI), multiple sclerosis (MS), demyelinating diseases, myelopathy, progressive muscular atrophy, amputations, or paralysis often benefit from complex rehabilitative technology. The assistive devices are individually configured to help each person with her or his own unique disability.

Section 48.2 | Artificial Pancreas Improves Type 1 Diabetes Management

This section includes text excerpted from "Artificial Pancreas Improves Type 1 Diabetes Management," National Institutes of Health (NIH), October 29, 2019.

Diabetes is a disease that happens when your blood glucose, or blood sugar, is too high. Glucose is the main source of energy of the body. Insulin, a hormone made by the pancreas, tells the body's cells to take in glucose. If you have type 1 diabetes, your body does not make insulin, and glucose builds up in your blood. Over time, high levels of blood glucose can cause serious health problems.

People with diabetes must test their blood glucose regularly with a fingerstick or use a continuous glucose monitor. They take insulin when needed by giving themselves injections or using an insulin pump. Researchers have developed all-in-one diabetes management systems. These "artificial pancreas" systems track blood glucose levels using a continuous glucose monitor, calculate when insulin is needed, and automatically deliver it using an insulin pump. Artificial pancreas systems do not entirely eliminate the need for patient input, but substantially reduce the level of effort.

Use of Technologies in Managing Diseases and Improving Health

To test the efficacy and safety of an artificial pancreas, a team led by Drs. Sue A. Brown and Boris Kovatchev at the University of Virginia and Dr. Roy W. Beck at the Jaeb Center for Health Research carried out a 6-month study of the Control-IQ technology system from Tandem Diabetes Care. They enrolled 168 people with type 1 diabetes. The study was funded by the National Institutes of Health's (NIH) National Institute of Diabetes and Digestive and Kidney Diseases (NIDDK). Results were published online on October 16, 2019, in the *New England Journal of Medicine.*

Participants were randomly assigned to use either the Control-IQ artificial pancreas or sensor-augmented pump (SAP) therapy. SAP uses a continuous glucose monitor and insulin pump, but still requires frequent input and decisions from the user about when and how much insulin to administer. The Control-IQ system uses advanced computer algorithms to automatically adjust insulin doses based on glucose levels.

People who used the artificial pancreas system showed a significant increase in the amount of time their blood glucose levels stayed in the target range of 70 to 180 mg/dL—from 61 percent at the start of the study to 71 percent. This translated to an additional 2.6 hours per day in range. In contrast, the control group remained unchanged at 59 percent. Artificial pancreas users also showed improvements in time spent with high and low blood glucose and other measurements related to diabetes control.

No severe low blood sugar (hypoglycemia) events occurred in either group. Diabetic ketoacidosis—a life-threatening complication—occurred in one participant in the artificial pancreas group due to an issue with the insulin pump setup called "pump infusion" set failure.

"This artificial pancreas system has several unique features that improve glucose control beyond what is achievable using traditional methods," says Kovatchev. "In particular, there is a special safety module dedicated to the prevention of hypoglycemia, and there is gradually intensified control overnight to achieve near-normal blood sugar levels every morning."

"Artificial pancreas technology has tremendous potential to improve the day-to-day lives of people with type 1 diabetes," says NIDDK director Dr. Griffin P. Rodgers. "By making management of type 1 diabetes easier and more precise, this technology could reduce the daily burden of this disease, while also potentially reducing diabetes complications including eye, nerve, and kidney diseases."

Section 48.3 | **Wearable Blood-Pressure Monitor**

This section includes text excerpted from "A Wearable Blood Pressure Monitor May Be in Our Future," MedlinePlus, National Institutes of Health (NIH), January 14, 2019.

More and more consumers are using health monitors they can wear. These wearables make it easier for patients to track their own health on a daily basis and stay motivated.

Soon, blood pressure may be something patients can track with wearables 24/7. Researchers supported by the National Institutes of Health (NIH) are testing a new wearable that can monitor a patient's blood pressure with a small, wearable skin patch.

The patch monitors a patient's blood pressure more accurately than other methods, such as an inflatable cuff around the arm. This is because it is able to record blood pressure in the central arteries and veins, which are located in our necks. The patch's ultrasound waves monitor subtle, real-time changes in the shape and size of pulsing blood vessels. These changes indicate when pressure rises and drops. The sensor can monitor pulses more than an inch beneath the skin. That is deeper than previous patches and other skin sensors.

The National Institutes of Health's (NIH) director Francis H. Collins, M.D., Ph.D., said the new technology shows great promise. "So far, the new device appears to function better than any commercially available, noninvasive device for measuring central blood pressure," he wrote in his blog.

As of now, the patch needs to be connected to wires to monitor central blood pressure, but the researchers hope to develop a wireless version. "The hope is that one day soon their device will offer round-the-clock monitoring of central blood pressure. That could utterly transform our management of hypertension," Dr. Collins added.

Section 48.4 | **Using Artificial Intelligence to Catch Irregular Heartbeats**

This section includes text excerpted from "Using Artificial Intelligence to Catch Irregular Heartbeats," National Institutes of Health (NIH), January 15, 2019.

Thanks to advances in wearable health technologies, it is now possible for people to monitor their heart rhythms at home for days, weeks, or even months via wireless electrocardiogram (EKG) patches. In fact, the Apple Watch makes it possible to record a real-time EKG whenever you want.

Use of Technologies in Managing Diseases and Improving Health

For true medical benefit, however, the challenge lies in analyzing the vast amounts of data—often hundreds of hours' worth per person—to distinguish reliably between harmless rhythm irregularities and potentially life-threatening problems. Now, the researchers at the National Institutes of Health (NIH)-funded researchers have found that artificial intelligence (AI) can help.

A powerful computer "studied" more than 90,000 EKG recordings, from which it "learned" to recognize patterns, form rules, and apply them accurately to future EKG readings. The computer became so "smart" that it could classify 10 different types of irregular heart rhythms, including atrial fibrillation (AFib). In fact, after just seven months of training, the computer-devised algorithm was as good—and in some cases even better than—cardiology experts at making the correct diagnostic call.

Electrocardiogram tests measure electrical impulses in the heart, which signals the heart muscle to contract and pump blood to the rest of the body. The precise, wave-like features of the electrical impulses allow doctors to determine whether a person's heart is beating normally. For example, in people with AFib, the heart's upper chambers (the atria) contract rapidly and unpredictably, causing the ventricles (the main heart muscle) to contract irregularly rather than in a steady rhythm. This is an important arrhythmia to detect, even if it may only be present occasionally over many days of monitoring. That is not always easy to do with current methods.

Here is where the team, led by computer scientists Awni Hannun and Andrew Ng of Stanford University in Palo Alto, California, saw an AI opportunity. As published in *Nature Medicine*, the Stanford team started by assembling a large EKG dataset from more than 53,000 people. The data included various forms of arrhythmia and normal heart rhythms from people who had worn the U.S. Food and Drug Administration (FDA)-approved Zio patch for about two weeks.

The Zio patch is a two-by-five-inch adhesive patch, worn much similar to a bandage, on the upper left side of the chest. It is water resistant and can be kept on around the clock while a person sleeps, exercises, or takes a shower. The wireless patch continuously monitors heart rhythms, storing EKG data for later analysis.

The Stanford researchers looked to machine learning to process all the EKG data. In machine learning, computers rely on large datasets of examples in order to learn how to perform a given task. The accuracy improves as the machine "sees" more data.

But the team's real interest was in utilizing a special class of machine learning called "deep neural networks," or "deep learning." Deep learning is inspired by how the human brain's neural networks process information, learning to focus on some details but not others.

In deep learning, computers look for patterns in data. As they begin to "see" complex relationships, some connections in the network are strengthened while others are weakened. The network is typically composed of multiple information-processing layers, which operate on the data and compute increasingly complex and abstract representations.

Those data reach the final output layer, which acts as a classifier, assigning each bit of data to a particular category or, in the case of the EKG readings, a diagnosis. In this way, computers can learn to analyze and sort highly complex data using both more obvious and hidden features.

Ultimately, the computer in the new study could differentiate between EKG readings representing 10 different arrhythmias as well as a normal heart rhythm. It could also tell the difference between irregular heart rhythms and background "noise" caused by interference of one kind or another, such as a jostled or disconnected Zio patch.

For validation, the computer attempted to assign a diagnosis to the EKG readings of 328 additional patients. Independently, several expert cardiologists also read those EKGs and reached a consensus diagnosis for each patient. In almost all cases, the computer's diagnosis agreed with the consensus of the cardiologists. The computer also made its calls much faster.

Next, the researchers compared the computer's diagnosis to those of six individual cardiologists who were not part of the original consensus committee. And, the results show that the computer actually outperformed these experienced cardiologists!

The findings suggest that AI can be used to improve the accuracy and efficiency of EKG readings. In fact, Hannun reports that iRhythm Technologies, maker of the Zio patch, has already incorporated the algorithm into the interpretation now being used to analyze data from real patients.

This surely is just the beginning of AI applications to health and healthcare. In recognition of the opportunities ahead, the NIH launched a working group on AI to explore ways to make the best use of existing data, and harness the potential of AI and machine learning to advance biomedical research and the practice of medicine.

Section 48.5 | Biosensors and Your Health

This section includes text excerpted from "Biosensors and Your Health," *NIH News in Health,* National Institutes of Health (NIH), July 2017.

Your body alerts you to many aspects of your health. Your stomach growling tells you when to eat. A powerful yawn lets you know you are tired. Your body gives off many other valuable signals, but requires technology to detect them. Scientists are looking for new ways to track and use your body's signals to improve your health and manage disease.

Physical activity trackers and step counters are now helping people develop and maintain healthy habits. These devices have also opened doors for people to participate in health research. Researchers are designing more advanced devices called "biosensors" that measure biological, chemical, and physical signs of health.

"The variety of biosensors used by researchers, clinicians, and people from every walk of life is growing," says Dr. Šeila Selimovic, a biosensors expert at the National Institutes of Health (NIH). "Some speed up test results so treatments can be started promptly. Others provide the benefits of continuous monitoring of health conditions. (Biosensors) function in fascinating ways. (They use) chemical attraction, electrical currents, light-detection systems, and compact wireless-sensing technologies."

The mercury thermometer is one of the earliest biosensor technologies used in medicine. In modern thermometers, mercury has been replaced by safer temperature-sensitive probes. But, the goal is still the same: to detect changes in your body temperature.

Another common biosensor used at home is the pregnancy test. Home pregnancy tests use color-changing strips to detect pregnancy hormones in urine. Pregnancy tests are still done in doctor's offices. But, the home test has become a reliable alternative since it was first introduced more than 40 years ago.

The rapid strep test is another commonly used biosensor. If you have a sore throat, your doctor may want to use one to test for bacteria called "*streptococci.*" The rapid strep test can provide results from a swab of the back of your throat in a few minutes—with 95 percent accuracy. Your doctor may still send a throat swab to a lab to confirm a positive test result. But they can use the rapid test results to start treatment immediately.

In parts of the world where public healthcare is not readily available, researchers hope to introduce rapid tests for people living in remote regions to test for infections such as influenza, human immunodeficiency virus (HIV), and hepatitis C. Biosensor technologies can now be combined with smartphone cameras and wireless signaling. These advances make health tests more portable and affordable than lab-based equipment.

Biosensors can also be used to continuously monitor a health condition. Blood-oxygen monitors are now found throughout hospitals and in patients' homes. These devices detect changes in the level of oxygen in the bloodstream. A rapid drop in oxygen can cause brain injury and requires quick medical attention. Blood oxygen monitors are ideal for people with lung and heart conditions, those undergoing anesthesia, or those being treated in intensive, neonatal, or emergency care. Other biosensors can be used to continuously monitor your blood sugar levels (for managing diabetes), blood pressure, or heart rate.

Flexible sensors are making even more types of monitoring possible. A team of engineers, led by Dr. Patrick Mercier and Dr. Joseph Wang at the University of California San Diego, is developing a flexible sensor that measures blood-alcohol levels. It looks similar to a temporary tattoo. The sensor releases a sweat-promoting chemical into the skin and detects alcohol in the sweat. The sensor then sends the information wirelessly to a laptop or mobile device. Similar devices are being developed by other groups to monitor cystic fibrosis (CF) and other diseases and conditions.

At the University of Minnesota, a group of researchers led by Dr. Michael McAlpine has developed inks for 3-D printing sensors that are flexible, stretchable, and sensitive. These sensors can be used to detect human movements, such as flexing a finger. They can be printed directly onto skin and used to detect body signals, such as a pulse. They can also detect chemicals in the environment and be used to warn of hazards.

The NIH also supports research to use sensors to gather data about environmental and other factors involved in childhood asthma. These sensor systems monitor what children are exposed to and their body's reactions. For example, Dr. Zhenyu Li, a biomedical engineer at George Washington University, is developing a sensor that can be worn on a child's wrist to detect formaldehyde, an air pollutant that can trigger asthma.

"Researchers do not have tools at the moment that can monitor environmental triggers, physiological responses, and behavior without interrupting normal activities," Li says. There are many different asthma triggers, he explains. He expects to have a wearable sensor prototype that he and his clinical partners can begin testing with patients. He is also working on a device that can be placed in a child's home to detect multiple air pollutants, just as those found in tobacco smoke and some manufactured wood products, such as flooring and furniture.

Biosensors can be placed inside your body as well. Dr. Natalie Wisniewski, a biomedical engineer at a medical-device company in San Francisco called "Profusa," is developing miniature sensors that can be injected under the skin. These sensors automatically track chemicals in your body without drawing blood. They continuously scan multiple factors at once. Normally, you need to stay in a hospital to have your body chemistry continuously monitored. With this technology, information about the chemicals in your body could be accessed around the clock, from anywhere.

Once placed under the skin, such biosensors can last for months to years. They can monitor various body functions through chemical changes. All this information can be collected on a cell phone app and shared with your physician, a caretaker, or anyone else you choose.

"Health sensors have the potential to dramatically improve the way we practice medicine and shift the focus away from reactive treatments to preventive maintenance," Wisniewski explains.

Use of Technologies in Managing Diseases and Improving Health

Biosensors are quickly becoming part of healthcare routines. New sensor technologies are opening avenues to better health. Researchers are working to develop the biosensors of tomorrow. These could provide access to better health in ways one can not yet imagine.

Section 48.6 | Beyond Games: Using Virtual Reality to Improve Health

This section includes text excerpted from "Beyond Games," *NIH News in Health*, National Institutes of Health (NIH), July 2019.

Virtual reality—often referred to as "VR"—used to be science fiction. Today, it is everywhere. All you need is a smartphone and a headset to immerse yourself in 3-D virtual worlds or games. This booming technology may also be useful for healthcare and research.

"In the last few years, there's been a huge expansion in the number of exciting clinical applications of virtual reality," says Dr. Andrew Huberman, a VR researcher at Stanford University.

The National Institutes of Health (NIH)-funded researchers are finding that VR may help with many areas of medicine. These include tailoring rehabilitation exercises, improving mental health, and reducing pain.

RESTORING MOVEMENT

Scientists have been testing VR to treat movement problems. These can be caused by a stroke, a brain injury, Parkinson disease (PD), or other conditions. Rehabilitation exercises can sometimes help people train their muscles to improve their movement. But, these exercises can be boring—especially to kids.

Dr. Amy Bastian, a movement specialist at the Kennedy Krieger Institute, is using VR to make rehabilitation exercises more engaging for kids. It also lets her team tailor the exercises to individual children's needs.

"With VR, we can do things that are really hard to do in real-world therapy," Bastian says. "If we want you to learn to reach and control your balance in one direction, we can make all the game components move things in that direction."

Virtual reality can also help kids who have trouble following directions, she explains. "We can say something like, 'just punch the red things.' This can get them to do all kinds of complex tasks."

Bastian is also developing VR exercises for adults who have damage to the cerebellum, the part of the brain that coordinates movement. This type of brain injury makes people's movements jerky and uncoordinated.

The team is testing whether other parts of the brain can be taught to coordinate movements instead. But this cannot happen if the eyes can see the body, because the damaged cerebellum tries to take over. That is why her team is putting people into a VR scene where their bodies do not exist. They must reach for targets with now-invisible limbs. Because the people cannot see their arms, other brain areas must take over to complete the task.

Coins fall from the virtual sky when the person makes a smooth movement to grab an object. This instant feedback for a successful movement is vital for the brain to forge new learning pathways, Bastian explains. "In VR, we can manipulate the environment in real time to help them learn to use another brain system."

FIGHTING FEAR

Huberman is using VR to test techniques to help people cope with fear and anxiety. VR is ideal for studying such mental states, he explains.

"Vision, more than any other sense, is the sense that humans use to navigate the world and survive. And, more than any other sense, it drives phobias and anxiety."

What you see can be easily manipulated using a virtual environment. His team is using this aspect of VR to help people learn to manage their fears.

"We can create experiences that are very realistic," Huberman explains. "We can create an experience that's a little bit threatening, or one that's very threatening."

Virtual reality can show people scenes of sharks or spiders, put them high on top of a building, or have them standing in front of a crowd to speak. After their participants have one of these VR experiences, the team teaches them ways to manage their stress and discomfort. These include focused breathing exercises and other techniques. The researchers then put people back into the stressful VR environment to see if the techniques can help them reduce their anxiety in the moment.

A unique advantage of VR, Huberman explains, is that researchers can directly measure signs of anxiety. These include changes in eye movements and pupil size. The study is still in progress, but Huberman says the training seems to be helping people with their anxiety.

DISTRACTING FROM PAIN

In addition to helping people process uncomfortable mental experiences, VR may help people cope with physical discomfort. Researchers are testing how VR can help reduce the pain from certain medical procedures.

Dr. Sam Sharar, a pain expert at the University of Washington, uses VR to distract children and adults who are recovering from burns.

"Burn pain can be really, really bad. It's hard to tolerate," Sharar says. For burns to heal, the wounds must be washed and covered again every day. These procedures are very painful. Drugs that reduce pain often provide only partial relief for people with burn injuries.

Sharar believes VR can relieve pain by distracting the brain. "People have a fixed amount of conscious attention," he says. "If you divert some of that from experiencing a painful procedure to another task, the brain experiences less pain. This happens even though the same pain signal is coming through the skin."

His team and others developed a VR program that places people in a freezing cold virtual world. It engages their eyes and ears to block out what is happening to their skin. It also has a game where people hit a target to distract more of their attention.

The team's studies have shown that the immersive program reduced people's pain during burn care by half compared with playing a regular video game.

Sharar and other researchers continue looking for ways to use virtual environments to provide more effective pain relief. For people with chronic pain, which lasts for more than three months, using VR distraction has not been found to be helpful. His team and others are now using VR to expand access to techniques that have proven to help people manage chronic pain, such as cognitive-behavioral therapy (CBT).

"If VR could be used to deliver this type of therapy in an immersive, virtual environment," Sharar says, "I think that would have tremendous potential to improve self-management of pain."

Virtual reality continues to drop in cost and grow in popularity, Huberman adds. He thinks the feedback it can provide to the senses will also continue to improve. Such improvements could potentially open doors to its use in more areas of healthcare.

Section 48.7 | Online Weight Management

This section contains text excerpted from the following sources: Text in this section begins with excerpts from "Losing Weight," Centers for Disease Control and Prevention (CDC), February 13, 2018; Text under the heading "The Body Weight Planner" is excerpted from "Online Weight Management Gets Personal," *NIH News in Health*, National Institutes of Health (NIH), January 2016. Reviewed December 2019.

It is natural for anyone trying to lose weight to want to lose it very quickly. But evidence shows that people who lose weight gradually and steadily (about 1 to 2 pounds per week) are more successful at keeping weight off. Healthy weight loss is not just about a "diet" or "program." It is about an ongoing lifestyle that includes long-term changes in daily eating and exercise habits.

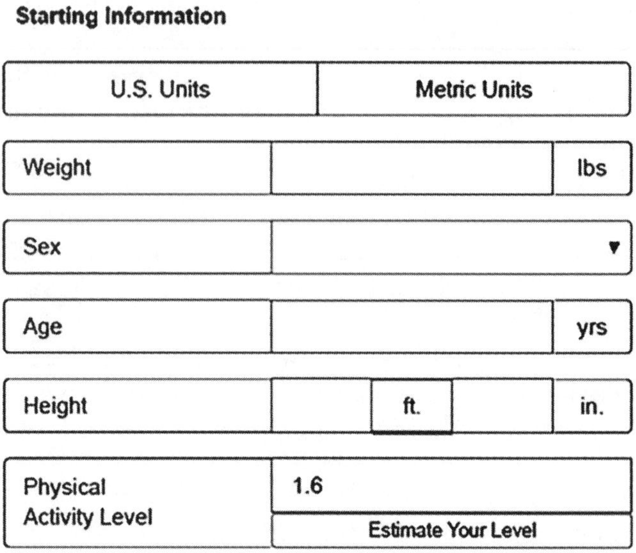

Starting Information

U.S. Units	Metric Units
Weight		lbs
Sex		▼
Age		yrs
Height	ft.	in.
Physical Activity Level	1.6
	Estimate Your Level

Figure 48.1. Body Weight Planner *(Source: "Body Weight Planner," National Institute of Diabetes and Digestive and Kidney Diseases (NIDDK))*

Once you have achieved a healthy weight, by relying on healthful eating and physical activity most days of the week (about 60 to 90 minutes, moderate intensity), you are more likely to be successful at keeping the weight off over the long term.

Losing weight is not easy, and it takes commitment. The good news is that no matter what your weight loss goal is, even a modest weight loss, such as 5 to 10 percent of your total body weight, is likely to produce health benefits, such as improvements in blood pressure, blood cholesterol, and blood sugars.

THE BODY WEIGHT PLANNER

It is always a good time to resolve to eat better, be more active, and lose weight. For the more than two out of three Americans who are either overweight or obese, there is now a free, research-based tool to help you reach your goals: the NIH Body Weight Planner (www.niddk.nih.gov/health-information/weight-management/body-weight-planner?dkrd=lgdmn0001).

"A lot of people want to change their lifestyle to lose weight and improve their overall health but really don't know what it takes," says Dr. Kevin Hall, a senior National Institutes of Health (NIH) researcher who created the Planner. "The Body Weight Planner is the first tool of its kind. It uses specific information about the diet and physical activity changes that are needed to help people reach and stay at their goal weight over time."

Use of Technologies in Managing Diseases and Improving Health

Keeping your body at a healthy weight may help you lower your risk of heart disease, type 2 diabetes, and certain types of cancer that can result from being overweight or obese.

To use the NIH Body Weight Planner, just enter your weight, sex, age, height, and physical activities during work and leisure. Then enter a target date for reaching your goal weight. You can also add details such as percent body fat and metabolic rate. The Planner will then calculate your personal calorie and physical activity targets to achieve your goal and maintain it over time.

"In the past, people have relied on simple rules of thumb, such as cutting 500 calories per day to lose 1 pound of body weight per week," Hall says. "It turns out that this rule overestimates how much weight people actually lose." The NIH Body Weight Planner uses technology based on years of scientific research to accurately calculate how your body adjusts to changes in your eating habits and physical activity.

The NIH Body Weight Planner "has changed my life," says one user. "At 280 pounds, I decided to make a change. I used the Body Weight Planner and set a goal to reach 220 pounds in 180 days. I tracked my calories, dropped weight, and hit the 220 goal. My doctor was really happy."

Hall says the Body Weight Planner is compatible with most web and mobile browsers. NIH is also working to develop mobile apps for tracking your body weight and physical activity, and for assessing how well you stick to your plan over time. This will help you change your plan or goals as needed.

Try the NIH Body Weight Planner to take charge of your weight and your health. Be sure to talk with your healthcare provider about setting realistic and healthy weight goals.

Reaching Weight Loss Goals
Eat Healthy

- Eat smaller portions.
- Select a mix of colorful vegetables each day.
- Choose whole grains.
- Go easy on fats and oils.
- Limit added sugars.

Be Active

- Stick with activities you enjoy.
- Go for a brisk walk, ride a bike, or do some gardening.
- Do strengthening activities. Lift canned food or books if you do not have weights.
- If you are short on time, get active for just 10 minutes, several times a day. Every little bit counts!

Build Healthy Habits

- Make a healthy shopping list and stick to it.
- Keep a food and physical activity diary to track your progress.
- Be realistic and aim for slow, modest weight loss.

Chapter 49 | **Home Improvement Assistance**

Home improvements, modifications, and repairs can help older adults maintain their independence and prevent accidents. Work can range from simple changes, such as replacing door knobs with pull handles, to major structural projects such as installing a wheelchair ramp.

Changes can improve the accessibility, adaptability, and/or universal design of a home. Improving accessibility involves things such as widening doorways and lowering countertop and light switch heights for someone who uses a wheelchair. Changes that do not require home redesign, such as installing grab bars in bathrooms, are adaptability features. Universal design is usually built in when a home is constructed. It includes features that are sturdy and reliable, easy for all people to use, and flexible enough to be adapted for special needs.

EVALUATING YOUR NEEDS

Before any changes are made to the home, evaluate your current and future needs room by room. Once you have explored all areas, make a list of potential problems and solutions. Prepare checklists which will help you to conduct an initial review.

FINANCIAL ASSISTANCE

Minor improvements and repairs can cost between $150 and $2,000. Many home remodeling contractors offer reduced rates or sliding-scale fees based on income and ability to pay.

Public and private financing options may also be available. Sources of support include the following.

- Modification and repair funds provided by the Older Americans Act (OAA) are distributed by Area Agencies on Aging (AAA). To contact your local AAA, contact the Eldercare Locator at 800-677-1116.

This chapter includes text excerpted from "Home Improvement Assistance," Administration for Community Living (ACL), October 18, 2015. Reviewed December 2019.

- Rebuilding Together, Inc., a national volunteer organization, is able to assist some low-income seniors through its local affiliates.
- Local energy and social service departments can assist through the U.S. Department of Energy's (DOE) Low-Income Home Energy Assistance Program (LIHEAP) and Weatherization Assistance Program (WAP).
- Many cities and towns make grant funds available through their local departments of community development.
- Lenders may offer home equity conversion mortgages or reverse mortgages that allow homeowners to utilize home equity to pay for improvements.

Older Americans Act*

Congress passed the OAA in 1965 in response to concern by policymakers about a lack of community social services for older persons. The original legislation established authority for grants to states for community planning and social services, research and development projects, and personnel training in the field of aging. The law also established the Administration on Aging (AoA) to administer the newly created grant programs and to serve as the federal focal point on matters concerning older persons. Although older individuals may receive services under many other federal programs, today the OAA is considered to be a major vehicle for the organization and delivery of social and nutrition services to this group and their caregivers. It authorizes a wide array of service programs through a national network of 56 state agencies on aging, 629 area agencies on aging, nearly 20,000 service providers, 244 Tribal organizations, and 2 Native Hawaiian organizations representing 400 Tribes. The OAA also includes community service employment for low-income older Americans; training, research, and demonstration activities in the field of aging; and vulnerable elder rights protection activities.

*Text excerpted from "Older Americans Act," Administration for Community Living (ACL), November 8, 2017

HIRING A CONTRACTOR

For some repairs and improvements, you may choose to hire a professional contractor without a public-assistance program. In that case, keep these important tips in mind.

- Make sure the contractor is licensed, bonded, and insured for the specific type of work.
- Check with your local Better Business Bureau (BBB) and Chamber of Commerce to see whether any complaints against the contractor are on file.

Home Improvement Assistance

- Talk with family and friends to get recommendations based on their experiences. Contractors with good reputations can usually be counted on to do a good job again.
- Ask for a written agreement that specifies the exact tasks and timeline.
- Your agreement should outline the total estimated cost and require only a small down payment. The terms should require balance payment when the job is completed.
- Consider asking a trusted friend or family member to help you review the contract and/or monitor work throughout the project.

Chapter 50 | **Transitional Care Planning**

When you learn that the disease you are having has reached an advanced stage, you are faced with many decisions about your end-of-life care. Talking about these decisions early can make it easier on you and your family later. The following are some questions you may want to think about:

- What is important to you during this time?
- Is it most important that you be as comfortable and alert as possible during the last stages of the disease?
- Is it most important to continue with treatments that may help you live longer but make you uncomfortable?

DECIDE WHAT QUALITY CARE AT THE END-OF-LIFE MEANS FOR YOU

Some patients choose to receive all possible treatments. Others choose to receive only some treatments or no treatment at all. Some choose to receive only care that will keep them comfortable. Having information about your options will help you make these choices. Together, you, your family, and your doctor can decide on a plan for your care during the advanced stages of the disease.

Your care continues even after all treatments have stopped. End-of-life care is more than what happens moments before dying. Care is needed in the days, weeks, and sometimes even months before death.

During this time, many patients feel it is important to:

- Have their pain and symptoms controlled
- Avoid a long process of dying
- Feel a sense of control over what is happening to them
- Cause less emotional and financial burden on the family
- Become closer with loved ones

Your doctors and family need to know the kind of end-of-life care you want.

This chapter includes text excerpted from "Planning the Transition to End-of-Life Care in Advanced Cancer (PDQ®)—Patient Version," National Cancer Institute (NCI), November 24, 2015. Reviewed December 2019.

MAKE END-OF-LIFE CARE DECISIONS EARLY

You may be able to think about your options more clearly if you talk about them before the decisions need to be made. It is a good idea to let your doctors, family, and caregivers know your wishes before there is an emergency.

TALKING WITH YOUR DOCTOR ABOUT END-OF-LIFE CARE
You May Need to Start the Conversation

Some doctors do not ask patients about end-of-life issues. If you want to make choices about these issues, talk with your doctors so that your wishes can be carried out. Open communication can help you and your doctors make decisions together and create a plan of care that meets your goals and wishes. If your doctor is not comfortable talking about end-of-life plans, you can talk to other specialists for help.

Understand Your Prognosis

Having a good understanding of your prognosis is important when making decisions about your care and treatment. You will probably want to know how long you have to live. That is a hard question for doctors to answer. It can be different for each person. Treatments can work differently for each person. Your doctor can talk about the treatment options with you and your family and explain the effects they may have on your quality of life (QOL). Knowing the benefits and risks of available treatments can help you decide on your goals of care.

Decide on Your Care Goals

Your care goals depends in part on whether QOL or length of life is more important to you. Your goals of care may change as your condition changes or if new treatments become available. Tell your doctor what your goals of care are, even if you are not asked. It is important that you and your doctor are working toward the same goals.

Take Part in Making Decisions

Do you want to take part in making the decisions about your care? Or would you rather have your family and your doctors make those decisions? This is a personal choice and your family and doctors need to know what you want.

Many patients who start talking with their doctors early about end-of-life issues report feeling better prepared. Better communication with your doctors may make it easier to deal with concerns about being older, living alone, relieving symptoms, spiritual well-being, and how your family will cope in the future.

THE TRANSITION TO END-OF-LIFE CARE

The word "transition" can mean a passage from one place to another. The transition or change from looking toward recovery to receiving end-of-life care is not an easy one and there are important decisions to be made. If you become too sick before you have made your wishes known, others will make care and treatment decisions for you, without knowing what you would have wanted. It may be less stressful for everyone if you, your family, and your healthcare providers have planned ahead for this time.

The goal of end-of-life care is to prevent suffering and relieve symptoms. The right time to transition to end-of-life care is when this supports your changing conditions and changing goals of care.

There are certain times when you may think about stopping treatment and transitioning to comfort care. These include:

- Finding out that the disease is not responding to treatment and that more treatment is not likely to help
- Having poor QOL due to the side effects or complications of treatment
- Being unable to carry out daily activities when the disease progresses

Together with your doctor, you and your family members can share an understanding about treatment choices and when transition to end-of-life care is the best choice. When you make the decisions and plans, doctors and family members can be sure they are doing what you want.

Chapter 51 | **Palliative and Hospice Care**

Many Americans die in facilities such as hospitals or nursing homes receiving care that is not consistent with their wishes. To make sure that does not happen, older people need to know what their end-of-life care options are and state their preferences to their caregivers in advance. For example, if an older person wants to die at home, receiving end-of-life care for pain and other symptoms, and makes this known to healthcare providers and family, it is less likely she or he will die in a hospital receiving unwanted treatments.

Caregivers have several factors to consider when choosing end-of-life care, including the older person's desire to pursue life-extending or curative treatments, how long she or he has left to live, and the preferred setting for care.

UNDERSTANDING PALLIATIVE CARE

Doctors can provide treatment to seriously ill patients in the hopes of a cure for as long as possible. These patients may also receive medical care for their symptoms, or palliative care, along with curative treatment.

A palliative care consultation team is a multidisciplinary team that works with the patient, family, and the patient's other doctors to provide medical, social, emotional, and practical support. The team is made of palliative care specialist doctors and nurses, and includes others, such as social workers, nutritionists, and chaplains.

Palliative care can be provided in hospitals, nursing homes, outpatient palliative care clinics, and certain other specialized clinics, or at home. Medicare, Medicaid, and insurance policies may cover palliative care. Veterans may be eligible for palliative care through the U.S. Department of Veterans Affairs (VA). Private health insurance might pay for some services. Health insurance providers can answer questions about what they will cover. Check to see if insurance will cover your particular situation.

This chapter includes text excerpted from "What Are Palliative Care and Hospice Care?" National Institute on Aging (NIA), National Institutes of Health (NIH), May 17, 2017.

In palliative care, you do not have to give up treatment that might cure a serious illness. Palliative care can be provided along with curative treatment and may begin at the time of diagnosis. Over time, if the doctor or the palliative care team believes ongoing treatment is no longer helping, there are two possibilities. Palliative care could transition to hospice care if the doctor believes the person is likely to die within six months.

UNDERSTANDING HOSPICE CARE

Increasingly, people are choosing hospice care at the end of life. Hospice can be provided in any setting—home, nursing home, assisted-living facility, or inpatient hospital.

At some point, it may not be possible to cure a serious illness, or a patient may choose not to undergo certain treatments. Hospice is designed for this situation. The patient beginning hospice care understands that her or his illness is not responding to medical attempts to cure it or to slow the disease's progress.

Like palliative care, hospice provides comprehensive comfort care as well as support for the family, but, in hospice, attempts to cure the person's illness are stopped. Hospice is provided for a person with a terminal illness whose doctor believes she or he has 6 months or less to live if the illness runs its natural course.

Hospice is an approach to care, so it is not tied to a specific place. It can be offered in two types of settings—at home or in a facility such as a nursing home, hospital, or even in a separate hospice center.

Hospice care brings together a team of people with special skills—among them nurses, doctors, social workers, spiritual advisors, and trained volunteers. Everyone works together with the person who is dying, the caregiver, and/or the family to provide the medical, emotional, and spiritual support needed.

A member of the hospice team visits regularly, and someone is always available by phone—24 hours a day, 7 days a week. Hospice may be covered by Medicare and other insurance companies; check to see if insurance will cover your particular situation.

It is important to remember that stopping treatment aimed at curing an illness does not mean discontinuing all treatment. A good example is an older person with cancer. If the doctor determines that the cancer is not responding to chemotherapy and the patient chooses to enter into hospice care, then the chemotherapy will stop. Other medical care may continue as long as it is helpful. For example, if the person has high blood pressure, she or he will still get medicine for that.

Although hospice provides a lot of support, the day-to-day care of a person dying at home is provided by family and friends. The hospice team coaches family members on how to care for the dying person and even provides respite care when caregivers need a break. Respite care can be for as short as a few hours or for as long as several weeks.

Families of people who received care through a hospice program are more satisfied with end-of-life care than are those of people who did not have hospice services. Also, hospice recipients are more likely to have their pain controlled and less likely to undergo tests or be given medicines they do not need, compared with people who do not use hospice care.

What Does the Hospice Six-Month Requirement Mean?

Some people misinterpret their doctors' suggestion to consider hospice. They think it means death is very near. But, that is not always the case. Sometimes, people do not begin hospice care soon enough to take full advantage of the help it offers. Perhaps they wait too long to begin hospice; they are too close to death. Or, some people are not eligible for hospice care soon enough to receive its full benefit.

In the United States, people enrolled in Medicare can receive hospice care if their healthcare provider thinks they have less than six months to live should the disease take its usual course. Doctors have a hard time predicting how long an older, sick person will live. Health often declines slowly, and some people might need a lot of help with daily living for more than six months before they die.

Talk to the doctor if you think a hospice program might be helpful. If she or he agrees, but thinks it is too soon for Medicare to cover the services, then you can investigate how to pay for the services that are needed.

What happens if someone under hospice care lives longer than six months? If the doctor continues to certify that that person is still close to dying, Medicare can continue to pay for hospice services. It is also possible to leave hospice care for a while and then later return if the healthcare provider still believes that the patient has less than six months to live.

Chapter 52 | **Tips for Caregivers**

It can be a labor of love, and sometimes a job of necessity. Millions of Americans provide unpaid care for someone with a serious health condition each year. These often-unsung heroes provide hours of assistance to others. Yet the stress and strain of caregiving can take a toll on their own health. The National Institutes of Health (NIH)-funded researchers are working to understand the risks these caregivers face. And scientists are seeking better ways to protect caregivers' health.

Many of us will end up becoming or needing a caregiver at some point in our lives. Chances are that we will be helping out older family members who cannot fully care for themselves. Caregiving responsibilities can include everyday tasks, such as helping with meals, schedules, and bathing and dressing. It can also involve managing medicines, doctor visits, health insurance, and money. Caregivers often give emotional support as well.

People who provide unpaid care for an elderly, ill, or disabled family member or friend in the home are called "informal caregivers." Most are middle-aged. Roughly two-thirds are women. Nearly half of informal caregivers assist someone who is age 75 or older. As the elderly population continues to grow nationwide, so will the need for informal caregivers.

Studies have shown that some people can thrive when caring for others. Caregiving may help to strengthen connections to a loved one. Some find joy, fulfillment, and a sense of being appreciated in looking after others. But, for many, the strain of caregiving can become overwhelming. Friends and family often take on the caregiving role without any training. They are expected to meet many complex demands without much help. Many caregivers hold down a full-time job and may also have children or others to care for.

"With all of its rewards, there is a substantial cost to caregiving—financially, physically, and emotionally," says Dr. Richard J. Hodes, director of the NIH's National Institute on Aging (NIA). "One important insight from our research is

This chapter includes text excerpted from "Coping with Caregiving," *NIH News in Health*, National Institutes of Health (NIH), December 6, 2017.

that because of the stress and time demands placed on caregivers, they are less likely to find time to address their own health problems."

Informal caregivers, for example, may be less likely to fill a needed prescription for themselves or get a screening test for breast cancer. "Caregivers also tend to report lower levels of physical activity, poorer nutrition, and poorer sleep or sleep disturbance," says Dr. Erin Kent, an NIH expert on cancer caregiving.

Studies have linked informal caregiving to a variety of long-term health problems. Caregivers are more likely to have heart disease, cancer, diabetes, arthritis, and excess weight. They are also at risk for depression or anxiety. And they are more likely to have problems with memory and paying attention.

"Caregivers may even suffer from physical health problems related to caregiving tasks, such as back or muscle injuries from lifting people," Kent adds.

Caregivers may face different challenges and risks depending on the health of the person they are caring for. Taking care of loved ones with cancer or dementia can be especially demanding. Research suggests that these caregivers bear greater levels of physical and mental burdens than caregivers of the frail elderly or people with diabetes.

"Cancer caregivers often spend more hours per day providing more intensive care over a shorter period of time," Kent says. "The health of cancer patients can deteriorate quickly, which can cause heightened stress for caregivers. And aggressive cancer treatments can leave patients greatly weakened. They may need extra care, and their medications may need to be monitored more often."

Cancer survivorship, too, can bring intense levels of uncertainty and anxiety. "A hallmark of cancer is that it may return months or even years later," Kent says. "Both cancer survivors and their caregivers may struggle to live with ongoing fear and stress of a cancer recurrence."

Dementia can also create unique challenges to caregivers. The healthcare costs alone can take an enormous toll. A study found that out-of-pocket spending for families of dementia patients during the last 5 years of life averaged more than $60,000, which was 81 percent higher than for older people who died from other causes.

Research has found that caregivers for people with dementia have particularly high levels of stress hormones. Caregivers and care recipients often struggle with the problems related to dementia, such as agitation, aggression, trouble sleeping, wandering, and confusion. These caregivers spend more days sick with an infectious disease, have a weaker immune response to the flu vaccine, and have slower wound healing.

One major successful and expanding effort to help ease caregiver stress is known as "REACH" (Resources for Enhancing Alzheimer's Caregiver Health). Just over a decade ago, NIH-funded researchers showed that a supportive, educational program for dementia caregivers could greatly improve their quality of life (QOL) and reduce rates of clinical depression. As part of the program, trained staff connected with caregivers over six months by making several home visits, telephone calls, and structured telephone support sessions.

"REACH showed that what caregivers need is support. They need to know that there are people out there and resources available to help them," says Dr. John Haaga, who oversees the NIH's behavioral and social research related to aging. REACH II, a follow-up intervention, was tailored for culturally diverse caregivers.

The REACH program is now being more widely employed. It has been adapted for use in free community-based programs, such as in local Area Agencies on Aging (AAA). It Is also being used by the U.S. Department of Veterans Affairs (VA) and by the Indian Health Service (IHS), in collaboration with the Administration for Community Living (ACL).

"We know how to support families caring for an older adult. But that knowledge is not easily accessible to the families who need it," says Dr. Laura Gitlin, a coauthor of the REACH study and an expert on caregiving and aging at Johns Hopkins University. "Caregivers need to know it's not only acceptable, but recommended, that they find time to care for themselves. They should consider joining a caregiver's support group, taking breaks each day, and keeping up with their own hobbies and interests."

To learn more about aging-related and dementia caregiver resources, contact the NIH's National Institute on Aging (NIA) at 800-222-2225 or niaic@nia.nih.gov. To learn about cancer-related caregiver resources, contact the NIH's National Cancer Institute (NCI) at 800-422-6237.

SELF-CARE FOR CAREGIVERS

Here are a few tips that will help you to fulfill your role as a caregiver.

- **Get organized.** Make to-do lists, and set a daily routine.
- **Ask for help.** Make a list of ways others can help. For instance, someone might pick up groceries or sit with the person while you do errands.
- **Have a break.** Take breaks each day, and spend time with your friends.
- **Follow your pastime interests.** Keep up with your hobbies and interests.
- **Join a caregiver's support group.** Meeting other caregivers may give you a chance to exchange stories and ideas.
- **Eat healthy.** Eat healthy foods, and exercise as often as you can.
- **See your doctor regularly.** Be sure to tell your healthcare provider that you are a caregiver, and mention if you have symptoms of depression or sickness.
- **Build your skills.** Some hospitals offer classes on how to care for someone with an injury or illness. To find these classes, ask your doctor or contact your local AAA at www.n4a.org.

Part 6 | **Children and Chronic Disease**

Chapter 53 | Caring for a Seriously Ill Child

WHAT IS PEDIATRIC PALLIATIVE CARE?[1]

A child's serious illness affects the entire family. Pediatric palliative care can support everyone. It can help with many serious illnesses, including genetic disorders, cancer, neurological disorders, heart and lung conditions, and others. Whether you are having difficulty managing your child's condition and care or simply want extra support, palliative care can help.

Pediatric palliative care is supportive care for children with serious illnesses and their families. It offers an added layer of support based on your unique needs. Because you are the expert on your child and family, palliative care provides services that you consider important. It can help:

- Ease your child's pain and other symptoms
- Provide emotional support and reduce stress
- Address family concerns
- Communicate with healthcare providers
- Coordinate care and appointments
- Explain complicated terms and care options
- Locate community resources to help your family

Many children need more than relief from symptoms. Palliative care can also help your child:

- Understand a diagnosis
- Communicate effectively with doctors
- Cope with concerns about school and friends
- Receive services, such as art or music therapy
- Find ways to relax and play

This chapter includes text excerpted from documents published by two public domain sources. Text under the headings marked 1 are excerpted from "Pediatric Palliative Care at a Glance," National Institute of Nursing Research (NINR), October 2019; Text under the headings marked 2 are excerpted from "Palliative Care for Children," National Institute of Nursing Research (NINR), July 2015. Reviewed December 2019.

DOES ACCEPTING PALLIATIVE CARE MEAN YOUR FAMILY IS GIVING UP ON OTHER TREATMENTS?[2]

No. The purpose of palliative care is to ease your child's pain and other symptoms and provide emotional and other support to your entire family. Palliative care can help children, from newborns to young adults, and their families—at any stage of a serious illness. Palliative care works alongside other treatments your child may be receiving. In fact, your child can start getting palliative care as soon as you learn about your child's illness.

HOW DO YOU KNOW IF YOUR CHILD OR FAMILY NEEDS PALLIATIVE CARE?[2]

Children living with a serious illness often experience physical and emotional distress related to their disease. Emotional distress is also common among their parents, siblings, and other family members. If your child has a genetic disorder, cancer, neurological disorder, heart or lung condition, or another serious illness, palliative care may help reduce pain and enhance quality of life.

Ask your child's healthcare provider about palliative care if your child or any member of your family (including you):

- Suffers from pain or other symptoms due to serious illness
- Experiences physical pain or emotional distress that is NOT under control
- Needs help understanding your child's health condition
- Needs support coordinating your child's care

HOW CAN YOUR FAMILY GET PALLIATIVE CARE?[2]

The palliative care process can begin when your child's healthcare provider refers you to palliative care services. Or, you or your child can ask your healthcare provider for a referral if you feel that palliative care would be helpful for your child, your family, or yourself.

IF YOUR CHILD IS PUT IN PALLIATIVE CARE, CAN YOUR CHILD STILL SEE THE SAME PRIMARY-HEALTHCARE PROVIDER?[2]

Yes. Your child does not have to change to a new primary-healthcare provider when starting palliative care. The palliative care team and your child's healthcare provider work together to help you and your child decide the best care plan for your child.

WHEN CAN CARE START?[1]

Palliative care can help children at any age or stage of a serious illness, from diagnosis forward. It is available at the same time as any other treatments that doctors may prescribe and can begin as soon as your child needs it. Care for your child and family can begin when your child's healthcare provider refers you to palliative care services. The healthcare provider may suggest a referral, or you can request one.

HOW DOES IT WORK?[1]

Palliative care surrounds your family with a team of specialists who will listen to your needs and work together to meet them.

Every palliative care team is different. Your team may include:

- Doctors
- Nurses
- Child life specialists
- Respite providers
- Art and music therapists
- Chaplains
- Case managers
- Counselors
- Home health aides
- Social workers
- Nutritionists
- Pharmacists

WHERE IS CARE PROVIDED?[1]

Palliative care can be provided in a hospital, during clinic visits, or at home. If palliative care starts in the hospital, your team can help your child make a successful move to your home or other healthcare setting. Depending on your child's condition and treatment, the care team may be able to find a nursing or community care agency to support care at home.

HOW CAN YOUR CHILD'S PAIN BE MANAGED?[2]

The palliative care team can bring your child comfort in many ways. Treating pain often involves medication, but there are also other methods to address a child's discomfort. Your child may feel better with changes such as low lighting, comfortable room temperatures, pleasant smells, guided relaxation, and deep breathing techniques. Your child may welcome additional activities such as video chats, social media, soothing music, and massage and art therapy that may help decrease pain and anxiety.

If your child has an illness that causes pain that is not relieved by drugs such as acetaminophen (Tylenol®) or ibuprofen (Motrin® or Advil®), your child's palliative care team may recommend trying stronger medicines. There is no reason to wait before beginning these medications. Should your child's pain increase, the dose may be safely increased over time to provide relief.

Pain relief can be offered in a hospital, at home, or in other healthcare settings. Your palliative care team will partner with you and your child to learn what is causing discomfort and how best to handle it.

WHO PAYS FOR CARE?[1]

Many insurance plans cover palliative care. Ask your healthcare team to put you in touch with a social worker, case manager, or financial advisor at your hospital or clinic to learn about payment options.

WHAT NEXT?[1]

Talk to your loved ones, including your child, about how palliative care can support your family. Remember, even young children can express their needs and preferences.

Talk to your child's healthcare provider. Prepare by writing down your family's questions about palliative care. It may also help to take notes during the conversation. Visit the Palliative Care Provider Directory of Hospitals to see whether a hospital in your area offers a palliative care program (www.getpalliativecare.org).

Chapter 54 | Questions and Answers about the Pediatric Intensive Care Unit

A stay in the hospital can be unnerving for anyone, especially parents with a seriously ill child in the pediatric intensive care unit (PICU). But both adults and children can benefit from a basic understanding of this specialized unit of the hospital. Knowing more about the PICU, what it is designed to do, how it operates, and who works there can help allay some concerns and better prepare parents and kids for a PICU stay.

WHAT IS PEDIATRIC INTENSIVE CARE UNIT?

The PICU is a section of a hospital devoted to providing the highest level of care to critically ill infants, children, and teenagers. With a much higher staff-to-patient ratio than other hospital areas, the PICU is able to ensure that children are monitored very closely and that help will be available immediately if a quick response is required. In addition, the PICU typically has its own dedicated array of medical technology—such as ventilators, dialysis equipment, medication pumps, and computerized monitoring devices—all of which has been designed for the particular needs of young patients.

WHAT CONDITIONS DO REQUIRE PEDIATRIC INTENSIVE CARE UNIT CARE?

Children with very serious illnesses or injuries are admitted to the PICU when their conditions cannot be treated in the hospital's emergency room, normal pediatric area, or general medical floors. Examples of such conditions include severe trauma from accidents or injuries, poisoning, pneumonia, childhood cancer, and congenital heart defects. Children are also sent to the PICU following certain surgeries, such as organ transplants, brain and heart surgery, and some reconstructive procedures. Depending on the severity of the condition and the treatment required, PICU stays can range from one day to several months.

WHO DOES TAKES CARE OF CHILDREN IN THE PEDIATRIC INTENSIVE CARE UNIT?

The PICU is staffed by a multidisciplinary team of medical professionals who are trained in intensive-care procedures and who specialize in treating and working with children. These include:

- **Attending physicians.** These are doctors who undertake a three-year residency after medical school to become a pediatric specialist and then go through several years of additional training in intensive care.
- **Other PICU physicians.** This includes fellows undergoing advanced pediatric training, residents who are completing their education in pediatrics, and specialists in various medical areas such as cardiology, neurology, and oncology.
- **Nurses.** Staff nurses, who have the most interaction with patients and their families, handle the daily care of patients, monitor and record progress, and work with doctors and other team members to plan and implement treatment. There are also charge nurses, nurse managers, and nurse practitioners, all of whom play a role in the daily operation of the PICU.
- **Other team members.** In addition to doctors and nurses, the PICU team may include pharmacists, medical therapists, technicians, social workers, chaplains, and secretaries or receptionists, all of whom contribute to patient care, family support, and the smooth running of the unit.

WHAT DOES HAPPEN IN THE PEDIATRIC INTENSIVE CARE UNIT?

At first, the PICU may seem hectic and scary. Patients do not always know what is going on; they are regularly disturbed by staff monitoring them or treating other patients; lights go on and off at all hours, and there is frequent noise and activity. Learning in advance about some of the PICU's procedures, routines, and equipment can help children and parents be prepared for their stay. These can include:

- **Admission.** Procedures for admission to the PICU vary depending on whether the child is arriving from a scheduled surgery or an emergency situation. In both instances, the patient will be examined by a team of doctors and nurses, and her or his condition will be assessed. In the case of a routine admission, this could be relatively brief, while in an emergency it may be followed by an intense period of treatment and other attention.

- **Morning rounds.** Almost every PICU has regularly scheduled morning rounds, generally beginning around 7:30. Here the medical team visits each patient, discusses progress, and makes plans for the day's activities. Some PICU units also have formal afternoon rounds, and many of these same types of discussions take place during staff shift changes.

- **Daily routine.** Throughout the day, numerous staff members—physicians, nurses, respiratory therapists, dietitians, pharmacists, and social workers—care for the children on the unit. Some medical procedures are performed right in the PICU, and sometimes patients are moved to other parts of the hospital for testing and treatment.

- **Communication.** In addition to discussing patient status and treatment plans among themselves, PICU staff ensure that they give frequent updates to parents. In some hospitals, parents are invited to observe morning rounds and in others there are formal discussions scheduled with members of the medical team. In all cases, parents are encouraged to ask questions and participate as much as possible in their child's care.

- **Monitors and alarms.** All children in the PICU are attached to monitors that keep track of such functions as breathing, heart rate, and blood pressure, and these often make noises that can be unsettling, such as humming and beeping. On occasion, an alarm might sound. Obviously, this is to alert the staff that something could be wrong, so it is not unusual for them to come rushing in, ask visitors to leave, and begin examining the patient. Although this can be an indication of a serious medical situation, it is just as likely that the alarm has sounded because a child moved, a sensor wire has come loose, or a technician has made an adjustment to the equipment.

- **Intravenous.** Most children in the PICU have intravenous (IV) lines inserted into the veins of their hands or arms to administer medication and other fluids. In some cases, a larger tube is needed to deliver greater volumes of fluid. These are called "central lines" and are inserted into larger blood vessels, such as those in the chest, neck, or groin. There are also arterial lines, which are similar to IVs but are inserted into arteries rather than veins, and may be used to monitor blood pressure and blood oxygen levels.

- **Ventilators.** When kids in the PICU need extra help breathing, they are usually fitted with an oxygen mask on their faces or tubes in their noses. But some patients who need even more help are connected to a ventilator, a machine that actually breathes for them. In these instances, a plastic tube is inserted into the trachea (windpipe) and connected to the ventilator at the other end.

- **Tests.** Since patients in the unit are seriously ill, and treatment must be adjusted frequently, careful monitoring is a vital part of ensuring proper care. Doctors may routinely order tests of the child's blood, urine, and spinal fluid, as well as x-rays, ultrasounds, CT or CAT (computerized tomography) scans, and magnetic resonance imaging (MRI) scans.

- **Medications.** Almost everyone in the PICU is on some kind of medication, and dosages and types might be altered from time to time. Some drugs are given at intervals, such as every few hours, and some are administered continuously through IVs. Because of injury, surgery or medical conditions, children in the PICU may experience pain, so pain medication is frequently given to provide relief. Sedation might also be administered to lessen anxiety and keep the child relaxed.

WHAT IS THE ROLE OF PARENTS IN THE PEDIATRIC INTENSIVE CARE UNIT?

Parents play a critical role in comforting and supporting their children during their stay in the PICU. One important task is to communicate with doctors and nurses and, with older children, explain their condition and prepare them for tests and other procedures. In some hospitals, parents may be able to help bathe young children or change infants' diapers. But just as crucial to the patients' well-being is talking to them, touching them, playing their favorite games, coloring, listening to music, reading stories, or watching videos.

It is also important for parents to take care of themselves during the child's stay. Being with a child in the PICU continuously for more than a few days can be both physically and emotionally exhausting, so it is a good idea for parents to leave the unit frequently to visit the cafeteria or watch television or read in a waiting room. Many hospitals provide comfortable sleeping arrangements for parents with children in the PICU, and it is a good idea to take advantage of these facilities to get some much-needed rest.

WHAT DOES HAPPEN WHEN CHILDREN LEAVE THE PEDIATRIC INTENSIVE CARE UNIT?

Upon leaving the PICU, some patients are sent directly home, but more often they are moved to a regular hospital room where more routine treatment and monitoring will take place for a period of time. Although this is an indication that the child's condition is improving, it can actually be a traumatic experience for some parents who become concerned that their child may not be ready for a reduced level of care. Hospital staff can be a source of support at this time, giving parents detailed updates on progress and providing reassurance. Discharge from

Questions and Answers about the Pediatric Intensive Care Unit

the PICU is a significant milestone on the road to recovery, and generally, both parents and children are relieved to be in a less intense environment.

References

1. "Pediatric Intensive Care Unit (PICU)," Cincinnati Children's Hospital Medical Center, n.d.
2. "PICU Family Guide," Monroe Carell Jr. Children's Hospital at Vanderbilt, June 1, 2016.
3. "PICU Parents Guide," Pediatric Critical Care Unit (PICU), Duke University Medical Center, n.d.
4. Torres, Adalberto, Jr., MD. "When Your Child's in the Pediatric Intensive Care Unit," The Nemours Foundation/KidsHealth®, September 2015.

Chapter 55 | The Civil Rights of Students with Hidden Disabilities

If you are a student with a hidden disability or have interest to know more about how students with hidden disabilities are protected against discrimination by federal law, this chapter is for you.

Section 504 of the Rehabilitation Act of 1973 protects the rights of persons with handicaps in programs and activities that receive federal financial assistance. Section 504 protects the rights not only of individuals with visible disabilities but also those with disabilities that may not be apparent.

Section 504 provides that: "No otherwise qualified individual with handicaps in the United States . . . shall, solely by reason of her or his handicap, be excluded from the participation in, be denied the benefits of, or be subjected to discrimination under any program or activity receiving federal financial assistance...."

The U.S. Department of Education (ED) enforces Section 504 in programs and activities that receive financial assistance from ED. Recipients of this assistance include public-school districts, institutions of higher education, and other state and local education agencies. ED maintains an Office for Civil Rights (OCR), with 10 regional offices and a headquarters office in Washington, D.C., to enforce Section 504 and other civil rights laws that pertain to recipients of ED funds.

DISABILITIES COVERED UNDER SECTION 504

The ED Section 504 regulation defines an "individual with handicaps" as any person who has a physical or mental impairment which substantially limits one or more major life activities, has a record of such an impairment, or is regarded as having such an impairment. The regulation further defines a physical or mental impairment as any physiological disorder or condition, cosmetic disfigurement,

This chapter includes text excerpted from "The Civil Rights of Students with Hidden Disabilities under Section 504 of the Rehabilitation Act of 1973," U.S. Department of Education (ED), 2001. September 25, 2018.

or anatomical loss affecting one or more of the following body systems: neurological; musculoskeletal; special sense organs; respiratory, including speech organs; cardiovascular; reproductive; digestive; genitourinary; hemic and lymphatic; skin; and endocrine; or any mental or psychological disorder, such as mental retardation, organic brain syndrome, emotional or mental illness, and specific learning disabilities. The definition does not set forth a list of specific diseases and conditions that constitute physical or mental impairments because of the difficulty of ensuring the comprehensiveness of any such list.

The key factor in determining whether a person is considered an "individual with handicaps" covered by Section 504 is whether the physical or mental impairment results in a substantial limitation of one or more major life activities. "Major life activities," as defined in the regulation, include functions such as caring for one's self, performing manual tasks, walking, seeing, hearing, speaking, breathing, learning, and working.

The impairment must have a material effect on one's ability to perform a major life activity. For example, an individual who has a physical or mental impairment would not be considered a person with handicaps if the condition does not in any way limit the individual, or only results in some minor limitation. However, in some cases, Section 504 also protects individuals who do not have a handicapping condition but are treated as though they do because they have a history of, or have been misclassified as having, a mental or physical impairment that substantially limits one or more major life activities. For example, if you have a history of a handicapping condition but no longer have the condition, or have been incorrectly classified as having such a condition, you too are protected from discrimination under Section 504. Frequently occurring examples of the first group are persons with histories of mental or emotional illness, heart disease, or cancer; of the second group, persons who have been misclassified as mentally retarded. Persons who are not disabled may be covered by Section 504 also if they are treated as if they are handicapped, for example, if they are infected with the human immunodeficiency virus (HIV).

WHAT ARE HIDDEN DISABILITIES?

Hidden disabilities are physical or mental impairments that are not readily apparent to others. They include such conditions and diseases as specific learning disabilities, diabetes, epilepsy, and allergy. A disability, such as a limp, paralysis, total blindness, or deafness is usually obvious to others. But, hidden disabilities, such as low vision, poor hearing, heart disease, or chronic illness may not be obvious. A chronic illness involves a recurring and long-term disability, such as diabetes, heart disease, kidney and liver disease, high blood pressure, or ulcers.

Approximately 4 million students with disabilities are enrolled in public elementary and secondary schools in the United States. Of these 43 percent are students classified as learning disabled, 8 percent as emotionally disturbed, and 1 percent as other health impaired. These hidden disabilities often cannot be readily known without the administration of appropriate diagnostic tests.

THE RESPONSIBILITIES OF U.S. DEPARTMENT OF EDUCATION RECIPIENTS IN PRESCHOOL, ELEMENTARY, SECONDARY, AND ADULT EDUCATION

For coverage under Section 504, an individual with handicaps must be "qualified" for service by the school or institution receiving ED funds. For example, the ED Section 504 regulation defines a "qualified handicapped person" with respect to public preschool, elementary, secondary, or adult education services, as a person with a handicap who is:

- Of an age during which persons without handicaps are provided such services
- Of any age during which it is mandatory under state law to provide such services to persons with handicaps
- A person for whom a state is required to provide a free appropriate public education under the Individuals with Disabilities Education Act (IDEA)

Under the Section 504 regulation, a recipient that operates a public elementary or a secondary education program has a number of responsibilities toward qualified handicapped persons in its jurisdiction. These recipients must:

- Undertake annually to identify and locate all unserved handicapped children
- Provide a "free appropriate public education" to each student with handicaps, regardless of the nature or severity of the handicap. This means providing regular or special education and related aids and services designed to meet the individual educational needs of handicapped persons as adequately as the needs of nonhandicapped persons are met.
- Ensure that each student with handicaps is educated with nonhandicapped students to the maximum extent appropriate to the needs of the handicapped person
- Establish nondiscriminatory evaluation and placement procedures to avoid the inappropriate education that may result from the misclassification or misplacement of students
- Establish procedural safeguards to enable parents and guardians to participate meaningfully in decisions regarding the evaluation and placement of their children
- Afford handicapped children an equal opportunity to participate in nonacademic and extracurricular services and activities

A recipient that operates a preschool education or day care program, or an adult education program may not exclude qualified handicapped persons and must take into account their needs of qualified handicapped persons in determining the aid, benefits, or services to be provided under those programs and activities.

Students with hidden disabilities frequently are not properly diagnosed. For example, a student with an undiagnosed hearing impairment may be unable to understand much of what a teacher says; a student with a learning disability may be unable to process oral or written information routinely; or a student with an emotional problem may be unable to concentrate in a regular classroom setting. As a result, these students, regardless of their intelligence, will be unable to fully demonstrate their ability or attain educational benefits equal to that of nonhandicapped students. They may be perceived by teachers and fellow students as slow, lazy, or as discipline problems.

Whether a child is already in school or not, if her/his parents feel the child needs special education or related services, they should get in touch with the local superintendent of schools. For example, a parent who believes her or his child has a hearing impairment or is having difficulty understanding a teacher may request to have the child evaluated so that the child may receive an appropriate education. A child with behavior problems, or one who is doing poorly academically, may have an undiagnosed hidden disability. A parent has the right to request that the school determine whether the child is handicapped and whether special education or related services are needed to provide the child with an appropriate education. Once it is determined that a child needs special education or related services, the recipient school system must arrange to provide appropriate services.

THE RESPONSIBILITIES OF DEPARTMENT OF EDUCATION RECIPIENTS IN POSTSECONDARY EDUCATION

The ED Section 504 regulation defines a qualified individual with handicaps for postsecondary education programs as a person with a handicap who meets the academic and technical standards requisite for admission to, or participation in, the college's education program or activity.

A college has no obligation to identify students with handicaps. In fact, Section 504 prohibits a postsecondary education recipient from making a pre-admission inquiry as to whether an applicant for admission is a handicapped person. However, a postsecondary institution is required to inform applicants and other interested parties of the availability of auxiliary aids, services, and academic adjustments, and the name of the person designated to coordinate the college's efforts to carry out the requirements of Section 504. After admission (including the period between admission and enrollment), the college may make confidential inquiries as to whether a person has a handicap for the purpose of determining whether certain academic adjustments or auxiliary aids or services may be needed.

Many students with hidden disabilities, seeking college degrees, are provided with special education services during their elementary and secondary school years. It is especially important for these students to understand that postsecondary institutions also have responsibilities to protect the rights of students with disabilities. In elementary and secondary school, their school district was responsible for identifying, evaluating, and providing individualized special education and related services to meet their needs. At the postsecondary level, however, there are some important differences. The key provisions of Section 504 at the postsecondary level are highlighted below.

At the postsecondary level, it is the student's responsibility to make her or his handicapping condition known and to request academic adjustments. This should be done in a timely manner. A student may choose to make her or his needs known to the Section 504 Coordinator, to an appropriate dean, a faculty advisor, or to each professor on an individual basis.

A student who requests academic adjustments or auxiliary aids because of a handicapping condition may be requested by the institution to provide documentation of the handicap and the need for the services requested. This may be especially important to an institution attempting to understand the nature and extent of a hidden disability.

The requested documentation may include the results of medical, psychological, or emotional diagnostic tests, or other professional evaluations to verify the need for academic adjustments or auxiliary aids.

HOW THE NEEDS OF STUDENTS WITH HIDDEN DISABILITIES CAN BE ADDRESSED

The following examples illustrate how schools can address the needs of their students with hidden disabilities.

- A student with a long-term, debilitating medical problem such as cancer, kidney disease, or diabetes may be given special consideration to accommodate the student's needs. For example, a student with cancer may need a class schedule that allows for rest and recuperation following chemotherapy.
- A student with a learning disability that affects the ability to demonstrate knowledge on a standardized test or in certain testing situations may require modified test arrangements, such as oral testing or different testing formats.
- A student with a learning disability or impaired vision that affects the ability to take notes in class may need a notetaker or tape recorder.

- A student with a chronic medical problem such as kidney or liver disease may have difficulty in walking distances or climbing stairs. Under Section 504, this student may require special parking space, sufficient time between classes, or other considerations, to conserve the student's energy for academic pursuits.
- A student with diabetes, which adversely affects the body's ability to manufacture insulin, may need a class schedule that will accommodate the student's special needs.
- An emotionally or mentally ill student may need an adjusted class schedule to allow time for regular counseling or therapy.
- A student with epilepsy who has no control over seizures, and whose seizures are stimulated by stress or tension, may need accommodation for such stressful activities as lengthy academic testing or competitive endeavors in physical education.
- A student with arthritis may have persistent pain, tenderness or swelling in one or more joints. A student experiencing arthritic pain may require a modified physical education program.

These are just a few examples of how the needs of students with hidden disabilities may be addressed. If you are a student (or a parent or guardian of a student) with a hidden disability, or represent an institution seeking to address the needs of such students, you may wish to seek further information from OCR.

Chapter 56 | Managing Chronic Health Conditions in Schools

Section 56.1 | Major Chronic Health Conditions

This section contains text excerpted from the following sources: Text under the heading "Asthma" is excerpted from "Asthma," Centers for Disease Control and Prevention (CDC), May 29, 2019; Text under the heading "Diabetes" is excerpted from "Diabetes in Schools," Centers for Disease Control and Prevention (CDC), May 9, 2017; Text under the heading "Epilepsy" is excerpted from "Epilepsy," Centers for Disease Control and Prevention (CDC), May 29, 2019; Text under the heading "Food Allergies" is excerpted from "Food Allergies," Centers for Disease Control and Prevention (CDC), May 29, 2019; Text under the heading "Oral Health" is excerpted from "Oral Health," Centers for Disease Control and Prevention (CDC), May 29, 2019.

ASTHMA

Asthma is a leading chronic illness among children and adolescents in the United States. It is also one of the leading causes of school absenteeism. On average, in a classroom of 30 children, about 3 are likely to have asthma. Low-income populations, minorities, and children living in inner cities experience more emergency department visits, hospitalizations, and deaths due to asthma than the general population.

When children and adolescents are exposed to things in the environment—such as dust mites, and tobacco smoke—an asthma episode can occur. These are called "asthma triggers." Asthma symptoms can be controlled by avoiding triggers and taking medications prescribed by a healthcare provider, if needed. Asthma is common but treatable: using treatment based on current scientific knowledge reduces illness and future episodes.

Managing Asthma in Schools

Asthma-friendly schools are those that make the effort to create a safe and supportive learning environment for students with asthma. They have policies and

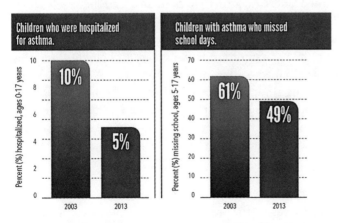

Figure 56.1. Asthma-Related Hospitalizations and Missed School Days Were Fewer than in 2013 *(Source: "Asthma in Children," Centers for Disease Control and Prevention (CDC))*

procedures that allow students to successfully manage their asthma. Research and case studies that looked at ways to best manage asthma in schools found that successful school-based asthma programs:

- Establish strong links with asthma care clinicians to ensure appropriate and ongoing medical care.
- Target students who are the most affected by asthma at school to identify and intervene with those in greatest need.
- Get administrative buy-in and build a team of enthusiastic people, including a full-time school nurse, to support the program.
- Use a coordinated, multi-component and collaborative approach that includes school nursing services, asthma education for students and professional development for school staff.
- Provide appropriate school health services for students with asthma, ensuring that students take their medicines and learn to use them when appropriate.
- Provide asthma education for students with asthma and awareness programs for students, school staff, parents, and families.
- Provide a safe and healthy school environment to reduce asthma triggers
- Offer safe and enjoyable physical education and activities for students with asthma.
- Support evaluation of school-based programs and use adequate and appropriate outcome measures.

DIABETES
Diabetes Facts
Diabetes (type 1 or type 2) affects about 208,000 (0.25%) of all people younger than 20 years in the United States. According to estimates for 2008–2009, about 23,500 persons in this age group were newly diagnosed with diabetes annually.

Ensuring that students with diabetes have the health services they need in school to manage their chronic condition is important in helping them stay healthy and ready to learn. Managing diabetes at school is most effective when there is a partnership among students, parents, school nurse, healthcare providers, teachers, counselors, coaches, transportation, food service employees, and administrators. Support may include helping a student take medications, check blood sugar levels, choose healthy foods in the cafeteria, and be physically active.

Managing Diabetes at School
Diabetes does not have to get in the way of a good experience at school. Remember, parents and schools have the same goal: to ensure that students with diabetes are safe and that they are able to learn in a supportive environment. Schools should:

Managing Chronic Health Conditions in Schools

- Develop a plan to help students care for diabetes and handle any diabetes-related emergencies.
- Work with a child's parents, doctor and school staff to create a Diabetes Medical Management Plan including information on services the school will provide and how to recognize high and low blood sugar levels.
- Ensure all physician and emergency contacts are updated and provided to school staff.
- Be sure school workers have a glucagon emergency kit and know how to use it if a student experiences a low blood sugar emergency. School staff should be given the National Diabetes Education Program (NDEP) School Guide hypoglycemia and hyperglycemia emergency care plans.

Diabetes Self-Management

Help students to manage diabetes at a level right for her or his age:

- If a child is going to monitor her or his blood sugar, ensure that she or he feels comfortable doing so.
- If a trained school employee will do the monitoring, be sure the student knows where and when to go for testing.
- Encourage students to eat healthy foods, including a healthy breakfast, which will help students stay focused and active. Students and parents should look at the school menus together to help them make choices for a healthy meal plan.
- Having diabetes does not mean that a child cannot be physically active or participate in physical education classes. They should get at least 60 minutes of physical activity every day. In fact, being active can help a child improve her or his blood sugar control.
- If a child with diabetes gets sick, she or he can take longer to recover than children without diabetes. Talk to the student's parents to make sure their child has all the vaccinations they need before starting the school year.
- Encourage students to wash their hands regularly, especially before eating and after using the bathroom.

EPILEPSY

Epilepsy is a common disorder of the brain that causes recurring seizures. Epilepsy affects people of all ages, but children and older adults are more likely to have epilepsy. Seizures are the main sign of epilepsy and most people can control this with treatment. Some seizures can resemble staring spells while other seizures can cause a person to collapse, stiffen or shake, and become unaware of what is going on around them. Many times, the cause is unknown.

Picture a school with 1,000 students—that means about 6 students would have epilepsy. For many children, epilepsy is easily controlled with medication and they can do what all the other kids can do, and perform as well academically. For others, it can be more challenging.

Compared with students with other health concerns, a Centers for Disease Control and Prevention (CDC) study shows that students aged 6 to 17 years with epilepsy were more likely to miss 11 or more days of school in the past year. Also, students with epilepsy were more likely to have difficulties in school, use special education services, and have activity limitations, such as less participation in sports or clubs compared with students with other medical conditions.

Managing Epilepsy at School

Managing epilepsy while at school may involve:

- Educating the school nurse, teachers, staff, and students about epilepsy and its treatment, seizure first aid, and possible stigma associated with epilepsy
- Following the seizure action plan and administering first aid (including the use of rescue medications)
- Understanding the importance of medication adherence and supporting students who take daily medications
- Helping students avoid seizure triggers, such as flashing lights, or other triggers identified in the seizure action plan
- Monitoring and addressing any related medical conditions, including mental-health concerns such as depression
- Providing case management services for students whose medical condition disrupts their school attendance or academic performance
- Referring students with uncontrolled seizures to medical services within the community or to the Epilepsy Foundation
- Understanding the laws related to disability, medical conditions, and special education to ensure that children with epilepsy are able to access the free and appropriate education afforded to them under the law
- Monitoring student behavior to prevent bullying of students with epilepsy

What Is a Seizure Action Plan?

A Seizure Action Plan contains the essential information school staff may need to know in order to help a student who has seizures. It includes information on first aid, parent and healthcare provider contacts, and medications specifically for that child. Seizure Action Plans are an important tool that helps parents and schools partner to keep children safe and healthy during the school day.

FOOD ALLERGIES

Food allergies are a growing food safety and public-health concern that affect an estimated 8 percent of children in the United States. That is 1 in 13 children, or about 2 students per classroom. A food allergy occurs when the body has a specific and reproducible immune response to certain foods. The body's immune response can be severe and life-threatening, such as anaphylaxis. Although the immune system normally protects people from germs, in people with food allergies, the immune system mistakenly responds to food as if it were harmful.

There is no cure for food allergies. Strict avoidance of the food allergen is the only way to prevent a reaction. However, because it is not always easy or possible to avoid certain foods, staff in schools, out-of-school time, and early care and education programs (ECE) should develop plans for preventing an allergic reaction and responding to a food allergy emergency, including anaphylaxis. Early and quick recognition and treatment can prevent serious health problems or death.

Eight foods or food groups account for most serious allergic reactions in the United States: milk, eggs, fish, crustacean shellfish, wheat, soy, peanuts, and tree nuts.

The symptoms and severity of allergic reactions to food can be different between individuals, and can also be different for one person over time. Anaphylaxis is a sudden and severe allergic reaction that may cause death. Not all allergic reactions will develop into anaphylaxis.

- Children with food allergies are two to four times more likely to have asthma or other allergic conditions than children without food allergies.
- The prevalence of food allergies among children increased 50 percent between 1997 to 2011, and allergic reactions to foods have become the most common cause of anaphylaxis in community health settings.

Managing Food Allergies at School

The CDC, in consultation with the U.S. Department of Education (ED), several federal agencies, and many stakeholders, developed *Voluntary Guidelines for Managing Food Allergies* to provide practical information and recommendations for each of the five priority areas that should be addressed in each school's or ECE program's Food Allergy Management Prevention Plan to:

- Ensure the daily management of food allergies in individual children
- Prepare for food allergy emergencies
- Provide professional development on food allergies for staff members
- Educate children and family members about food allergies
- Create and maintain a healthy and safe educational environment

ORAL HEALTH

Tooth decay (cavities) is one of the most common chronic conditions of childhood in the United States. About 1 in 5 (20%) children aged 5 to 11 years have at least 1 untreated decayed tooth. The percentage of children and adolescents aged 5 to 19 years with untreated tooth decay is twice as high for children from low-income families (25%) compared with children from higher-income households (12%).

Poor oral health can have a detrimental effect on children's quality of life (QOL), their performance at school, and their success later in life. Tooth decay is preventable and ensuring that students have the preventive oral health services they need in school is important in helping them stay healthy and ready to learn. Dental sealants prevent tooth decay and also stop cavities from growing—they result in a large reduction in tooth decay among school-aged children aged 5 to 16 years.

Addressing Oral Health in School

School sealant programs provide sealants to children in a school setting, and school-linked programs screen the children in school and refer them to private dental practices or public-dental clinics that place the sealants. These programs have been shown to increase the number of children who receive sealants at school, and are especially important for reaching children from low-income families who are less likely to receive private dental care. Programs that offer oral healthcare to students should:

- Use evidence-based practices in preventing dental caries through school-based sealant programs
- Voice support for policies that allow the use of dental personnel to the top of their licensure when dentists are not required to be on site, as per state or local regulations
- Develop referral networks with dental practitioners in the community

Section 56.2 | Chronic Health Conditions and the Whole School, Whole Community, Whole Child Model

This section contains text excerpted from the following sources: Text in this section begins with excerpts from "Managing Chronic Health Conditions in Schools," Centers for Disease Control and Prevention (CDC), September 18, 2018; Text beginning with the heading "What Is the Whole School, Whole Community, Whole Child Model?" is excerpted from "Whole School, Whole Community, Whole Child (WSCC)," Centers for Disease Control and Prevention (CDC), May 29, 2019.

About 25 percent of children in the United States aged 2 to 8 years have a chronic health condition such as asthma, obesity, other physical conditions, and behavior/learning problems. The healthcare needs of children with chronic illness can be complex and continuous and includes both daily management and addressing potential emergencies.

Health services in schools are a key component of the Whole School, Whole Community, Whole Child model (WSCC). Ensuring that students have the health services they need in school to manage their chronic condition is important in helping them stay healthy and ready to learn.

WHAT IS THE WHOLE SCHOOL, WHOLE COMMUNITY, WHOLE CHILD MODEL?

The WSCC model is the Centers for Disease Control and Prevention's (CDC) framework for addressing health in schools. The WSCC model is

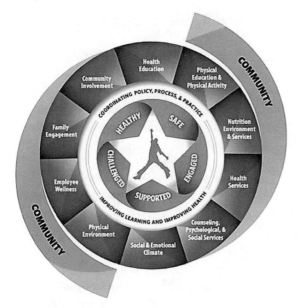

Figure 56.2. WSCC Model

student-centered and emphasizes the role of the community in supporting the school, the connections between health and academic achievement and the importance of evidence-based school policies and practices. The WSCC model has 10 components:

- Physical education and physical activity
- Nutrition environment and services
- Health education
- Social and emotional school climate
- Physical environment
- Health services
- Counseling, psychological, and social services
- Employee wellness
- Community involvement
- Family engagement

HOW DOES THE WHOLE SCHOOL, WHOLE COMMUNITY, WHOLE CHILD MODEL HELP TO IMPROVE LEARNING AND HEALTH?

The WSCC model meets the need for greater emphasis on both the psychosocial and physical environment as well as the increasing roles that community agencies and families play in improving childhood health behaviors and development. The WSCC model also addresses the need to engage students as active participants in their learning and health.

HOW CAN SCHOOLS USE THE WHOLE SCHOOL, WHOLE COMMUNITY, WHOLE CHILD MODEL?

Establishing healthy behaviors during childhood is easier and more effective than trying to change unhealthy behaviors during adulthood. Schools play a critical role in promoting the health and safety of young people and helping them establish lifelong healthy behaviors. Every school has a unique set of needs. To better serve their students, school leaders and staff can incorporate the WSCC model components as they see fit.

WHAT ROLE DO FAMILIES AND COMMUNITY AGENCIES PLAY IN THE WHOLE SCHOOL, WHOLE COMMUNITY, WHOLE CHILD MODEL APPROACH?

Family and community involvement in schools is important to the learning, development and health of students. When schools engage families in meaningful ways to improve student health and learning, families can support and reinforce healthy behaviors in multiple settings—at home, in school, in out-of-school programs, and in the community. With help from school leaders, community agencies and groups can collaborate with schools to provide valuable resources for student health and learning. In turn, schools, students, and their families can contribute to the community through service-learning opportunities and by sharing school facilities with community members (e.g., school-based community health centers and fitness facilities).

Section 56.3 | Chronic Health Conditions and Academic Achievement

This section includes text excerpted from "Research Brief: Chronic Health Conditions and Academic Achievement," Centers for Disease Control and Prevention (CDC), 2017.

STUDENTS AND CHRONIC HEALTH CONDITIONS

About 25 percent of children in the United States aged 2 to 8 years have a chronic health condition, such as asthma, obesity, other physical conditions, and behavior/learning problems. Although it is difficult to estimate and there is not 1 single source of information for chronic conditions in school-aged children, various studies state that for children aged less than 18 years, about 16 percent have poor oral health, 7 to 10 percent have asthma, 4 percent have food allergies, 0.7 percent have seizure disorders, and 0.3 percent have diabetes.

Students with chronic health conditions may face lower academic achievement, increased disability, fewer job opportunities and limited community interactions as they enter adulthood. Because these youth spend a significant amount of their time in schools, it is important to understand the relationship between chronic health conditions and academic achievement. Previous reports show that students who are able to manage their chronic health conditions tend to have better academic outcomes.

Studies show that some students with chronic health conditions have lower academic achievement than students who do not have such conditions, although this relationship varies by condition and can be influenced by additional factors. In this section, "academic achievement" refers to academic performance, education-related behavior, and cognitive skills. "Academic performance" refers to class grades, grade point average (GPA), standardized test scores, and graduation rates. "Education-related behavior" includes attendance, dropout rate, and behavior problems. "Cognitive skills" include students' concentration, language ability, and short- and long-term memory.

WHAT THE RESEARCH SHOWS

Most of the studies (47 of the 54) focused on asthma or seizure disorders/epilepsy, and their relationship to academic achievement. Seven studies covered more than one condition or chronic health conditions in general. Many studies have noted that students with chronic health conditions miss more school (absenteeism) than students who do not have such conditions. Absenteeism, in turn, is associated with lower academic achievement.

Epilepsy/Seizure Disorders

Epilepsy/seizure disorders were the focus of 24 studies. Of these, 20 reported significant associations, usually negative, with academic measures, such as cognitive ability, scores on intelligence tests, and school performance. Measures of students' performance and cognitive ability came from reports by teachers or parents and from tests administered to students. The following sections highlight the results from the studies.

Asthma

Asthma is one of the most prevalent chronic health conditions among children and adolescents. Of the five chronic health conditions in this review, asthma was most frequently associated with school days missed. Having asthma alone, however, was not related to academic risk. As reported in the included studies, both asthma education programs and having a full-time school nurse-led to improved symptom management and fewer school absences.

Diabetes

Three studies focused on diabetes and academic performance and showed that most students with diabetes achieve at least as well as their siblings and classmates in test scores, verbal performance, and academic behavior.

Poor Oral Health

Three studies addressed the association of oral health and academic performance. All concluded that poor oral health was associated with more school absences and reductions in affected students' overall ability to learn.

Food Allergies

No studies met inclusion criteria for this section, however, research has shown an association between having food allergies and experiencing bullying. Bullying, in turn, can lead to students' feeling less connected to their school and to lower grades.

Some chronic health conditions may compromise students' academic performance. However, many students with chronic health conditions can still achieve at a high level, especially when they have appropriate support at home, at school, and in their communities.

Section 56.4 | **Promoting Health for Children and Adolescents**

This section includes text excerpted from "Promoting Health for Children and Adolescents," Centers for Disease Control and Prevention (CDC), September 10, 2019.

Establishing healthy behaviors to prevent chronic disease is easier and more effective during childhood and adolescence than trying to change unhealthy behaviors during adulthood. The Centers for Disease Control and Prevention's (CDC), National Center for Chronic Disease Prevention and Health Promotion (NCCDPHP) works with parents, early care and education (ECE) facilities, schools, health systems, and communities to keep children healthy by:

- Reducing obesity risk for children in ECE facilities
- Improving healthy food options and nutrition education in school
- Improving physical education and physical activity opportunities in school
- Preventing use of all tobacco products
- Helping children and adolescents manage their chronic health conditions in school
- Promoting the use of dental sealants to prevent cavities
- Promoting adequate sleep

REDUCING OBESITY RISK IN EARLY CARE AND EDUCATION FACILITIES

Childhood obesity is a serious national problem. In the United States, the rate of obesity is 13.9 percent among children aged 2 to 5. Children's health behaviors are shaped by influences in multiple settings, including home, ECE facilities, schools, and communities.

The ECE settings—which include day care, preschool, pre-K facilities, and care provided in homes—are ideal places to encourage good nutrition and physical activity for early obesity prevention.

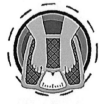

20.6% OF ADOLESCENTS
aged 12 to 19 have obesity.

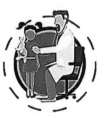

1 IN 4 STUDENTS
has a chronic condition.

27.1% OF HIGH SCHOOL STUDENTS
use at least one tobacco product.

Figure 56.3. Health Conditions of Students in the United States

431

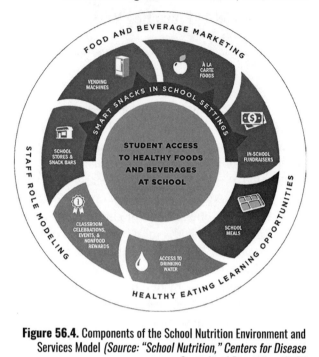

Figure 56.4. Components of the School Nutrition Environment and Services Model *(Source: "School Nutrition," Centers for Disease Control and Prevention (CDC))*

IMPROVING HEALTHY FOOD OPTIONS IN SCHOOL

The percentage of obesity is 18.4 percent among children aged 6 to 11 and rises to 20.6 percent for adolescents aged 12 to 19. Children who have obesity are at higher risk of obesity as adults. School is an ideal setting for children to learn and practice healthy eating.

Most U.S. children attend school for at least 6 hours a day and consume as much as half of their daily calories at school. The CDC's Healthy Schools in the Division of Population Health recommends that schools create an environment that helps students make healthy choices about food and beverages.

Some examples of CDC-recommended actions to improve nutrition in schools are given below.

- Promote access to and participation in school breakfast and lunch.
- Ensure that all foods and beverages sold or served outside of school meal programs are nutritious and appealing.
- Offer healthy foods and beverages at school celebrations and events and only nonfood items as rewards.
- Provide more access to drinking water.
- Promote healthy foods and beverages—for example, by pricing them lower than less healthy items.

- Include nutrition education in health education, throughout the school day, and in after-school programs—for example, through school gardens and farm-to-school activities.

IMPROVING PHYSICAL EDUCATION AND PHYSICAL ACTIVITY OPPORTUNITIES IN SCHOOL

About one-quarter of adolescents get the recommended 60 minutes a day of physical activity. The CDC's Healthy Schools program recommends that schools use all available opportunities for students to get physical activity and learn how to be physically active for a lifetime. Schools are encouraged to:

- Offer physical education to increase students' knowledge, skills, and confidence to be physically active and improve their health and academic outcomes, such as increased physical activity, improved grades and standardized test scores, and better classroom behavior
- Offer recess at all grade levels to encourage students to be physically active and engaged with their peers in activities of their choice
- Integrate physical activity into classroom instruction
- Promote before- and after-school opportunities to be physically active, through walking or biking programs, physical activity clubs, intramural programs, and competitive sports

PREVENTING YOUTH USE OF TOBACCO PRODUCTS

Nearly 9 in 10 adult cigarette smokers in the United States first tried a cigarette before age 18. Every day, about 2,000 young people under 18 try their first cigarette, and more than 300 become daily cigarette smokers. About 7 of every 100 middle school students and about 27 of every 100 high school students report current use of some type of tobacco product.

Any tobacco use among young people—whether burned, electronic, or smokeless—is unsafe because nicotine is addictive and can harm the developing brain. Nicotine exposure during adolescence affects learning, memory, and attention and primes the brain for addiction.

HELPING CHILDREN AND ADOLESCENTS MANAGE CHRONIC CONDITIONS

As many as one in four U.S. students has a chronic health condition, such as asthma, diabetes, or epilepsy. Managing students' chronic health conditions can be a challenge for school personnel. A coordinated effort that involves family members, community groups, social service agencies, and medical providers working with teachers, school nurses, and staff is crucial.

The healthcare needs of children with chronic health conditions can be complex and continuous and include both daily management and potential emergencies. Ensuring that students have the health services they need to manage their chronic conditions while at school is important in helping them stay healthy and ready to learn.

The CDC funds state education agencies to improve the delivery of health services in schools and increase the number of students who can effectively manage their chronic health conditions.

PROMOTING THE USE OF DENTAL SEALANTS

Dental sealants are protective coatings applied to the chewing surfaces of the back teeth, where most cavities start. Although use of sealants has increased, this effective intervention remains underused. Less than half of children aged 6 to 11 have dental sealants. The use of dental sealants varies among racial and ethnic groups, as does the prevalence of treated and untreated cavities. In addition, children from lower-income families are twice as likely to have untreated cavities as those from higher-income families, but they are less likely to have dental sealants.

School sealant programs provide dental sealants at no charge to children who are less likely to receive private dental care. These programs provide sealants to students during the school day using mobile dental equipment. Providing these services at school is especially effective at reaching children at risk of developing cavities.

Programs funded by the CDC's Division of Oral Health (DOH) focus on schools that serve children at high risk of cavities. The CDC provides guidance to state and community programs to help them plan, set up, and evaluate school sealant programs and to complement the services provided by private dentists. An online data collection tool called "SEALS" allows programs to evaluate the cost-effectiveness of their efforts.

PROMOTING BETTER SLEEP

Sleep is increasingly recognized as a component of good health. Getting enough sleep can help children to prevent obesity, type 2 diabetes, attention and behavior problems, poor mental health, and injuries. Children aged 6 to 12 need 9 to 12 hours of sleep a night. Teens aged 13 to 18 need 8 to 10 hours of sleep a night.

The CDC works to increase parents' awareness about their children's need for good sleep and how they can help their children get enough—for example, by setting the same bed and wake-up times each day, including on weekends, and by modeling good sleep behaviors.

Section 56.5 | Addressing the Needs of Students with Chronic Health Conditions: Strategies for Schools

This section includes text excerpted from "Addressing the Needs of Students with Chronic Health Conditions: Strategies for Schools," Centers for Disease Control and Prevention (CDC), 2017.

Children and adolescents with chronic health conditions spend many hours in school and depend on trained school staff and a healthy school environment to help them manage these conditions. A good working partnership between students, school nurses, clinicians, school staff, and administrators, can help reduce absenteeism and improve academic achievement.

About 25 percent of children aged 2 through 8 years have a chronic health condition, including asthma, obesity, other physical conditions, and behavior or learning problems. Although it is difficult to estimate and there is not one single source of information for chronic conditions in school-aged children, various studies state that for children and teens younger than 18, about 16 percent have poor oral health conditions, 7 to 10 percent have asthma, 4 percent have food allergies, 0.7 percent have seizure disorders and 0.3 percent have diabetes.

Studies show that for some students, chronic health conditions are associated with lower academic achievement, but this finding varies by condition and can be influenced by other factors. Schools are responsible for helping students manage chronic health conditions for two reasons. First, students may rely on the school for clinical services, such as those provided by a school nurse or at a school-based health center, because of barriers to healthcare access. Second, federal and state regulations require schools to provide services and accommodations for students with chronic health conditions.

This section describes strategies for school-based management of students' chronic health conditions, for example, seizure disorders/epilepsy, asthma, diabetes, poor oral health, and food allergies. It also summarizes current scientific knowledge from a systematic literature review on the relationship between the role of school-health services in the health and academic outcomes of students with chronic health conditions. It also reflects position statements and guidelines from national organizations with expertise in school health, and the Whole School, Whole Community, Whole Child (WSCC) approach for comprehensive school health. School districts and schools can use the following strategies and activities to address the needs of students with chronic health conditions.

PLANNING AND DEVELOPING A COORDINATED SYSTEM TO MEET THE NEEDS OF STUDENTS WITH CHRONIC HEALTH CONDITIONS

A coordinated system based on the WSCC framework is one that reinforces the connection between health and learning. It can help facilitate collaboration across several disciplines—for example, nursing, mental health or counseling services, nutrition services, and physical activity—to better support students with chronic health conditions. School districts and schools can:

- Assess existing school health policies and practices to determine strengths and weaknesses related to supporting students with chronic health conditions. The Centers for Disease Control and Prevention (CDC) offers an easy-to-use online tool, the School Health Index, for this purpose.
- Designate a leader at the district level to address policies and practices that meet the needs of students with chronic health conditions. Likely candidates include the school health coordinator or a nursing supervisor. This person can help the school system coordinate and integrate policies and programs and can advocate for community resources that can benefit these students.
- Identify a person in the school building to coordinate the implementation of policies, practices, and systems that support students with chronic health conditions
- Ensure that policies and procedures are consistent with federal and state laws and regulations, such as the Individuals with Disabilities Education Act (IDEA), Section 504 of the Rehabilitation Act of 1973, Americans with Disabilities Act (ADA), the Health Insurance Portability and Accountability Act (HIPAA), and the Family Educational Rights and Privacy Act (FERPA)
- Get support for policies, practices, and systems from school nurses, parents, administrators, and community members. Leveraging community resources can strengthen school-community connections and improve health and educational outcomes for students.

PROVIDING SCHOOL-BASED HEALTH SERVICES AND CARE COORDINATION FOR STUDENTS WITH CHRONIC HEALTH CONDITIONS

School health services and care coordination for students with chronic health conditions can improve health outcomes and academic achievement, and reduce absenteeism. Direct health education for students and their caregivers can have similar positive effects. Using a multi-tiered approach based on the WSCC model that includes mental-health services, appropriate nutrition and physical activity, a safe physical environment, and appropriate staff professional development, can help students with chronic health conditions succeed.

PROVIDING SPECIFIC AND AGE-APPROPRIATE EDUCATION TO STUDENTS AND THEIR FAMILIES TO IMPROVE SELF-MANAGEMENT OF CHRONIC HEALTH CONDITIONS

Disease-specific education programs are associated with better school attendance and higher grades. For example, asthma education programs for children or their caregivers can increase asthma control, improve inhaler skills, and decrease hospital stays. Education programs such as Kickin' Asthma that focus on appropriate medication use, for example, when to take a reliever medication versus a controller medication, lead to improvements in symptoms and decrease emergency room and inpatient admissions:

- Offer bilingual or culturally appropriate education and programs for children and their families.
- If in-person classes are not available, consider using web-based education or an external organization to monitor student gains in knowledge or application to their daily lives.
- Provide psychosocial support for families when possible—this has been associated with a larger average gain in grade point average (GPA) when this need is met for individual students compared to when it is not.

PROVIDING PROFESSIONAL DEVELOPMENT OPPORTUNITIES FOR SCHOOL STAFF ON IMPROVING HEALTH AND ACADEMIC OUTCOMES OF STUDENTS WITH CHRONIC HEALTH CONDITIONS

Students who are able to manage their chronic health conditions tend to have better academic outcomes. School administrators and staff need to be aware of the connection between learning and health. In the case of asthma, for example, comprehensive education interventions that include training for staff, along with case management and education for students, have been associated with better control of symptoms.

- Provide training for appropriate school staff on resources that support students with chronic health conditions.
- Consider allowing staff time to participate in off-site learning opportunities, e-learning modules, or webinars.

PROVIDING APPROPRIATE COUNSELING, PSYCHOLOGICAL, AND SOCIAL SERVICES FOR STUDENTS AFFECTED BY CHRONIC HEALTH CONDITIONS

In addition to addressing physical health, it is important to identify the mental-health needs of students with chronic health conditions, who are at higher risk of bullying than other students—they may not want to draw attention to themselves or appear different from other students.

- Identify and track students with emotional, behavioral, and mental-health needs.
- Provide or refer students and families to school- and community-based counseling services.
- Help students with chronic health conditions during transitions, such as changes in schools or in family structure.
- Promote a positive school climate where respect is encouraged and students can seek help from trusted adults.

PROVIDING A SAFE PHYSICAL ENVIRONMENT WITH APPROPRIATE NUTRITION, PHYSICAL EDUCATION, AND PHYSICAL ACTIVITY OPPORTUNITIES

Schools are responsible for the safety of their students during the school day. Students with certain chronic health conditions, such as asthma, for example, may have increased sensitivity to their surroundings. The school nutrition environment can help shape lifelong eating behaviors, and students with certain diet-related chronic health conditions, such as food allergies or diabetes, should have the opportunity to make healthy choices while at school.

- Provide a safe physical environment, both outside and inside school buildings, for example, with proper cleaning and maintenance, ventilation, and limited exposure to chemicals and pollutants.
- Ensure that foods are labeled and that menus are available to students and their families. In addition, food allergens, such as peanuts, should be prohibited in the classroom.
- Encourage all students to participate in physical activity, regardless of ability, unless medical needs prevent it.
- Align activities with provisions in local wellness policies and with national or state physical education standards.

School health services and care coordination for students with chronic health conditions can improve health outcomes and academic achievement, and reduce absenteeism. Direct health education for students and their caregivers can have similar positive effects. Using a multi-tiered approach based on the WSCC model that includes mental-health services, appropriate nutrition and physical activity, a safe physical environment, and appropriate staff professional development, can help students with chronic health conditions succeed.

Chapter 57 | Finding a Camp for a Child with Chronic Health Needs

For many families, summer camp has been an annual tradition and a rite of passage for both children and parents. Kids enjoy the chance to gain some independence, experience nature, take part in fun activities, learn new skills, and form new relationships that may last a lifetime. Parents, meanwhile, not only get a bit of a break but also appreciate the lasting positive effect that camp will have on their children.

This holds true for kids with chronic health needs and their families, as well. But of course, there are some special considerations in these cases, and both parents and children should be prepared to do considerable research in order to select the most appropriate camp and plan for the child's time away from home. There are more camps for kids with special needs now than ever before, all of which offer a wide array of appropriate physical, mental, social, and therapeutic activities and many that specialize in particular disorders. Learning about the available options and doing a bit of advance preparation can help ensure that camp is a rewarding experience for the entire family.

TYPES OF CAMPS
There are three primary types of camps that parents of children with chronic health conditions will need to consider: general (or mainstream) camps, those designed for children with a variety of special needs, and those aimed at specific conditions or health requirements.

- **General camps.** Under the Americans with Disabilities Act (ADA), all camps are required to take reasonable steps to accommodate children with special needs. Parents will have to do some research to find out exactly what is available at any given camp, but such accommodations could include wheelchair ramps, medical staff, and special activities. The advantage of this kind of camp is that kids with chronic conditions interact with "mainstream" kids for a potentially more well-rounded experience.

- **Special-needs camps.** These camps welcome children with a wide variety of special needs and conditions. They generally have a broad range of activities designed to accommodate many kinds of disabilities and disorders—physical, behavioral, dietary, allergy, or medical. Another advantage is that they usually have a larger medical team and a better-equipped infirmary than mainstream camps.
- **Camps for specific conditions.** Since the 1970s there has been a dramatic increase in the number of camps aimed at specific chronic disorders. These include cancer, cerebral palsy, epilepsy, diabetes, human immunodeficiency virus (HIV)/acquired immunodeficiency syndrome (AIDS), neurological conditions, and spina bifida, among many others. Not only do these camps tailor activities to the needs and abilities related to that particular condition, but they often include sessions with trained professionals to help kids learn to deal with their disorders successfully. And their medical staff and facilities are prepared to handle these children's special requirements.

BENEFITS OF CAMP

Some of the benefits of summer camp are the same for children with chronic health needs as for other kids, and some are unique. These can include:

- **Fun.** An obvious benefit, but one that is certain to be at the top of the child's list. Camp gives kids struggling with chronic conditions a chance to get involved in new activities and enjoy themselves.
- **Independence.** Children with health issues are routinely dependent on parents and medical professionals for care and treatment. The camp provides them with a measure of self-sufficiency that they most likely do not experience on a day-to-day basis.
- **Exercise.** Depending on their condition, kids can get involved in a number of physical activities at camp that can improve coordination, cardiovascular health, and muscle development.
- **Achievement.** Children participating in camp activities gain a sense of accomplishment as they meet goals and learn new skills. This both increases self-confidence and develops abilities that last beyond the duration of camp.
- **Sense of community.** At mainstream camps, kids with chronic issues interact with all sorts of people, become part of a team, and feel less isolated. And at special-needs camps, they not only realize these

benefits but also meet others with similar disorders and recognize that they are not alone but are part of a larger community.

- **Learning.** Attending any camp gives children the chance to learn new skills and try new activities, but special-needs camps provide the opportunity to learn more about their particular condition and develop techniques for improving their quality of life.

SEARCHING FOR A CAMP

There are a number of ways to begin looking for a camp for a child with chronic health needs. An Internet search is one way to start. Camps have a lot of useful information on their websites, such as the special needs they can accommodate, available activities, daily menus, and photos of the staff and facilities. Another good idea is to ask the child's doctor or other medical professional for a recommendation. Hospital departments and associations devoted to specific conditions often run their own camps or, if not, can make some recommendations. Parents or kids in support groups are another good source of ideas.

As the search proceeds, there are a number of questions to consider while trying to sort through the options. These include:

- How far is the camp from home?
- How long has it been in operation?
- Does the physical layout to accommodate wheelchairs, crutches, etc.?
- What medical care and facilities are available?
- What provisions are made for emergencies?
- Can special dietary needs be accommodated?
- How many kids are at the camp at any given time?
- What is the age range of the campers?
- What is the camper-to-counselor ratio?
- What training and certification do counselors have?
- Have background checks conducted on the staff?
- How are the days structured?
- What indoor and outdoor activities are available?
- What kind of educational sessions take place?
- Is transportation available?
- What is the cost, and what is included?

When exploring camp options, it is important to involve the child in the research and selection process. Make a list of her or his likes and dislikes, priorities, and questions, and be sure to include these in the search.

A final step is to visit the camp with the child who will be attending. Arrange a tour, inspect the living arrangements, meet the administrators and medical staff, and talk to several counselors. If possible, observe a few of the activities and speak with some of the campers and their parents. It is just as important that both the parents and the child have a good feeling about the camp as it is to ensure that the facilities meet the child's special needs.

References

1. Bachrach, Steven J., MD. "Camps for Kids with Special Needs," The Nemours Foundation/KidsHealth®, January 2014.
2. Grand, Lillieth. "How to Find Just the Right Camp for Special Needs Kids," PDXParent.com, March 10, 2015.
3. McCarthy, Alicia, MSN, CPNP. "Summer Camp for Children and Adolescents with Chronic Conditions," Medscape.com, 2015.
4. Waltari, Mary L., Esq. "Choosing Summer Camp for Kids with Disabilities," Special Needs Alliance (SNA), March 3. 2016.

Chapter 58 | **Robotic Device for Kids with Cerebral Palsy**

WHAT IS CEREBRAL PALSY?

Cerebral palsy (CP) is a group of disorders that affect a person's ability to move and maintain balance and posture. CP is the most common motor disability in childhood. "Cerebral" means having to do with the brain. "Palsy" means weakness or problems with using the muscles. CP is caused by abnormal brain development or damage to the developing brain that affects a person's ability to control her or his muscles.

The symptoms of CP vary from person to person. A person with severe CP might need to use special equipment to be able to walk, or might not be able to walk at all and might need lifelong care. A person with mild CP, on the other hand, might walk a little awkwardly, but might not need any special help. CP does not get worse over time, though the exact symptoms can change over a person's lifetime.

All people with CP have problems with movement and posture. Many also have related conditions, such as intellectual disability; seizures; problems with vision, hearing, or speech; changes in the spine (such as scoliosis); or joint problems (such as contractures).

There is no cure for CP, but treatment can improve the lives of those who have the condition. It is important to begin a treatment program as early as possible.

After a CP diagnosis is made, a team of health professionals works with the child and family to develop a plan to help the child reach her or his full potential. Common treatments include medicines; surgery; braces; and physical, occupational, and speech therapy. No single treatment is the best one for all children with CP. Before deciding on a treatment plan, it is important to talk with the child's doctor to understand all the risks and benefits.

This chapter contains text excerpted from the following sources: Text under the heading "What Is Cerebral Palsy?" is excerpted from "What Is Cerebral Palsy?" Centers for Disease Control and Prevention (CDC), April 30, 2019; Text under the heading "How Robotic Device Can Help Kids with Cerebral Palsy" is excerpted from "Robotic Device Helps Kids with Cerebral Palsy," *NIH News in Health*, National Institutes of Health (NIH), October 2017.

HOW ROBOTIC DEVICE CAN HELP KIDS WITH CEREBRAL PALSY

Researchers at the National Institutes of Health (NIH) have been developing a robotic device to help improve the way children with CP walk.

One of the most common signs of CP is crouch gait, an excessive bending of the knees while walking. Leg braces, muscle injections, physical therapy, and leg surgery can help children with CP improve their walking ability, but long-term problems often remain.

Dr. Thomas Bulea and his team of researchers at the NIH Clinical Center (CC) created a wearable robotic device, called an "exoskeleton," to help kids straighten their legs as they walk.

Seven children, ages 5 to 19 years old, helped test the device. Each was able to walk at least 30 feet without a walking aid. After putting on the device, 6 of the 7 children were better able to extend their knees. The children used their own muscles while walking with the device. They were not letting the exoskeleton do all the work to straighten their legs.

"The improvements in their walking, along with their preserved muscle activity, make us optimistic that our approach could train a new walking pattern in these children if deployed over an extended time," Bulea says.

Chapter 59 | Telemedicine for Children

WHAT IS TELEMEDICINE?

When thinking about healthcare, most of us conjure up images of office visits or trips to the emergency room (ER). Whether it is for a routine check-up, lab tests, an outpatient procedure or major surgery, the norm is for patients and caregivers to leave their homes (often sitting in traffic or rushing from work) to meet their doctor at a healthcare facility of some kind. But things are changing.

Based on advances in information and communications technologies, medical professionals as well as other "health and care" providers can now offer increasingly robust, remote (from their location to another), interactive (two-way) services to consumers, patients, and caregivers.

Telemedicine can be defined as "using telecommunications technologies to support the delivery of all kinds of medical, diagnostic and treatment-related services usually by doctors." For example, this includes conducting diagnostic tests, closely monitoring a patient's progress after treatment or therapy, and facilitating access to specialists that are not located in the same place as the patient.

TELEMEDICINE AND PATIENT HEALTH

Telemedicine seeks to improve a patient's health by permitting two-way, real-time interactive communication between the patient, and the physician or practitioner at the distant site. This electronic communication means the use of interactive telecommunications equipment that includes, at a minimum, audio and video equipment.

This chapter contains text excerpted from the following sources: Text under the heading "What Is Telemedicine?" is excerpted from "Telehealth, Telemedicine, and Telecare: What's What?" Federal Communications Commission (FCC), November 26, 2014. Reviewed December 2019; Text under the heading "Telemedicine and Patient Health" is excerpted from "Telemedicine," Centers for Medicare & Medicaid Services (CMS), December 3, 2011. Reviewed December 2019; Text under the heading "Telemedicine and Quality of Care" is excerpted from "Telemedicine May Affect Quality of Care," *NIH News in Health*, National Institutes of Health (NIH), June 2019.

Telemedicine is viewed as a cost-effective alternative to the more traditional face-to-face way of providing medical care (e.g., face-to-face consultations or examinations between the healthcare provider and patient) that states can choose to cover under Medicaid. This definition is modeled on Medicare's definition of telehealth services (42 CFR 410.78).

Note. The federal Medicaid statute does not recognize telemedicine as a distinct service.

TELEMEDICINE AND QUALITY OF CARE

A study suggests that in-person doctor visits provide better care for children with certain infections.

Researchers used claims data from a health plan to look at visits for children with respiratory illnesses. These included colds, sore throats, and ear infections. More than 5,000 children received care via telemedicine. About 88,000 visited an urgent care clinic. More than a million saw primary-care doctors.

The team counted the antibiotics prescribed within two days for each type of visit.

Children were given antibiotics most often after telemedicine visits. They received these drugs after 52 percent of telemedicine, 42 percent of urgent care, and 31 percent of primary-care visits.

The team looked at whether doctors followed guidelines for giving antibiotics. These drugs can treat bacterial infections such as strep throat. But they cannot treat viral infections such as colds and flu.

Only 59 percent of telemedicine visits met the guidelines, compared with 67 percent of urgent-care visits and 78 percent of primary care visits.

"As a pediatrician and a parent, I understand the appeal of telemedicine when a child is sick, since it offers the promise of connecting with a doctor in a way that is convenient and timely," says Dr. Kristin Ray at the University of Pittsburgh. "But, it is important to make sure that the quality of care that children receive remains high."

Part 7 | Legal, Financial, and Insurance Issues That Impact Disease Management

Chapter 60 | The Americans with Disabilities Act

WHAT IS THE AMERICANS WITH DISABILITIES ACT?

The Americans with Disabilities Act (ADA) is a federal law guaranteeing equal opportunity for individuals with disabilities in public accommodations, employment, transportation, state and local government services, and telecommunications.

SIGNIFICANCE OF THE AMERICANS WITH DISABILITIES ACT

July 26, 2019, marked the 29th anniversary of ADA, a civil rights law that promotes the inclusion of people with disabilities at work, school, or other community settings. An estimated 61 million people are living with a disability in the United States, and many people will experience a disability at some time during the course of their lives. Disabilities limit how a child or adult functions. Limitations may include difficulty walking or climbing stairs; hearing; seeing; or concentrating, remembering, or making decisions.

Enacted on July 26, 1990, the goals of the ADA are to promote equal opportunity, full participation, independent living, and economic self-sufficiency for people with disabilities, as well as protect individuals with disabilities from discrimination. The ADA has made a positive difference in the lives of people with disabilities by providing better access to buildings, transportation, and employment; however, challenges remain with access to healthcare, as well as the inclusion of people with disabilities in health promotion and disease prevention programs.

This chapter contains text excerpted from the following sources: Text under the heading "What Is the Americans with Disabilities Act?" is excerpted from "What Is the Americans with Disabilities Act (ADA)?" U.S. Department of Health and Human Services (HHS), September 11, 2014. December 2019; Text under the heading "Significance of the Americans with Disabilities Act" is excerpted from "Disability-Inclusive Communities," Centers for Disease Control and Prevention (CDC), July 22, 2019; Text under the heading "An Overview of the Americans with Disabilities Act" is excerpted from "A Guide to Disability Rights Laws," ADA.gov, U.S. Department of Justice (DOJ), July 2009. Reviewed December 2019.

Additionally, people with disabilities continue to face significant differences in health compared to people who do not have disabilities. For example:

- Adults with disabilities are three times more likely to have heart disease, stroke, diabetes, or cancer than adults without disabilities.
- Adults with disabilities are more likely to smoke, to have obesity, and to be physically inactive than adults without disabilities.
- Women with disabilities are less likely to have received a mammogram in the previous two years than women without disabilities.

AN OVERVIEW OF THE AMERICANS WITH DISABILITIES ACT

The ADA prohibits discrimination on the basis of disability in employment, state and local government, public accommodations, commercial facilities, transportation, and telecommunications. It also applies to the U.S. Congress.

To be protected by the ADA, one must have a disability or have a relationship or association with an individual with a disability. An individual with a disability is defined by the ADA as "a person who has a physical or mental impairment that substantially limits one or more major life activities, a person who has a history or record of such an impairment, or a person who is perceived by others as having such an impairment." The ADA does not specifically name all of the impairments that are covered.

Americans with Disabilities Act Title I: Employment

Title I requires employers with 15 or more employees to provide qualified individuals with disabilities an equal opportunity to benefit from the full range of employment-related opportunities available to others. For example, it prohibits discrimination in recruitment, hiring, promotions, training, pay, social activities, and other privileges of employment. It restricts questions that can be asked about an applicant's disability before a job offer is made, and it requires that employers make reasonable accommodation to the known physical or mental limitations of otherwise qualified individuals with disabilities, unless it results in an undue hardship. Religious entities with 15 or more employees are covered under Title I.

Title I complaints must be filed with the U.S. Equal Employment Opportunity Commission (EEOC) within 180 days of the date of discrimination, or 300 days if the charge is filed with a designated state or local fair employment practice agency. Individuals may file a lawsuit in federal court only after they receive a "right-to-sue" letter from the EEOC.

Charges of employment discrimination on the basis of disability may be filed at any EEOC field office. Field offices are located in 50 cities throughout the U.S. and are listed in most telephone directories under "U.S. Government." For the appropriate EEOC field office in your geographic area.

Americans with Disabilities Act Title II: State and Local Government Activities

Title II covers all activities of state and local governments regardless of the government entity's size or receipt of federal funding. Title II requires that state and local governments give people with disabilities an equal opportunity to benefit from all of their programs, services, and activities (e.g., public education, employment, transportation, recreation, healthcare, social services, courts, voting, and town meetings).

State and local governments are required to follow specific architectural standards in the new construction and alteration of their buildings. They also must relocate programs or otherwise provide access to inaccessible older buildings, and communicate effectively with people who have hearing, vision, or speech disabilities. Public entities are not required to take actions that would result in undue financial and administrative burdens. They are required to make reasonable modifications to policies, practices, and procedures where necessary to avoid discrimination unless they can demonstrate that doing so would fundamentally alter the nature of the service, program, or activity being provided.

Complaints of Title II violations may be filed with the U.S. Department of Justice (DOJ) within 180 days of the date of discrimination. In certain situations, cases may be referred to a mediation program sponsored by the Department. The Department may bring a lawsuit where it has investigated a matter and has been unable to resolve violations. Title II may also be enforced through private lawsuits in federal court. It is not necessary to file a complaint with the DOJ or any other federal agency, or to receive a "right-to-sue" letter, before going to court.

Americans with Disabilities Act Title II: Public Transportation

The transportation provisions of Title II cover public-transportation services, such as city buses and public-rail transit (e.g., subways, commuter rails, Amtrak). Public-transportation authorities may not discriminate against people with disabilities in the provision of their services. They must comply with requirements for accessibility in newly purchased vehicles, make good faith efforts to purchase or lease accessible used buses, remanufacture buses in an accessible manner, and unless it would result in an undue burden, provide paratransit where they operate fixed-route bus or rail systems. Paratransit is a service where individuals who are unable to use the regular transit system independently (because of physical or mental impairment) are picked up and dropped off at their destinations.

Americans with Disabilities Act Title III: Public Accommodations

Title III covers businesses and nonprofit service providers that are public accommodations, privately operated entities offering certain types of courses and examinations, privately operated transportation, and commercial facilities.

451

Public accommodations are private entities who own, lease, lease to, or operate facilities, such as restaurants, retail stores, hotels, movie theaters, private schools, convention centers, doctors' offices, homeless shelters, transportation depots, zoos, funeral homes, day care centers, and recreation facilities including sports stadiums and fitness clubs. Transportation services provided by private entities are also covered by Title III.

Public accommodations must comply with basic nondiscrimination requirements that prohibit exclusion, segregation, and unequal treatment. They also must comply with specific requirements related to architectural standards for new and altered buildings; reasonable modifications to policies, practices, and procedures; effective communication with people with hearing, vision, or speech disabilities; and other access requirements. Additionally, public accommodations must remove barriers in existing buildings where it is easy to do so without much difficulty or expense, given the public accommodation's resources.

Courses and examinations related to professional, educational, or trade-related applications, licensing, certifications, or credentialing must be provided in a place and manner accessible to people with disabilities, or alternative accessible arrangements must be offered.

Commercial facilities, such as factories and warehouses, must comply with the ADA's architectural standards for new construction and alterations.

Complaints of Title III violations may be filed with the DOJ. In certain situations, cases may be referred to a mediation program sponsored by the Department. The Department is authorized to bring a lawsuit where there is a pattern or practice of discrimination in violation of Title III, or where an act of discrimination raises an issue of general public importance. Title III may also be enforced through private lawsuits. It is not necessary to file a complaint with the DOJ (or any federal agency) or to receive a "right-to-sue" letter, before going to court.

Americans with Disabilities Act Title IV: Telecommunications Relay Services

Title IV addresses telephone and television access for people with hearing and speech disabilities. It requires common carriers (telephone companies) to establish interstate and intrastate telecommunications relay services (TRS) 24 hours a day, 7 days a week. TRS enables callers with hearing and speech disabilities who use a text telephone (TTY) (also known as "telecommunications device for the deaf" (TDD)), and callers who use voice telephones to communicate with each other through a third-party communications assistant. The Federal Communications Commission (FCC) has set minimum standards for TRS services. Title IV also requires closed captioning of federally funded public-service announcements.

Chapter 61 | The Family and Medical Leave Act

The Family and Medical Leave Act (FMLA) entitles eligible employees of covered employers to take unpaid, job-protected leave for specified family and medical reasons. This chapter provides general information about which employers are covered by the FMLA, when employees are eligible and entitled to take FMLA leave, and what rules apply when employees take FMLA leave.

COVERED EMPLOYERS

The FMLA only applies to employers that meet certain criteria. A covered employer is a:
- Private-sector employer, with 50 or more employees in 20 or more workweeks in the current or preceding calendar year, including a joint employer or successor in interest to a covered employer
- Public agency, including a local, state, or federal government agency, regardless of the number of employees it employs
- Public or private elementary or secondary school, regardless of the number of employees it employs

ELIGIBLE EMPLOYEES

Only eligible employees are entitled to take FMLA leave. An eligible employee is one who:
- Works for a covered employer
- Has worked for the employer for at least 12 months
- Has at least 1,250 hours of service for the employer during the 12-month period immediately preceding the leave*

Special hours of service eligibility requirements apply to airline flight crew employees.

This chapter includes text excerpted from "The Family and Medical Leave Act," U.S. Department of Labor (DOL), 2012. Reviewed December 2019.

- Works at a location where the employer has at least 50 employees within 75 miles

The 12 months of employment do not have to be consecutive. That means any time previously worked for the same employer (including seasonal work) could, in most cases, be used to meet the 12-month requirement. If the employee has a break in service that lasted seven years or more, the time worked prior to the break will not count unless the break is due to service covered by the Uniformed Services Employment and Reemployment Rights Act (USERRA), or there is a written agreement, including a collective bargaining agreement, outlining the employer's intention to rehire the employee after the break-in service.

LEAVE ENTITLEMENT

Eligible employees may take up to 12 workweeks of leave in a 12-month period for one or more of the following reasons:

- The birth of a son or daughter or placement of a son or daughter with the employee for adoption or foster care
- To care for a spouse, son, daughter, or parent who has a serious health condition
- For a serious health condition that makes the employee unable to perform the essential functions of her or his job
- For any qualifying exigency arising out of the fact that a spouse, son, daughter, or parent is a military member on covered active duty or call to covered active duty status

An eligible employee may also take up to 26 workweeks of leave during a "single 12-month period" to care for a covered servicemember with a serious injury or illness, when the employee is the spouse, son, daughter, parent, or next of kin of the servicemember. The "single 12-month period" for military caregiver leave is different from the 12-month period used for other FMLA leave reasons.

Under some circumstances, employees may take FMLA leave on an intermittent or reduced schedule basis. That means an employee may take leave in separate blocks of time or by reducing the time she or he works each day or week for a single qualifying reason. When leave is needed for planned medical treatment, the employee must make a reasonable effort to schedule treatment so as not to unduly disrupt the employer's operations. If FMLA leave is for the birth, adoption, or foster placement of a child, use of intermittent or reduced schedule leave requires the employer's approval.

Under certain conditions, employees may choose, or employers may require employees to "substitute" accrued paid leave, such as sick or vacation leave, to cover some or all of the FMLA leave period. An employee's ability to substitute accrued paid leave is determined by the terms and conditions of the employer's leave policy.

NOTICE

Employees must comply with their employer's usual and customary requirements for requesting leave and provide enough information for their employer to reasonably determine whether the FMLA may apply to the leave request. Employees generally must request leave 30 days in advance when the need for leave is foreseeable. When the need for leave is foreseeable less than 30 days in advance or is unforeseeable, employees must provide notice as soon as possible and practicable under the circumstances.

When an employee seeks leave for a FMLA-qualifying reason for the first time, the employee need not expressly assert FMLA rights or even mention the FMLA. If an employee later requests additional leave for the same qualifying condition, the employee must specifically reference either the qualifying reason for leave or the need for FMLA leave.

Covered employers must:

- Post a notice explaining rights and responsibilities under the FMLA (and may be subject to a civil money penalty of up to $110 for willful failure to post);
- Include information about the FMLA in their employee handbooks or provide information to new employees upon hire;
- When an employee requests FMLA leave or the employer acquires knowledge that leave may be for an FMLA-qualifying reason, provide the employee with notice concerning her or his eligibility for FMLA leave and her or his rights and responsibilities under the FMLA; and
- Notify employees whether leave is designated as FMLA leave and the amount of leave that will be deducted from the employee's FMLA entitlement.

CERTIFICATION

When an employee requests FMLA leave due to her or his own serious health condition or a covered family member's serious health condition, the employer may require certification in support of the leave from a healthcare provider. An employer may also require second or third medical opinions (at the employer's expense) and periodic recertification of a serious health condition.

JOB RESTORATION AND HEALTH BENEFITS

Upon return from FMLA leave, an employee must be restored to her or his original job or to an equivalent job with equivalent pay, benefits, and other terms and conditions of employment. An employee's use of FMLA leave cannot be counted against the employee under a "no-fault" attendance policy. Employers are also required to continue group health insurance coverage for an employee on FMLA leave under the same terms and conditions as if the employee had not taken leave.

OTHER PROVISIONS

Special rules apply to employees of local education agencies. Generally, these rules apply to intermittent or reduced schedule FMLA leave or the taking of FMLA leave near the end of a school term.

Salaried executive, administrative, and professional employees of covered employers who meet the Fair Labor Standards Act (FLSA) criteria for exemption from minimum wage and overtime under the FLSA regulations, 29 CFR Part 541, do not lose their FLSA-exempt status by using any unpaid FMLA leave. This special exception to the "salary basis" requirements for FLSA's exemption extends only to an eligible employee's use of FMLA leave.

ENFORCEMENT

It is unlawful for any employer to interfere with, restrain, or deny the exercise of or the attempt to exercise any right provided by the FMLA. It is also unlawful for an employer to discharge or discriminate against any individual for opposing any practice, or because of involvement in any proceeding, related to the FMLA. The Wage and Hour Division (WHD) is responsible for administering and enforcing the FMLA for most employees. Most federal and certain congressional employees are also covered by the law but are subject to the jurisdiction of the U.S. Office of Personnel Management (OPM) or Congress. If you believe that your rights under the FMLA have been violated, you may file a complaint with the WHD or file a private lawsuit against your employer in court.

Chapter 62 | Advance Directives

Advance directives explain how you want medical decisions to be made when you are too ill to speak for yourself. These legal documents tell your family, friends, and healthcare professionals what kind of healthcare you want and who you want to make decisions for you.

TYPES OF ADVANCE DIRECTIVES

A healthcare proxy is a document that names someone you trust to make health decisions if you cannot. This is also called "a durable power of attorney."

A living will tells which treatment you want if your life is threatened, including:

- Dialysis and breathing machines
- Resuscitation, if you stop breathing, or if your heart stops
- Tube feeding
- Organ or tissue donation after you die

HOW TO GET ADVANCE DIRECTIVES

Get an advance directive from any of these:

- Your healthcare provider
- Your attorney
- Your local Area Agency on Aging (AAA)
- Your state health department

This chapter contains text excerpted from the following sources: Text in this chapter begins with excerpts from "Advance Directives and Long-Term Care," Centers for Medicare & Medicaid Services (CMS), February 20, 2018; Text under the heading "Behavioral Health Advance Directive" is excerpted from "Advance Directives for Behavioral Health," Substance Abuse and Mental Health Services Administration (SAMHSA), May 17, 2019; Text beginning with the heading "Making Your Healthcare Directives Official" is excerpted from "Advance Care Planning: Healthcare Directives," National Institute on Aging (NIA), National Institutes of Health (NIH), January 15, 2018.

WHAT TO DO WITH YOUR ADVANCE DIRECTIVES

You should:

- Keep the original copies of your advance directives where you can easily find them
- Give a copy to your healthcare proxy, healthcare providers, hospital, nursing home, family, and friends
- Carry a card in your wallet that says you have an advance directive
- Review your advance directives each year

BEHAVIORAL-HEALTH ADVANCE DIRECTIVE

In a behavioral-health advance directive, people are able to express their preferences on where to receive care and what treatments they are willing to undergo. They are also able to identify an agent or representative who is trusted and legally empowered to make healthcare decisions on their behalf. These decisions may include the use of all or certain medications, preferred facilities, and listings of visitors allowed in facility-based care. Advance directive laws may vary across states. Therefore, it is important to be sure that any advance directive form meets the requirements of a given state.

Common Components of a Behavioral-Health Advance Directive

A behavioral-health advance directive should have:

- A statement of one's intent in creating an advance directive for behavioral-healthcare decision-making
- The designation of another person to make decisions for an individual if she or he is determined to be legally incompetent to make choices. Generally, this designation also includes provisions for who should be appointed as guardian if a court decides to name one.
- Specific instructions about preferences for hospitalization and alternatives to hospitalization, medications, electroconvulsive therapy (ECT), and emergency interventions, including seclusion, restraint, medication, and participation in experimental studies or drug trials
- Instructions about who should be notified immediately if and when the person is admitted to a psychiatric facility. Instructions should also include who should be prohibited from visiting and who should have temporary custody of minor children or pets.
- Personal rights to suspend or terminate an advance directive while incapacitated, if allowed by the law in the state
- A signature page with two witnesses and a notary who sign the advance directive

MAKING YOUR HEALTHCARE DIRECTIVES OFFICIAL

Once you have talked with your doctor and have an idea of the types of decisions that could come up in the future and whom you would prefer as a proxy, if you want one at all, the next step is to fill out the legal forms detailing your wishes. A lawyer can help but is not required. If you decide to use a lawyer, do not depend on her or him to help you understand different medical treatments. Start the planning process by talking with your doctor.

Many states have their own advance directive forms. Your local AAA can help you locate the right forms. You can find your area agency phone number by calling the Eldercare Locator toll-free at 800-677-1116, or by visiting www. eldercare.acl.gov.

Some states require your advance directive to be witnessed; a few require your signature to be notarized. A notary is a person licensed by the state to witness signatures. You might find a notary at your bank, post office, or local library, or call your insurance agent. Some notaries charge a fee.

Some states have registries that can store your advance directive for quick access by healthcare providers, your proxy, and anyone else to whom you have given permission. Private firms also will store your advance directive. There may be a fee for storing your form in a registry. If you store your advance directive in a registry and later make changes, you must replace the original with the updated version in the registry.

Some people spend a lot of time in more than one state—for example, visiting children and grandchildren. If that is your situation, consider preparing an advance directive using forms for each state—and keep a copy in each place, too.

WHAT TO DO AFTER YOU SET UP YOUR ADVANCE DIRECTIVE

Give copies of your advance directive to your healthcare proxy and alternate proxy. Give your doctor a copy for your medical records. Tell close family members and friends where you keep a copy. If you have to go to the hospital, give staff there a copy to include in your records. Because you might change your advance directive in the future, it is a good idea to keep track of who receives a copy.

Review your advance care planning decisions from time to time—for example, every 10 years, if not more often. You might want to revise your preferences for care if your situation or your health changes. Or, you might want to make adjustments if you receive a serious diagnosis; if you get married, separated, or divorced; if your spouse dies; or if something happens to your proxy or alternate. If your preferences change, you will want to make sure your doctor, proxy, and family know about them.

Talking about Your Advance Care Wishes

It can be helpful to have conversations with the people close to you about how you want to be cared for in a medical emergency or at the end of life. These talks can help you think through the wishes you want to put in your advance directive.

It is especially helpful to talk about your thoughts, beliefs, and values with your healthcare proxy. This will help prepare her or him to make medical decisions that best reflect your values.

After you have completed your advance directive, talk about your decisions with your healthcare proxy, loved ones, and your doctor to explain what you have decided. This way, they are not surprised by your wishes if there is an emergency.

Another way to convey your wishes is to make a video of yourself talking about them. This lets you express your wishes in your own words. Videos do not replace an advance directive, but they can be helpful for your healthcare proxy and your loved ones.

BE PREPARED

What happens if you have no advance directive or have made no plans and you become unable to speak for yourself? In such cases, the state where you live will assign someone to make medical decisions on your behalf. This will probably be your spouse, your parents if they are available, or your children if they are adults. If you have no family members, the state will choose someone to represent your best interests.

Always remember an advance directive is only used if you are in danger of dying and need certain emergency or special measures to keep you alive, but you are not able to make those decisions on your own. An advance directive allows you to make your wishes about medical treatment known.

It is difficult to predict the future with certainty. You may never face a medical situation where you are unable to speak for yourself and make your wishes known. But, having an advance directive may give you and those close to you some peace of mind.

Chapter 63 | Legal and Financial Planning for People with a Chronic Disease

Many people are unprepared to deal with the legal and financial consequences of a serious illness, such as Alzheimer disease (AD). Legal and medical experts encourage people diagnosed with a serious illness—particularly one that is expected to cause declining mental and physical health—to examine and update their financial and healthcare arrangements as soon as possible. Basic legal and financial documents, such as a will, a living trust, and advance directives, are available to ensure that the person's late-stage or end-of-life healthcare and financial decisions are carried out.

A complication of diseases such as AD is that the person may lack or gradually lose the ability to think clearly. This change affects her or his ability to make decisions and participate in legal and financial planning.

People with early-stage chronic disease can often understand many aspects and consequences of legal decision making. However, legal and medical experts say that many forms of planning can help the person and her or his family even if the person is diagnosed with later-stages of a chronic disease.

There are good reasons to retain a lawyer when preparing advance planning documents. For example, a lawyer can help interpret different state laws and suggest ways to ensure that the person's and family's wishes are carried out. It is important to understand that laws vary by state, and changes in a person's situation—for instance, a divorce, relocation, or death in the family—can influence how documents are prepared and maintained.

This chapter includes text excerpted from "Legal and Financial Planning for People with Alzheimer" National Institute on Aging (NIA), National Institutes of Health (NIH), November 15, 2017.

Table 63.1. Overview of Medical Documents

Medical Document	How It Is Used
Living will	Describes and instructs how the person wants end-of-life healthcare managed
Durable power of attorney for healthcare	Gives a designated person the authority to make healthcare decisions on behalf of the person with Alzheimer
Do not resuscitate (DNR) order	Instructs healthcare professionals not to perform Search Results Web results cardiopulmonary resuscitation (CPR) in case of stopped heart or stopped breathing

LEGAL, FINANCIAL, AND HEALTHCARE PLANNING DOCUMENTS

Families beginning the legal planning process should discuss a number of strategies and legal documents. Depending on the family situation and the applicable state laws, a lawyer may introduce some or all of the following terms and documents to assist in this process:

- Documents that communicate the healthcare wishes of someone who can no longer make healthcare decisions
- Documents that communicate the financial management and estate plan wishes of someone who can no longer make financial decisions

ADVANCE HEALTHCARE DIRECTIVES FOR PEOPLE WITH CHRONIC DISEASE

Advance directives for healthcare are documents that communicate the healthcare wishes of a person with chronic disease. These decisions are then carried out after the person no longer can make decisions. In most cases, these documents must be prepared while the person is legally able to execute them.

A living will records a person's wishes for medical treatment near the end of life or if the person is permanently unconscious and cannot make decisions about emergency treatment.

A durable power of attorney for healthcare designates a person, sometimes called an "agent" or "proxy," to make healthcare decisions when the person with chronic disease no longer can do so.

A do not resuscitate (DNR) order instructs healthcare professionals not to perform cardiopulmonary resuscitation (CPR) if a person's heart stops or if she or he stops breathing. A DNR order is signed by a doctor and put in a person's medical chart.

ADVANCE DIRECTIVES FOR FINANCIAL AND ESTATE MANAGEMENT

Advance directives for financial and estate management must be created while the person with chronic disease still can make these decisions (sometimes referred to as "having legal capacity" to make decisions). These directives may include the following:

Legal and Financial Planning for People with a Chronic Disease

Table 63.2. Overview of Legal and Financial Documents

Legal/Financial Document	How It Is Used
Will	Indicates how a person's assets and estate will be distributed among beneficiaries after her/his death
Durable power of attorney for finances	Gives a designated person the authority to make legal/financial decisions on behalf of the person with Alzheimer
Living trust	Gives a designated person (trustee) the authority to hold and distribute property and funds for the person with Alzheimer

- A **will** indicates how a person's assets and estate will be distributed upon death. It also can specify:
  - Arrangements for the care of minors
  - Gifts
  - Trusts to manage the estate
  - Funeral and/or burial arrangements

Medical and legal experts say that the newly diagnosed person with chronic disease and her or his family should move quickly to make or update a will and secure the estate.

- A **durable power of attorney** for finances names someone to make financial decisions when the person with chronic disease no longer can. It can help people with the disease and their families avoid court actions that may take away control of financial affairs.
- A **living trust** provides instructions about the person's estate and appoints someone, called the "trustee," to hold title to property and funds for the beneficiaries. The trustee follows these instructions after the person with chronic disease no longer can manage her or his affairs. The person with chronic disease also can name the trustee as the healthcare proxy through the durable power of attorney for healthcare. A living trust can:
  - Include a wide range of property
  - Provide a detailed plan for property disposition
  - Avoid the expense and delay of probate (in which the courts establish the validity of a will)
  - State how property should be distributed when the last beneficiary dies and whether the trust should continue to benefit others

WHERE CAN YOU GET HELP WITH LEGAL AND FINANCIAL PLANNING?

Healthcare providers cannot act as legal or financial advisers, but they can encourage planning discussions between patients and their families. Qualified clinicians can also guide patients, families, the care team, attorneys, and judges regarding the patient's ability to make decisions. Discussing advance care planning decisions with a doctor is free through Medicare during the annual wellness visit. Private health insurance may also cover these discussions.

An elder law attorney helps older people and families interpret state laws, plan how their wishes will be carried out, understand their financial options, and learn how to preserve financial assets while caring for a loved one.

The National Academy of Elder Law Attorneys (NAELA) and the American Bar Association (ABA) can help families find qualified attorneys.

Geriatric care managers are trained social workers or nurses who can help people with chronic disease and their families.

ADVANCE PLANNING ADVICE FOR PEOPLE WITH CHRONIC DISEASE
Start Discussions Early

The rate of decline differs for each person with chronic disease, and her or his ability to be involved in planning will decline over time. People in the early stages of the disease may be able to understand the issues, but they may also be defensive or emotionally unable to deal with difficult questions. Remember that not all people are diagnosed at an early stage. Decision making already may be difficult when chronic disease is diagnosed.

Review Plans over Time

Changes in personal situations—such as a divorce, relocation, or death in the family—and in state laws can affect how legal documents are prepared and maintained. Review plans regularly, and update documents as needed.

Reduce Anxiety about Funeral and Burial Arrangements

Advance planning for the funeral and burial can provide a sense of peace and reduce anxiety for both the person with chronic disease and the family.

LEGAL AND FINANCIAL PLANNING RESOURCES FOR LOW-INCOME FAMILIES

Families who cannot afford a lawyer still can do advance planning. Samples of basic health planning documents are available online. Area Agency on Aging (AAA) officials may provide legal advice or help. Other possible sources of legal assistance and referral include state legal aid offices, state bar associations, local nonprofit agencies, foundations, and social service agencies.

Chapter 64 | Medicaid and Hill-Burton Free and Reduced-Cost Healthcare

Section 64.1 | Medicaid

This section contains text excerpted from the following sources: Text in this section begins with excerpts from "What Is the Medicaid Program?" Health Resources and Services Administration (HRSA), February 12, 2014. Reviewed December 2019; Text under the heading "Mandatory and Optional Medicaid Benefits" is excerpted from "Mandatory and Optional Medicaid Benefits," Centers for Medicare & Medicaid Services (CMS), October 12, 2016. Reviewed December 2019.

Good health is important to everyone. If you cannot afford to pay for medical care right now, Medicaid can make it possible for you to get the care that you need so that you can get healthy and stay healthy.

Medicaid is available only to certain low-income individuals and families who fit into an eligibility group that is recognized by federal and state law. Medicaid does not give money directly to you; instead, it sends payments directly to your healthcare providers. Depending on your state's rules, you may also be asked to pay a small part of the cost (a "copayment") for some medical services. In general, you should apply for Medicaid if you have limited income and resources and match one of the descriptions discussed below.

PREGNANT WOMEN
Apply for Medicaid if you think you are pregnant. You may be eligible if you are married or single. If you are on Medicaid when your child is born, both you and your child will be covered.

CHILDREN AND TEENAGERS
Apply for Medicaid if you are the parent or guardian of a child who is 18 years old or younger and your family's income is limited, or if your child is sick enough to need nursing-home care, but could stay home with good quality care at home. If you are a teenager living on your own, the state may allow you to apply for Medicaid on your own behalf or allow any adult to apply for you. Many states also cover children up to the age of 21.

PEOPLE WHO ARE AGED, BLIND, AND/OR DISABLED
Apply if you are 65 years of age or older, blind, or disabled and have limited income and resources. Apply if you are terminally ill and want to receive hospice services. Apply if you are elderly, blind, or disabled; live in a nursing home, and have limited income and resources. Apply if you are elderly, blind, or disabled and need nursing-home care, but can stay at home with special community care services. Apply if you are eligible for Medicare and have limited income and resources.

OTHER SITUATIONS
Apply if you are losing welfare coverage and need health coverage. Apply if you are a family with children under age 18 and have limited income and resources.

(You do not need to be receiving a welfare check to qualify.) Apply if you have very high medical bills that you cannot pay and you are pregnant, under the age of 18 or over the age of 65, blind, or disabled.

Medicaid is a state-administered program and each state sets its own guidelines regarding eligibility and services.

MANDATORY AND OPTIONAL MEDICAID BENEFITS

Following are the mandatory Medicaid benefits, which states are required to provide under federal law, and optional benefits that states may cover if they choose.

Mandatory Benefits

- Inpatient hospital services
- Outpatient hospital services
- Early and periodic screening, diagnostic, and treatment services (EPSDT)
- Nursing facility services
- Home health services
- Physician services
- Rural health clinic services
- Federally qualified health center (FQHC) services

Optional Benefits

- Prescription drugs
- Clinic services
- Physical therapy
- Occupational therapy
- Speech, hearing, and language disorder services
- Respiratory care services
- Other diagnostic, screening, preventive, and rehabilitative services
- Podiatry services
- Optometry services
- Dental Services
- Dentures
- Prosthetics
- Eyeglasses
- Chiropractic services
- Other practitioner services
- Private-duty nursing services
- Personal care
- Hospice
- Case management

- Services for Individuals age 65 or older in an institution for mental disease (IMD)
- Services in an intermediate care facility for individuals with intellectual disability
- State plan home and community-based services-1915(i)
- Self-directed personal assistance services-1915(j)
- Community first choice option-1915(k)
- Tuberculosis (TB)-related services
- Inpatient psychiatric services for individuals under age 21
- Other services approved by the Secretary*
- Health homes for enrolees with chronic conditions–Section 1945

This includes services furnished in a religious nonmedical healthcare institution, emergency hospital services by a non-Medicare certified hospital, and critical access hospital (CAH).

Section 64.2 | Hill-Burton Free and Reduced-Cost Healthcare

This section contains text excerpted from the following sources: Text in this section begins with excerpts from "Hill-Burton Free and Reduced-Cost Healthcare," Health Resources and Services Administration (HRSA), April 2019; Text under the heading "Frequently Asked Questions about Hill-Burton Free and Reduced-Cost Healthcare" is excerpted from "Frequently Asked Questions," Health Resources and Services Administration (HRSA), April 2017.

In 1946, Congress passed a law that gave hospitals, nursing homes, and other health facilities grants and loans for construction and modernization. In return, they agreed to provide a reasonable volume of services to people unable to pay for medical care and to make their services available to all persons residing in the facility's area.

The Hospital Survey and Construction (or Hill-Burton) Act, which is commonly referred to as "Hill-Burton," stopped providing these funds in 1997, but about 140 healthcare facilities nationwide are still obligated to provide free or reduced-cost care. Since 1980, more than $6 billion in uncompensated services have been provided to eligible patients through Hill-Burton.

FREQUENTLY ASKED QUESTIONS ABOUT HILL-BURTON FREE AND REDUCED-COST HEALTHCARE
What Services Does the Hill-Burton Program Cover?
Each facility chooses which services it will provide at no or reduced cost. The covered services are specified in a notice which is published by the facility and also in a notice provided to all persons seeking services in the facility. Services

fully covered by third-party insurance or a government program (e.g., Medicare and Medicaid) are not eligible for Hill-Burton coverage. However, Hill-Burton may cover services not covered by government programs.

Can I Receive Hill-Burton Assistance to Cover My Medicare Deductible and Coinsurance Amounts or Medicaid Copay and Spend Down Amounts?

Medicare deductible and coinsurance amounts are not eligible under the program. However, Medicaid copayment amounts are eligible, except in a long-term care facility. In addition, Medicaid spend down amounts (the liability a patient must incur before being eligible for Medicaid) are eligible in all Hill-Burton facilities.

Where Can I Get Hill-Burton Free or Reduced-Cost Care?

Hill-Burton obligated facilities must provide a certain amount of free or reduced-cost healthcare each year. Obligated facilities may be hospitals, nursing homes, clinics, or other types of healthcare facilities. You may apply for free or reduced-cost care before or after they are provided at the Admissions Office, Business Office, or Patient Accounts Office at the obligated facility.

Who Can Receive Free or Reduced-Cost Care through the Hill-Burton Program?

Eligibility for Hill-Burton free or reduced-cost care is based on a person's family size and income. Income is calculated based on your actual income for the last 12 months or your last 3 month's income times four, whichever is less. You may qualify if your income falls within the U.S. Department of Health and Human Services (HHS) poverty guidelines or, at some facilities, if your income is as much as twice (or triple for nursing-home services) the poverty guidelines.

What Does "Income" Include?

Gross income (before taxes), interest/dividends earned, and child support payments are examples of income. Assets, food stamps, gifts, loans, or one-time insurance payments are examples of items not included as income when considering eligibility. For self-employed people, income is determined after deductions for business expenses.

When Can I Apply for Hill-Burton Assistance?

You may apply for Hill-Burton assistance at any time, before or after you receive care. You may even apply after a bill has been sent to a collection agency. If a hospital obtains a court judgment before you applied for Hill-Burton assistance, the solution must be worked out within the judicial system. However, if you applied for Hill-Burton before a judgment was rendered and are found eligible, you will receive Hill-Burton even if a judgment was rendered while you were waiting for a response to your application.

Medicaid and Hill-Burton Free and Reduced-Cost Healthcare

Must I Be a U.S. Citizen for Hill-Burton Eligibility?

No. However, to determine your Hill-Burton eligibility, you must have lived in the United States for at least three months.

Can I Apply for Hill-Burton Assistance on Behalf of an Uninsured Relative or Friend?

Yes. You can apply for Hill-Burton assistance on behalf of any patient for whom you can provide the information required to establish eligibility (i.e., you must be able to provide information regarding the patient's family size and income).

Do I Have to Wait Until I Am Sick Before I Can Apply for Hill-Burton Assistance?

Hill-Burton is not health insurance. To apply for Hill-Burton assistance, you must have already received services or know that you will require a specific service in the near future.

What Are Some Reasons I Could Be Denied Hill-Burton Care?

The facility may deny your request if:

- For nonnursing homes, your income is more than the current poverty guidelines, or more than twice the guidelines if specified in the facility's allocation plan
- For nursing-home services, your income is more than the poverty guidelines, or double or triple the guidelines, if specified in the facility's allocation plan
- The facility has given out its required amount of free care as specified in its allocation plan; the services you requested or received are not covered in the facility's allocation plan
- The services you requested or received are to be paid by Medicare/Medicaid, insurance or other financial assistance program
- The facility asks you to first apply for Medicaid/Medicare or a financial assistance program, and you do not cooperate
- You do not give the facility requested proof of your income, such as a pay stub

What Can I Do If I Have a Complaint against a Hill-Burton Facility?

If you feel you were unfairly denied free care or reduced-cost care, a complaint must be filed in writing to the central office.

You must include:

- The name and address of the person making the complaint
- The name and location of the facility
- A statement of the actions that the complainant considers to violate the requirements of the Hill-Burton program

Division of Poison Control and Healthcare Facilities
Parklawn Bldg.
5600 Fishers Ln.
Rm. 16C-17
Rockville, MD 20857

What Other Service Obligation Does a Hill-Burton Facility Have?

Under the community service assurance, Hill-Burton facilities are responsible for providing emergency treatment and for treating all persons residing in the service area, regardless of race, color, national origin, creed or Medicare or Medicaid status. This assurance is in effect for the life of the facility. If you feel you were unfairly denied services or discriminated against, you should contact the Office for Civil Rights (OCR) at 800-368-1019.

How Do I Apply for Free Care?

You should contact the Admissions, Business or Patient Accounts Office at a Hill-Burton obligated facility to find out if you qualify for assistance and whether or not a facility provides the specific services needed.

How Can I Find Out Which Facilities in My Area Are Hill-Burton Facilities?

Check the Hill-Burton Obligated Facilities List for a facility in your state. Be aware that although a facility may be listed, you still need to call the facility to be certain that it still has funds available and that the service you desire would be covered.

Chapter 65 | **Paying for Complementary and Integrative Health Approaches**

USE OF COMPLEMENTARY HEALTH APPROACHES IN THE UNITED STATES

Data from the 2012 National Health Interview Survey (NHIS) show that 33 percent of adults and almost 12 percent of children use complementary health approaches, and that the most commonly used approach is natural products

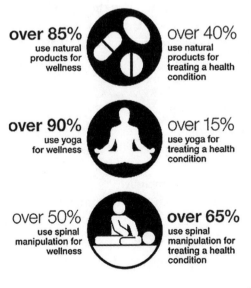

over 85%
use natural products for wellness

over 40%
use natural products for treating a health condition

over 90%
use yoga for wellness

over 15%
use yoga for treating a health condition

over 50%
use spinal manipulation for wellness

over 65%
use spinal manipulation for treating a health condition

Figure 65.1. Popularity of Complementary and Alternative Medicine in the United States *(Source: "Wellness-Related Use of Natural Product Supplements, Yoga, and Spinal Manipulation among Adults," National Center for Complementary and Integrative Health (NCCIH))*

This chapter includes text excerpted from "Paying for Complementary and Integrative Health Approaches," National Center for Complementary and Integrative Health (NCCIH), November 20, 2018.

(dietary supplements other than vitamins and minerals). Fish oil is the natural product most often used by adults and children. As for mind and body practices, adults and children most often turn to chiropractic or osteopathic manipulation, yoga, meditation, and massage therapy.

OUT-OF-POCKET SPENDING ON COMPLEMENTARY HEALTH APPROACHES

People seem to be willing to pay "out-of-pocket" (not through insurance) for certain complementary health approaches. In fact, out-of-pocket spending on these approaches for Americans ages 4 and older amounts to an estimated $30.2 billion per year, according to the 2012 NHIS. This includes:

- $14.7 billion out-of-pocket for visits to complementary and integrative health practitioners, such as chiropractors, acupuncturists, and massage therapists
- $12.8 billion out-of-pocket on natural products
- About $2.7 billion on self-care approaches (homeopathic medicines and self-help materials, such as books or CDs, related to complementary health topics)

This out-of-pocket spending for complementary health approaches represents 9.2 percent of all out-of-pocket spending by Americans on healthcare ($328.8 billion) and 1.1 percent of total healthcare spending ($2.82 trillion).

INSURANCE COVERAGE OF COMPLEMENTARY HEALTH APPROACHES

Many Americans use complementary health approaches, but the type of health insurance they have affects their decisions to use these practices. In a study, researchers analyzed 2012 NHIS data on acupuncture, chiropractic, and massage, and compared that with data from 2002. While use rates for all three approaches rose, the increase was much more pronounced among those who did not have health insurance. For those who had health insurance, coverage for these three approaches were more likely to be partial than full.

If you want to try a complementary or integrative approach and do not know if your health insurance will cover it, you should contact your health insurance provider to find out.

Some questions to ask your insurance provider include:

- Is this complementary or integrative approach covered for my health condition?
- Does it need to be:
  - Preauthorized or preapproved?
  - Ordered by a prescription?
- Do I need a referral?
- Does coverage require seeing a practitioner in the network?

Paying for Complementary and Integrative Health Approaches

- Do I have coverage if I go out-of-network?
- Are there any limits and requirements—for example, on the number of visits or the amount you will pay?
- How much do I have to pay out-of-pocket?

Keep records of all contacts you have with your insurance company, including notes on calls and copies of bills, claims, and letters. This may help if you have a claim dispute.

If you are choosing a new health insurance plan, ask the insurance provider about coverage of complementary or integrative health approaches. You should find out if you need a special "rider" or supplement to the standard plan for these approaches to be covered. You should also find out if the insurer offers a discount program in which plan members pay for fees and products out-of-pocket but at a lower rate.

Sources of Information on Insurers

Your state insurance department may be able to help you determine which insurance companies cover specific complementary or integrative health approaches. The USA.gov provides contact information for state and local consumer agencies, including insurance regulators.

Professional associations for complementary health specialties may monitor insurance coverage and reimbursement in their field. You can ask a reference librarian for help or search for them on the Internet.

ASKING PRACTITIONERS ABOUT PAYMENT

If you are planning to see a complementary or integrative practitioner, it is important to understand about payment. Here are some questions to ask:

- **Costs.** What does the first appointment cost? What do follow-up appointments cost? Is there a sliding scale based on income? How many appointments am I likely to need? Are there other costs (e.g., tests, equipment, supplements)?
- **Insurance.** Do you accept my insurance plan? What has been your experience with my plan's coverage for people with my condition? Do I file the claims, or do you take care of that?

FEDERAL HEALTH BENEFIT PROGRAMS

The federal government helps with some health expenses of people who are eligible for federal health benefit programs, such as programs for veterans, people aged 65 and older (Medicare), and people who cannot afford healthcare (Medicaid, funded jointly with the states).

Information on health benefits for veterans is available from the U.S. Department of Veterans Affairs (VA). Information on Medicare and Medicaid is available from the Centers for Medicare & Medicaid Services (CMS). A handbook, *Medicare & You,* explains what services Medicare covers.

Two other Internet resources—Benefits.gov and the Health and Insurance page on the Office of Personnel Management (OPM) website—explain federal health benefit programs. Benefits.gov has a benefits-finder that can help you learn more about qualifying for programs.

Chapter 66 | **Medicare's Preventive Services**

An easy and important way to stay healthy is to get disease prevention and early detection services. Disease prevention and early detection services can keep you from getting certain diseases or can help you find health problems early, when treatment works best. Talk with your doctor or healthcare provider to find out what tests or other services you may need, as described below, and how often you need them to stay healthy. If you have Medicare Part B, you will be able to get many preventive services at no cost to you.

PREVENTIVE SERVICES THAT COMES UNDER MEDICARE COVERAGE
Abdominal Aortic Aneurysm Screening
A one-time screening ultrasound for people at risk. If you have a family history of abdominal aortic aneurysms, or you are a man 65 to 75 and have smoked at least 100 cigarettes in your lifetime, you are considered at risk.

Alcohol Misuse Screening and Counseling
Medicare covers one alcohol misuse screening per year for adults with Medicare (including pregnant women) to identify those who misuse alcohol but are not alcohol dependent. If you screen positive, you can get up to four brief face-to-face counseling sessions per year (if you are competent and alert during counseling). A qualified primary-care doctor or other primary-care practitioner must provide counseling in a primary-care setting (such as a doctor's office).

Bone Mass Measurement
These tests help to see if you are at risk for broken bones. Medicare covers these tests once every 24 months (more often if medically necessary) for certain people at risk for osteoporosis.

This chapter includes text excerpted from "Staying Healthy—Medicare's Preventive Services," Centers for Medicare & Medicaid Services (CMS), September 2019.

Cardiovascular Disease

Medicare will cover one visit per year with your primary-care doctor to help lower your risk for cardiovascular disease. During this visit, your doctor may discuss aspirin use (if appropriate), check your blood pressure, and give you tips to make sure you are eating well.

Cardiovascular Disease Screenings

Ask your doctor to test your cholesterol, lipid, and triglyceride levels to help determine if you are at risk for a heart attack or stroke. If you are at risk, there are steps you can take to prevent these conditions. Medicare covers tests for cholesterol, lipid, and triglyceride levels every five years.

Colorectal Cancer Screenings

These tests help find colorectal cancer early, when treatment works best. If you are 50 or older, or are at high risk for colorectal cancer, Medicare covers one or more of these tests: fecal occult blood test, flexible sigmoidoscopy, screening colonoscopy, barium enema, and multi-target stool deoxyribonucleic acid (DNA) test (such as Cologuard™). How often Medicare pays for these tests depends on the test and your level of risk for this cancer. You and your doctor decide which test is best for you.

Depression Screening

Medicare covers one depression screening per year for all people with Medicare. The screening must be done in a primary-care setting (such as a doctor's office) that can provide follow-up treatment and referrals, if needed.

Diabetes Screenings

Medicare covers tests to check for diabetes or prediabetes. These tests are available if you have any of these risk factors: high blood pressure, history of abnormal cholesterol and triglyceride levels (dyslipidemia), obesity, or a history of high blood sugar. Tests are also covered if you have 2 or more of these: 65 or older, overweight, family history of diabetes (parents, brothers, sisters), a history of gestational diabetes (diabetes during pregnancy), or you delivered a baby weighing more than 9 pounds. Based on the results of these tests, you may be eligible for up to 2 screenings each year. Talk to your doctor for more information.

Diabetes Self-Management Training

This training helps teach you to cope with and manage your diabetes. The program may include tips for eating healthy, being active, monitoring blood sugar, taking medication, and reducing risks. You must have diabetes and a written order from your doctor or other healthcare providers.

Medicare's Preventive Services

Flu Shots
These shots help prevent influenza or flu virus. Medicare covers these shots once per flu season.

Glaucoma Tests
These tests help find the eye disease glaucoma. Medicare covers these tests once every 12 months for people at high risk for glaucoma.

Hepatitis B Shots
This series of shots helps protect people from getting hepatitis B. Medicare covers these shots for people at medium or high risk for hepatitis B.

Hepatitis B Virus Infection Screening
Medicare covers hepatitis B virus (HBV) infection screenings if you are at high risk for HBV infection or you are pregnant. Medicare will only cover these screenings if they are ordered by a primary-care provider. HBV infection screenings are covered annually only for those with continued high risk who do not get a hepatitis B vaccination. And for pregnant women at the first prenatal visit for each pregnancy, at the time of delivery for those with new or continued risk factors, at the first prenatal visit for future pregnancies, even if previously given the hepatitis B shot or had negative HBV screening results.

Hepatitis C Screening
Medicare covers a one-time hepatitis C screening test for those born between 1945 and 1965. Medicare also covers repeat screening annually for certain people at high risk who continue to engage in high-risk behavior. People with Medicare who are at high risk meet at least one of these conditions: current or past history of illicit injection drug use, or have had a blood transfusion before 1992.

HIV Screening
Medicare covers human immunodeficiency virus (HIV) screenings if you are 15 to 65, not at risk and ask for the screening or you are younger than 15 or older than 65, at an increased risk and ask for the screening. Medicare covers this test once every 12 months or up to 3 times during a pregnancy.

Lung Cancer Screening Test
Medicare covers lung cancer screening with low dose computed tomography (LDCT) once per year if you meet all of these: age 55 to 77, a current smoker or have quit smoking within the last 15 years, have a tobacco smoking history of at least 30 "pack years" (an average of 1 pack a day for 30 years), and get a written order from your physician or qualified nonphysician practitioner. Before your first lung cancer screening, you will need to schedule an appointment with your

doctor to discuss the benefits and risks of lung cancer screening. You and your doctor can decide whether lung cancer screening is right for you.

Breast Cancer Screening

Medicare covers mammograms once every 12 months for all women 40 and older. Medicare also covers 1 baseline mammogram for women between 35 and 39.

Medical Nutrition Therapy Services

Medicare may cover medical nutrition therapy and certain related services if you have diabetes or kidney disease, or you have had a kidney transplant in the last 36 months, and your doctor or other qualified nondoctor practitioner refers you for the service.

Medicare Diabetes Prevention Program

If you have Medicare Part B, have prediabetes, and meet other criteria, Medicare covers a once-per-lifetime proven health behavior change program to help you prevent type 2 diabetes. The program begins with at least 16 core sessions offered in a group setting over a 6-month period. After the core sessions, you may be eligible for additional monthly sessions that will help you maintain healthy habits.

Obesity Screening and Counseling

If you have a body mass index (BMI) of 30 or more, Medicare covers behavioral therapy sessions to help you lose weight. This counseling may be covered if you get it in a primary-care setting (such as a doctor's office), where it can be coordinated with your other care and a personalized prevention plan.

Pap Test, Pelvic Exam, and Breast Exam

These lab tests and exams check for cervical and vaginal cancers. Medicare covers these tests and exams every 24 months for all women and once every 12 months for women at high risk. Medicare also covers human papillomavirus (HPV) tests (when given with a Pap test) once every 5 years if you are age 30 to 65 without HPV symptoms.

Pneumococcal Shots

Medicare covers a pneumococcal shot to help prevent pneumococcal infections (such as certain types of pneumonia). Medicare also covers a different second shot if it is given one year (or later) after the first shot. Talk with your doctor or other healthcare provider to see if you need these shots.

Preventive Visits

One-time "Welcome to Medicare" preventive visit—Medicare covers a review of your health and education and counseling about preventive services, including certain screenings, shots, and referrals for other care, if needed. Medicare covers this visit only in the first 12 months of Medicare Part B (Medical Insurance) coverage.

Yearly "Wellness" visit—If you have had Part B for longer than 12 months, you are eligible for a yearly wellness visit to develop or update a personalized prevention plan based on your current health and risk factors. Medicare covers this visit once every 12 months.

Prostate Cancer Screenings

These tests help find prostate cancer. Medicare covers a digital rectal exam and a prostate-specific antigen (PSA) lab test once every 12 months for all men over 50 with Medicare (coverage begins the day after your 50th birthday).

Sexually Transmitted Infections Screening and Counseling

Medicare covers sexually transmitted infection (STI) screenings for chlamydia, gonorrhea, syphilis, and hepatitis B. These screenings are covered for people with Medicare who are pregnant and for certain people who are at increased risk for an STI when the tests are ordered by a primary-care doctor or other primary-care practitioner. Medicare covers these tests once every 12 months or at certain times during pregnancy. Medicare also covers up to two individual 20 to 30 minute, face-to-face high-intensity behavioral counseling sessions each year for sexually active adults at increased risk for STIs. Medicare will only cover these counseling sessions if they are provided by a primary-care provider and take place in a primary-care setting, such as a doctor's office. Counseling conducted in an inpatient setting, such as a skilled nursing facility, would not be covered as a preventive benefit.

Counseling to Prevent Tobacco Use and Tobacco-Caused Disease

Medicare covers up to 8 face-to-face visits in a 12-month period. All people with Medicare who use tobacco are covered. These visits must be provided by a qualified doctor or other Medicare-recognized provider.

WHAT YOU PAY

You will pay nothing for many preventive services if you get them from a qualified doctor or other healthcare provider who accepts assignment. For some preventive services, you might have to pay a deductible, coinsurance, and/or copayment. These amounts vary depending on the type of services you need and the kind of Medicare health plan you have.

Chapter 67 | Healthcare Benefit Laws: The Health Insurance Portability and Accountability Act and Consolidated Omnibus Budget Reconciliation Act

HEALTH INSURANCE PORTABILITY AND ACCOUNTABILITY ACT

The Health Insurance Portability and Accountability Act (HIPAA) offers protections for millions of America's workers that improve portability and continuity of health insurance coverage.

The Health Insurance Portability and Accountability Act Protects Workers and Their Families By

- Providing additional opportunities to enroll in group health plan coverage when they lose other health coverage, get married, or add a new dependent.
- Prohibiting discrimination in enrollment and in premiums charged to employees and their dependents, based on any health factors.

This chapter contains text excerpted from the following sources: Text under the heading "Health Insurance Portability and Accountability Act" is excerpted from "Health Insurance Portability and Accountability Act (HIPAA)," U.S. Department of Labor (DOL), July 3, 2019; Text under the heading "Consolidated Omnibus Budget Reconciliation Act Continuation Coverage" is excerpted from "COBRA Continuation Coverage," U.S. Department of Labor (DOL), November 2016. Reviewed December 2019.

- Preserving the states' role in regulating health insurance, including the states' authority to provide greater protections than those available under federal law.

Special Enrollment Rights

Special enrollment allows individuals who previously declined health coverage to enroll for coverage outside of a plan's open enrollment period. There are two types of special enrollment:

- **Loss of eligibility for other coverage.** Employees and dependents who decline coverage due to other health coverage and then lose eligibility or employer contributions have special enrollment rights. For example, an employee who turns down health benefits for herself/himself and her/his family because the family already has coverage through her/his spouse's plan can request special enrollment for her/his family in her/his own company's plan.
- **Certain life events.** Employees, spouses, and new dependents are permitted to special enroll because of marriage, birth, adoption, or placement for adoption.

For both types, the employee must request enrollment within 30 days of the loss of coverage or life event triggering the special enrollment.

Nondiscrimination Prohibitions

Employees and their family members cannot be denied eligibility or benefits based on certain health factors. They also cannot be charged more than similarly situated individuals based on any health factors. Health factors include medical conditions, claims experience, and genetic information.

The Health Insurance Portability and Accountability Act, and the Affordable Care Act (ACA) also provide protections from impermissible discrimination based on a health factor in wellness programs related to group health plan coverage (such as those that encourage employees to work out, stop smoking or meet certain health standards such as a target cholesterol level).

Preserving the States' Role

If a health plan provides benefits through an insurance company or health maintenance organization (HMO) (an insured plan), the HIPAA may be complemented by state laws that offer additional protections. For example, states may increase the number of days parents have to enroll newborns, adopted children, and children placed for adoption or require additional special enrollment circumstances.

Preexisting Condition Exclusions

The ACA prohibits plans from imposing preexisting condition exclusions for plan years beginning on or after January 1, 2014. For prior years, the HIPAA limited these exclusions and required plans to offset preexisting condition exclusion periods if the individual had prior health coverage.

CONSOLIDATED OMNIBUS BUDGET RECONCILIATION ACT CONTINUATION COVERAGE

Throughout a career, workers will face multiple life events, job changes or even job losses. The continuation coverage provisions of the Consolidated Omnibus Budget Reconciliation Act (COBRA)—help workers and their families keep their group health coverage during times of voluntary or involuntary job loss, reduction in the hours worked, transition between jobs and in certain other cases.

- The Consolidated Omnibus Budget Reconciliation Act generally requires that group health plans offer employees and their families the opportunity for a temporary extension of health coverage (called "continuation coverage") in certain instances where coverage under the plan would otherwise end.
- The law generally applies to all group health plans maintained by employers (private-sector and state/local government) that have at least 20 employees on more than 50 percent of its typical business days in the previous calendar year. Both full- and part-time employees are counted to determine whether a plan is subject to COBRA. The law does not apply to plans sponsored by the federal government or by churches and certain church-related organizations.
- Several events that can cause workers and their family members to lose group health coverage may result in the right to COBRA coverage. These include:
    - Termination of the covered employee's employment for any reason other than gross misconduct
    - Reduction in the covered employee's hours of employment
    - Covered employee becomes entitled to Medicare
    - Divorce or legal separation of the spouse from the covered employee
    - Death of the covered employee
    - Loss of dependent child status under the plan rules
- Under COBRA, the employee or family member may qualify to keep their group health plan benefits for a set period of time, depending on the reason for losing the health coverage. The following represents some basic information on periods of continuation coverage:

Table 67.1. Consolidated Omnibus Budget Reconciliation Act Continuation Coverage

Qualifying Event	Qualified Beneficiaries	Maximum Period of Continuation Coverage
Termination (for reasons other than gross misconduct) or reduction in hours of employment	Employee Spouse Dependent Child	18 months (In certain circumstances, qualified beneficiaries may become entitled to a disability extension of an additional 11 months or an extension of an additional 18 months due to the occurrence of a second qualifying event.)
Employee enrollment in Medicare	Spouse Dependent Child	36 months (The actual period of continuation coverage may vary depending on factors such as whether the Medicare entitlement occurred prior to or after the end of the covered employee's employment or reduction in hours.)
Divorce or legal separation	Spouse Dependent Child	36 months
Death of employee	Spouse Dependent Child	36 months
Loss of "dependent child" status under the plan	Dependent Child	36 months

- However, COBRA also provides that your continuation coverage may be cut short in certain cases.

Notification Requirements

- A general notice must be furnished to covered employees and spouses, within the first 90 days of coverage under the plan, informing them of their rights under COBRA and describing provisions of the law. COBRA information also is required to be contained in the plan's Summary Plan Description (SPD).
- Under COBRA, the covered employee or a family member has the responsibility to inform the plan administrator of a divorce, legal separation, disability, or a child losing dependent status under the plan.
- Employers have a responsibility to notify the plan administrator of the employee's death, termination of employment or reduction in hours, Medicare entitlement, or bankruptcy of a private-sector employer.
- When the plan administrator is notified that a qualifying event has happened (by the covered employee or family member, or by the employer), it must in turn notify each qualified beneficiary of the right to choose continuation coverage.

Healthcare Benefit Laws: HIPPA and COBRA

- The Consolidated Omnibus Budget Reconciliation Act allows at least 60 days from the date the election notice is provided to inform the plan administrator that the qualified beneficiary wants to elect continuation coverage.

Premium Payments

- Qualified individuals may be required to pay the entire premium for coverage up to 102 percent of the cost to the plan. Premiums may be higher for persons exercising the disability extension provisions of COBRA. Failure to make timely payments may result in loss of coverage.
- Premiums may be increased by the plan; however, premiums generally must be set in advance of each 12-month premium cycle.

Chapter 68 | Eligibility for Medicare Coverage of Home Healthcare

WHO IS ELIGIBLE?

If you have Medicare, you can use your home health benefits if:

- You are under the care of a doctor, and you are getting services under a plan of care established and reviewed regularly by a doctor
- You need, and a doctor certifies that you need, one or more of these:
  - Intermittent skilled nursing care (other than drawing blood)
  - Physical therapy
  - Speech-language pathology services
  - Continued occupational therapy
  - The home health agency caring for you is approved by Medicare (Medicare-certified)
- You are homebound, and a doctor certifies that you are homebound. To be homebound means:
  - You have trouble leaving your home without help (such as using a cane, wheelchair, walker, or crutches; special transportation; or help from another person) because of an illness or injury, or leaving your home is not recommended because of your condition
  - You are normally unable to leave your home, but if you do it requires a major effort

You may leave home for medical treatment or short, infrequent absences for nonmedical reasons, such as an occasional trip to the barber, a walk around the

This chapter includes text excerpted from "Medicare and Home Healthcare," Centers for Medicare & Medicaid Services (CMS), October 2017.

block or a drive, or attendance at a family reunion, funeral, graduation, or other infrequent or unique event. You can still get home healthcare if you attend adult day-care or religious services.

As part of your certification of eligibility, a doctor, or certain healthcare professionals who work with a doctor (such as a nurse practitioner), must document that they have had a face-to-face encounter with you (such as an appointment with your primary care doctor) within required time frames and that the encounter was related to the reason you need home healthcare.

If you only need skilled nursing care, but you need more than intermittent skilled nursing care, you do not qualify for home health services. To determine if you are eligible for home healthcare based on a medically-predictable recurring need for skilled nursing, Medicare defines intermittent as skilled nursing care that is needed or given either:

- Fewer than 7 days each week
- Daily for less than 8 hours each day for up to 21 days. Medicare may extend the three-week limit in exceptional circumstances if your doctor can predict when your need for daily skilled nursing care will end.

If you are expected to need full-time skilled nursing care over an extended period of time, you would not usually qualify for home health benefits.

WHAT IS COVERED?

If you are eligible for Medicare-covered home healthcare, Medicare covers these services if they are reasonable and necessary for the treatment of your illness or injury. Skilled nursing and therapy services are covered when a personalized assessment of your clinical condition shows that the specialized judgment, knowledge, and skills of a nurse or therapist are necessary for the services to be safely and effectively provided.

- **Skilled nursing care.** Medicare covers skilled nursing care when the services you need require the skills of a nurse, are reasonable and necessary for the treatment of your illness or injury, and are given on a part-time or intermittent basis (visits solely for the purpose of getting your blood drawn are not covered by Medicare). Part-time or intermittent means you may be able to get home health aide and skilled nursing services (combined) any number of days per week as long as the services are provided:
  - Fewer than 8 hours each day
  - 28 or fewer hours each week (or up to 35 hours a week in some limited situations)
- **A registered nurse (RN) or a licensed practical nurse (LPN) can provide skilled nursing services.** If you get services from an LPN,

your care will be supervised by an RN. Home health nurses provide direct care and teach you and your caregivers about your care. They also manage, observe, and evaluate your care. Examples of skilled nursing care include: giving IV drugs, certain injections, or tube feedings; changing dressings; and teaching about prescription drugs or diabetes care. Any service that could be done safely and effectively by a nonmedical person (or by yourself) without the supervision of a nurse is not skilled nursing care.

- **Physical therapy, occupational therapy, and speech-language pathology services.** Your therapy services are considered reasonable and necessary in the home setting if:
  - They are a specific, safe, and effective treatment for your condition
  - They are complex such that your condition requires services that can only be safely and effectively performed by, or under the supervision of, qualified therapists
  - Your condition requires one of these:
    - Therapy that is reasonable and necessary to restore or improve functions affected by your illness or injury
    - A skilled therapist to safely and effectively establish a program and/or perform therapy under a maintenance program to help you maintain your current condition or to prevent your condition from getting worse
    - The amount, frequency, and duration of the services are reasonable
- **Home health aide services.** Medicare will pay for part-time or intermittent home health aide services (such as personal care), if needed to maintain your health or treat your illness or injury. Medicare does not cover home health aide services unless you are also getting skilled care. Skilled care includes:
  - Skilled nursing care
  - Physical therapy
  - Speech-language pathology services
  - Continuing occupational therapy, if you no longer need any of the above

"Part-time or intermittent" means you may be able to get home health aide and skilled nursing services (combined) any number of days per week, as long as the services are provided:

- Fewer than 8 hours each day
- 28 or fewer hours each week (or up to 35 hours a week in some limited situations)
- **Medical social services.** Medicare covers these services when a doctor orders them to help you with social and emotional concerns that may

interfere with your treatment or how quickly you recover. This might include counseling or help finding resources in your community. However, Medicare does not cover medical social services unless you are also getting skilled care.

- **Medical supplies.** Medicare covers supplies, such as wound dressings, when your doctor orders them as part of your care.

Medicare pays separately for durable medical equipment. The equipment must meet certain criteria and be ordered by a doctor. Medicare usually pays 80 percent of the Medicare-approved amount for certain pieces of medical equipment, such as a wheelchair or walker. If your home health agency does not supply durable medical equipment directly, the home health agency staff will usually arrange for a home equipment supplier to bring the items you need to your home.

Note. Before your home healthcare begins, the home health agency should tell you how much of your bill Medicare will pay. The agency should also tell you if any items or services they give you are not covered by Medicare, and how much you will have to pay for them. This should be explained by both talking with you and in writing.

The home health agency is responsible for meeting all of your medical, nursing, rehabilitative, social, and discharge planning needs, as noted in your home health plan of care. Home health agencies are required to perform a comprehensive assessment of each of your care needs when you are admitted to the home health agency, and communicate those needs to the doctor responsible for the plan of care. After that, home health agencies are required to routinely assess your needs.

WHAT IS NOT COVERED?

Here are some examples of what Medicare does not pay for:

- 24-hour-a-day care at home
- Meals delivered to your home
- Homemaker services, such as shopping, cleaning, and laundry
- Custodial or personal care, such as bathing, dressing, and using the bathroom when this is the only care you need

Talk to your doctor or the home health agency if you have questions about whether certain services are covered. You can also call 800-633-4227. TTY users can call 877-486-2048.

Note. If you have a Medigap (Medicare Supplement Insurance) policy or other health coverage, be sure to tell your doctor or other healthcare provider so your bills get paid correctly.

Chapter 69 | **Things to Know before You Choose a Health-Insurance Plan**

Choosing a health-insurance plan can be complicated. Knowing just a few things before you compare plans can make it simpler.

THE METAL CATEGORIES: BRONZE, SILVER, GOLD, AND PLATINUM

Plans in the Health Insurance Marketplace are presented in four metal categories: Bronze, Silver, Gold, and Platinum. (Catastrophic plans are also available to some people.)

How You and Your Insurance Plan Split Costs

Estimated averages for a typical population. Your costs will vary.

Which Metal Category Is Right for You?
Bronze

- Lowest monthly premium
- Highest costs when you need care

Table 69.1. Estimated Averages for a Typical Population

Plan Category	The Insurance Company Pays	You Pay
Bronze	60%	40%
Silver	70%	30%
Gold	80%	20%
Platinum	90%	10%

This chapter includes text excerpted from "3 Things to Know before You Pick a Health Insurance Plan," Centers for Medicare & Medicaid Services (CMS), July 23, 2013. Reviewed December 2019.

- Bronze plan deductibles—the amount of medical costs you pay yourself before your insurance plan starts to pay—can be thousands of dollars a year.
- Good choice if you want a low-cost way to protect yourself from worst-case medical scenarios, such as serious sickness or injury. Your monthly premium will be low, but you will have to pay for most routine care yourself.

Silver
- Moderate monthly premium
- Moderate costs when you need care
- Silver deductibles—the costs you pay yourself before your plan pays anything—are usually lower than those of Bronze plans.
- Good choice if you qualify for extra savings—or, if not, if you are willing to pay a slightly higher monthly premium than Bronze to have more of your routine care covered.

Gold
- High monthly premium
- Low costs when you need care
- Deductibles—the amount of medical costs you pay yourself before your plan pays—are usually low.
- Good choice if you are willing to pay more each month to have more costs covered when you get medical treatment. If you use a lot of care, a Gold plan could be a good value.

Platinum
- Highest monthly premium
- Lowest costs when you get care
- Deductibles are very low, meaning your plan starts paying its share earlier than for other categories of plans.
- Good choice if you usually use a lot of care and are willing to pay a high monthly premium, knowing nearly all other costs will be covered.

Your Premium Can Be Lower, Based on Your Income
No matter which metal category you choose, you can save a lot of money on your monthly premium based on your income.

YOUR TOTAL COSTS FOR HEALTHCARE: PREMIUM, DEDUCTIBLE AND OUT-OF-POCKET COSTS
When choosing a plan, it is a good idea to think about your total healthcare costs, not just the bill (the premium) you pay to your insurance company every month.

Things to Know before You Choose a Health-Insurance Plan

Other amounts, sometimes called ""out-of-pocket costs," have a big impact on your total spending on healthcare—sometimes more than the premium itself.

Beyond Your Monthly Premium: Deductible and Out-of-Pocket Costs

- **Deductible.** How much you have to spend for covered health services before your insurance company pays anything (except free preventive services).
- **Copayments and coinsurance.** Payments you make each time you get a medical service after reaching your deductible.
- **Out-of-pocket maximum.** The most you have to spend for covered services in a year. After you reach this amount, the insurance company pays 100 percent for covered services.

How to Estimate Your Yearly Total Costs of Care

In order to pick a plan based on your total costs of care, you will need to estimate the medical services you will use for the year ahead. Of course, it is impossible to predict the exact amount. So, think about how much care you usually use, or are likely to use.

- Before you compare plans when you are logged in to HealthCare.gov or preview plans and prices before you log in, you can choose each family member's expected medical use as low, medium, or high.
- When you view plans, you will see an estimate of your total costs—including monthly premiums and all out-of-pocket costs—based on your household's expected use of care.
- Your actual expenses will vary but the estimate is useful for comparing plans' total impact on your household budget.

Total Costs and Metal Categories

When you compare plans in the Marketplace, the plans appear in four metal categories: Bronze, Silver, Gold, and Platinum. The categories are based on how you and the health plan share the total costs of your care.

Generally speaking, categories with higher premiums (Gold, Platinum) pay more of your total costs of healthcare. Categories with lower premiums (Bronze, Silver) pay less of your total costs.

So how do you find a category that works for you?

- **If you do not expect to use regular medical services and do not take regular prescriptions.** You may want a Bronze plan. These plans can have very low monthly premiums, but have high deductibles and pay less of your costs when you need care.
- **If you qualify for cost-sharing reductions (CSRs).** Silver plans may offer good value. If you qualify, your deductible will be lower and you will pay less each time you get care. But, you get these extra savings

only if you enroll in Silver. If you do not qualify for CSRs, compare premiums and out-of-pocket costs of Silver and Gold prices to find your right plan.

- **If you expect a lot of doctor visits or need regular prescriptions.** You may want a Gold plan or Platinum plan. These plans generally have higher monthly premiums but pay more of your costs when you need care.

HEALTH INSURANCE PLAN AND NETWORK TYPES

There are different types of Marketplace health insurance plans designed to meet different needs. Some types of plans restrict your provider choices or encourage you to get care from the plan's network of doctors, hospitals, pharmacies, and other medical service providers. Others pay a greater share of costs for providers outside the plan's network.

Types of Marketplace Plans

Depending on how many plans are offered in your area, you may find plans of all or any of these types at each metal level—Bronze, Silver, Gold, and Platinum.

Some examples of plan types you will find in the Marketplace include:

- **Exclusive provider organization (EPO).** A managed care plan where services are covered only if you use doctors, specialists, or hospitals in the plan's network (except in an emergency).
- **Health maintenance organization (HMO).** A type of health insurance plan that usually limits coverage to care from doctors who work for or contract with the HMO. It generally would not cover out-of-network care except in an emergency. An HMO may require you to live or work in its service area to be eligible for coverage. HMOs often provide integrated care and focus on prevention and wellness.
- **Point of service (POS).** A type of plan where you pay less if you use doctors, hospitals, and other healthcare providers that belong to the plan's network. POS plans require you to get a referral from your primary care doctor in order to see a specialist.
- **Preferred provider organization (PPO).** A type of health plan where you pay less if you use providers in the plan's network. You can use doctors, hospitals, and providers outside of the network without a referral for an additional cost.

QUALITY RATINGS OF HEALTH PLANS ON HEALTHCARE.GOV

For the 2020 plan year, HealthCare.gov is expanding the health insurance plan quality ratings (or star ratings) program to all states.

For the 2019 plan year, plans in only Michigan, Montana, New Hampshire, Virginia, and Wisconsin featured the quality ratings.

Overall Health Insurance Plan Quality Ratings

Each rated health plan has an "Overall" quality rating of 1 to 5 stars (5 is highest), which accounts for member experience, medical care, and health plan administration.

This gives you an objective way to quickly compare plans based on quality, as you shop.

What the Health Plan Star Ratings Are Based On

The plans' overall rating is based on three categories, each with its own star rating:
- **Member experience:** Based on surveys of member satisfaction with:
  - Their healthcare and doctors
  - Ease of getting appointments and services
- **Medical care:** Based on how well the plans' network providers manage member healthcare, including:
  - Providing regular screenings, vaccines, and other basic health services
  - Monitoring some conditions
- **Plan administration:** Based on how well the plan is run, including:
  - Customer service
  - Access to needed information
  - Network providers ordering appropriate tests and treatment

All health plans ratings are calculated the same way, using the same information sources.

Chapter 70 | **Purchasing Health Insurance as an Individual**

SHORT- AND LONG-TERM DISABILITY INSURANCE

If you cannot work because you get sick or injured, disability insurance will pay part of your income. You may be able to get insurance through your employer. You can also buy your own policy.

Types of Disability Policies

There are two types of disability policies:

- **Short-term policies** may pay for up to two years. Most last for a few months to a year.
- **Long-term policies** may pay benefits for a few years or until the disability ends.

Employers who offer coverage may provide short-term coverage, long-term coverage, or both.

If you plan to buy your own policy, shop around and ask:

- How is disability defined?
- When do benefits begin?
- How long do benefits last?
- How much money will the policy pay?

Federal Disability Programs

Two U.S. Social Security Administration (SSA) programs pay benefits to people with disabilities. Learn about Social Security Disability Insurance (SSDI) and Supplemental Security Insurance (SSI).

This chapter includes text excerpted from "Personal Insurance," USA.gov, September 3, 2019.

HEALTH INSURANCE PLANS
What Is Health Coverage?

Health insurance helps you pay for medical services and sometimes prescription drugs. Once you purchase insurance coverage, you and your health insurer each agree to pay a part of your medical expenses—usually a certain dollar amount or percentage of the expenses.

How to Get Health Coverage

You can get healthcare coverage through:

- A group coverage plan at your job or your spouse or partner's job
- Your parents' insurance plan, if you are under 26 years old
- A plan you purchase on your own directly from a health insurance company or through the Health Insurance Marketplace
- Government programs, such as Medicare, Medicaid, or Children's Health Insurance Program (CHIP)
- The U.S. Veterans Administration (VA) or TRICARE for military personnel
- Your state, if it provides a health insurance plan
- Continuing employer coverage from your former employer, on a temporary basis under the Consolidated Omnibus Budget Reconciliation Act (COBRA)

Types of Health Insurance Plans

When purchasing health insurance, your choices typically fall into one of three categories:

- Traditional fee-for-service health insurance plans are usually the most expensive choice, but they offer you the most flexibility in choosing healthcare providers
- Health maintenance organizations (HMOs) offer lower co-payments and cover the costs of more preventive care, but your choice of healthcare providers is limited to those who are part of the plan
- Preferred provider organizations (PPOs) offer lower co-payments such as HMOs but give you more flexibility in selecting a provider

Choosing a Health Insurance Plan

Read the fine print when choosing among different healthcare plans. Also ask a lot of questions, such as:

- Do I have the right to go to any doctor, hospital, clinic, or pharmacy I choose?
- Are specialists, such as eye doctors and dentists, covered?
- Does the plan cover special conditions or treatments, such as pregnancy, psychiatric care, and physical therapy?

- Does the plan cover home care or nursing home care?
- Will the plan cover all medications my physician may prescribe?
- What are the deductibles? Are there any co-payments? Deductibles are the amount you must pay before your insurance company will pay a claim. These differ from co-payments, which are the amount of money you pay when you receive medical services or a prescription.
- What is the most I will have to pay out of my own pocket to cover expenses?
- If there is a dispute about a bill or service, how is it handled?

LIFE INSURANCE

A life insurance policy states that you will pay premiums to an insurance company over time, and, in exchange, the company will pay a lump sum amount to a designated beneficiary upon your death. The money from your life insurance policy can help pay bills and help support your surviving family members' living expenses. You may need to adjust the amount of your life insurance policy related to major life events, such as buying a home, getting married, or having a child.

There is no set amount of life insurance you need. If you have dependents you want to provide for or leave an inheritance to charities, you may need more life insurance than someone without dependents or charitable causes to support. Consider potential future expenses that your loved ones may need. The life insurance payout could be used to replace the money you would have earned to pay for their college education, moving expenses, or retirement. You can buy an individual life insurance policy from an insurance agent. You may also be part of a group life insurance policy through your employer or civic organization. If you are a veteran, you may be eligible for the VA life insurance benefits.

There are two main types of life insurance policies:
- **Whole (or universal) life insurance policies** are considered permanent. As long as you pay the premium, the policy is in effect. In addition to paying a benefit upon your death, whole life insurance policies also have an investment or savings component. This means that you accumulate cash value over the life of the policy, so you can borrow money from these types of policies if you need to.
- **Term life insurance policies** are in effect for a certain period of time or term. If you have this type of policy and pass away during the term that the policy is in effect, the insurance company will pay a benefit. If you live past the time that the policy is in effect, the insurance company will not pay a benefit or give you a refund.

Term life insurance policies are usually less expensive than whole life insurance policies. This is because term life insurance policies only cover a set amount of time, while whole life insurance policies are intended to be permanent and because part of the money you pay is put away for savings.

Lost Life Insurance Policies

If you have misplaced a life insurance policy, your state's insurance commission may be able to help you locate a copy of it. A policy locator service can search for it for a fee. If the insurance company knows that an insured person has died but cannot locate the beneficiary, the company must turn the benefits over to the state's unclaimed property office.

Chapter 71 | High Deductible Health Insurance and Health Savings Accounts

One way to manage your healthcare expenses is by enrolling in a High Deductible Health Plan (HDHP) in combination with opening a Health Savings Account (HSA).

HIGH DEDUCTIBLE HEALTH PLAN

High deductible health plan is a plan with a higher deductible than a traditional insurance plan. The monthly premium is usually lower, but you pay more health-care costs yourself before the insurance company starts to pay its share (your deductible). A HDHP can be combined with an HSA, allowing you to pay for certain medical expenses with money free from federal taxes.

For 2019, the IRS defines a "HDHP" as any plan with a deductible of at least $1,350 for an individual or $2,700 for a family. An HDHP's total yearly out-of-pocket expenses (including deductibles, copayments, and coinsurance) cannot be more than $6,750 for an individual or $13,500 for a family. (This limit does not apply to out-of-network services.)

HEALTH SAVINGS ACCOUNT

Health savings account is a type of savings account that lets you set aside money on a pretax basis to pay for qualified medical expenses. By using untaxed dollars in an HSA to pay for deductibles, copayments, coinsurance, and some other expenses, you may be able to lower your overall healthcare costs. HSA funds generally may not be used to pay premiums.

While you can use the funds in an HSA at any time to pay for qualified medical expenses, you may contribute to an HSA only if you have an HDHP—generally a

This chapter includes text excerpted from "High Deductible Health Plans (HDHPS)," Centers for Medicare & Medicaid Services (CMS), August 8, 2019.

health plan (including a Marketplace plan) that only covers preventive services before the deductible. For plan year 2019, the minimum deductible is $1,350 for an individual and $2,700 for a family. For plan year 2020, the minimum deductible for an HDHP is $1,400 for an individual and $2,800 for a family. When you view plans in the Marketplace, you can see if they're "HSA-eligible."

For 2019, if you have an HDHP, you can contribute up to $3,500 for self-only coverage and up to $7,000 for family coverage into an HSA. For 2020, if you have an HDHP, you can contribute up to $3,550 for self-only coverage and up to $7,100 for family coverage into an HSA. HSA funds roll over year to year if you do not spend them. An HSA may earn interest or other earnings, which are not taxable.

Some health insurance companies offer HSAs for their HDHPs. Check with your company. You can also open an HSA through some banks and other financial institutions.

High deductible health plan is a plan with a higher deductible than a traditional insurance plan. The monthly premium is usually lower, but you pay more healthcare costs yourself before the insurance company starts to pay its share (your deductible). A HDHP can be combined with an HSA, allowing you to pay for certain medical expenses with money free from federal taxes.

For 2019, the IRS defines a "HDHP" as any plan with a deductible of at least $1,350 for an individual or $2,700 for a family. An HDHP's total yearly out-of-pocket expenses (including deductibles, copayments, and coinsurance) cannot be more than $6,750 for an individual or $13,500 for a family. (This limit does not apply to out-of-network services.)

Health savings account is a type of savings account that lets you set aside money on a pretax basis to pay for qualified medical expenses. By using untaxed dollars in an HSA to pay for deductibles, copayments, coinsurance, and some other expenses, you may be able to lower your overall healthcare costs. HSA funds generally may not be used to pay premiums.

While you can use the funds in an HSA at any time to pay for qualified medical expenses, you may contribute to an HSA only if you have an HDHP—generally a health plan (including a Marketplace plan) that only covers preventive services before the deductible. For plan year 2019, the minimum deductible is $1,350 for an individual and $2,700 for a family. For plan year 2020, the minimum deductible for an HDHP is $1,400 for an individual and $2,800 for a family. When you view plans in the Marketplace, you can see if they're "HSA-eligible."

For 2019, if you have an HDHP, you can contribute up to $3,500 for self-only coverage and up to $7,000 for family coverage into an HSA. For 2020, if you have an HDHP, you can contribute up to $3,550 for self-only coverage and up to $7,100 for family coverage into an HSA. HSA funds roll over year to year if you do not spend them. An HSA may earn interest or other earnings, which are not taxable.

High Deductible Health Insurance and Health Savings Accounts

Table 71.1. What You Pay for Your High Deductible Health Plan

	Minimum Deductible (The Amount You Pay for Healthcare Items and Services before Your Plan Starts to Pay)	Maximum Out-of-Pocket Costs (The Most You Had Have to Pay If You Need More Healthcare Items and Services)
Individual high deductible health plan	$1,400	$6,900
Family high deductible health plan	$2,800	$13,800

Some health insurance companies offer HSAs for their HDHPs. Check with your company. You can also open an HSA through some banks and other financial institutions.

HOW HIGH DEDUCTIBLE HEALTH PLANS AND HEALTH SAVINGS ACCOUNTS CAN REDUCE YOUR COSTS

High deductible health plans and HSAs can help you in reducing your healthcare costs. They can be of help for you in the following ways.

- If you enroll in an HDHP, you may pay a lower monthly premium but have a higher deductible (meaning you pay for more of your healthcare items and services before the insurance plan pays).
- If you combine your HDHP with an HSA, you can pay that deductible, plus other qualified medical expenses, using the money you set aside in your tax-free HSA.
- So, if you have an HDHP and do not need many healthcare items and services, you may benefit from a lower monthly premium. If you need more care, you will save by using the tax-free money in your HSA to pay for it.
- Your HSA balance rolls over year to year, so you can build up reserves to pay for healthcare items and services you need later.

WHAT IS CONSIDERED A HIGH DEDUCTIBLE HEALTH PLAN?

Under tax law, HDHPs must set a minimum deductible and a limit, or maximum, on out-of-pocket costs.

Table 71.1 shows the amount you need to pay for HDHPs for calendar year 2020.

High deductible health plan deductibles are often significantly higher than the minimums shown above and can be as high as the maximum out-of-pocket costs shown above.

Table 71.2. Amount of High Deductible Health Plan

Benefits of High Deductible Health Plans with Health Savings Accounts	But Also Consider...
High Deductible Health Plans (HDHPs) may have lower monthly premiums than non-HDHPs.	Your deductible—the costs you pay before the HDHP starts to pay—is higher than for many non-HDHPs.
You can deduct the amount you deposit in a Health Savings Accounts (HSA) from the income you pay federal income tax on.	If you have money in your HSA when you turn 65, you can spend it on anything you want—but if you are not spending it for a qualified medical expense it will be taxed as income at your then current tax rate.
You can use HSA funds to pay for deductibles, copayments, coinsurance, and other qualified medical expenses. Withdrawals to pay eligible medical expenses are tax-free.	
Unspent HSA funds roll over from year to year, allowing you to build tax-free savings to pay for medical care later. HSAs may earn interest, which is not subject to taxes.	
HDHPs are available in most areas, and may be available as qualified health plans at the Bronze, Silver, or Gold levels on HealthCare.gov. HDHPs may also be available for enrollment directly through health insurance companies and may be offered by your employer.	HDHPs may not be available in your area. You will find out when you compare plans on HealthCare.gov, or when you contact an agent, broker, or insurance company.
An HDHP may provide certain preventive care benefits without a deductible or with a deductible less than the minimum annual deductible.	

HOW HEALTH SAVINGS ACCOUNTS WORK WITH HIGH DEDUCTIBLE HEALTH PLAN?

An HSA is an account that lets you set aside money on a pretax basis to pay for qualified medical expenses, as defined in the tax law.

By using pretax dollars in an HSA to pay for deductibles, copayments, coinsurance, and other qualified expenses, including some dental, drug, and vision expenses, you can lower your overall healthcare costs. You can contribute to an HSA only if you have an HSA-eligible HDHP.

FINDING AND USING HEALTH SAVINGS ACCOUNTS-ELIGIBLE HIGH DEDUCTIBLE HEALTH PLANS

There are yearly limits for deposits into an HSA. These limits for 2020 are:

High Deductible Health Insurance and Health Savings Accounts

- $3,550 for self-only HDHP coverage
- $7,100 for family HDHP coverage

Amounts are adjusted yearly for inflation. If you are age 55 or older at the end of your tax year, your contribution limit is increased by $1,000.

How to Find a Health Savings Accounts-Eligible High Deductible Health Plans

- When you compare plans on HealthCare.gov, HSA-eligible HDHPs are identified on plan cards by an HSA-eligible flag in the upper left-hand corner.
- You can also filter to see only HSA-eligible plans by using the Filter option in the right-hand corner and selecting the Health Savings Account (HSA) Eligible Plans filter.

SETTING UP HEALTH SAVINGS ACCOUNTS

After you enroll in an HSA-eligible HDHP, you will need to open an HSA separately to get started.

How to Find a Health Savings Accounts Financial Institution

- Research HSA providers online. Use HSA comparison websites such as HSA search to help narrow your search.
- Check with your health insurance company to see if they partner with HSA financial institutions.
- Ask your bank if they offer an HSA option that meets your needs.

Things to Think about When Choosing a Health Savings Accounts

- Some HSAs have fees associated with them, such as a charge for opening or closing the account and monthly maintenance fees
- Banking options, services, and features, such as debit cards and online banking, may differ by HSA provider
- How you will make your pretax dollar deposits into your HSA may also vary

Chapter 72 | Medical Discount Plans—Service or Scam?

Looking for health insurance? Make sure that is what you are buying, or you could find yourself on the hook for big medical bills with no way to pay them.

Dishonest marketers make it sound like they are selling affordable health insurance, when really, it is a medical discount plan instead. Medical discount plans can be a way for some people to save money on their healthcare costs, but discount plans are not health insurance, and are not a substitute for it.

HEALTH INSURANCE VERSUS DISCOUNT PLANS

If you buy a health insurance plan, it generally covers a broad range of services and pays you or your healthcare provider for a portion of your medical bills.

With a medical discount plan, you generally pay a monthly fee to get discounts on specific services or products from a list of participating providers. Medical discount plans do not pay your healthcare costs.

Suspect a Healthcare Scam?*

Someone contacts you, offering discounts on health services and products. They might say the discount plan will save you money and that it meets the minimum coverage required under "Obamacare" so you would not have to pay a penalty or look at other plans.

Medical discount plans are not health insurance. Sometimes, medical discount plans illegally pretend to be insurance. Ask specific questions and do not pay until you read the terms. Your state insurance commissioner's office can tell you if a health plan is insurance. Most medical discount plans are a membership

This chapter contains text excerpted from the following sources: Text in this chapter begins with excerpts from "Discount Plan or Health Insurance?" Federal Trade Commission (FTC), November 2014. Reviewed December 2019; Text under the heading "Tips to Save Yourself from Scams" is excerpted from "Medical Discount Scams Bookmark," Federal Trade Commission (FTC), April 2013. Reviewed December 2019.

in a "club" that claims to offer reduced prices from certain doctors, certain pharmacies, and on some procedures. Some medical discount plans provide legitimate discounts, but others are scams that do not deliver on the medical services promised. Others are attempts to get your personal or financial information, so the scammer can use it to commit identity fraud.

Text excerpted from "Suspect a Healthcare Scam?" Federal Trade Commission (FTC), September 2013

MEDICAL DISCOUNT SCAMS

While there are medical discount plans that provide legitimate discounts, others take people's money and offer very little in return. Dishonest marketers sometimes make it sound like they are selling you health insurance, or lie about what their plans really offer. Here are some ways to ensure you do not get caught up in a discount scam

Beware of "Up-To Discounts"

"Discounts of up to 70 percent!"—but how often will you save that much? Savings with discount plans typically are a lot less. When you consider a discount plan's monthly premiums and enrollment fees, there may be no discount at all. What is more, if you have major health problems or an emergency, you will have to cover most, or all, of the bills if you do not have health insurance.

Confirm the Details

Medical discount plans are not a substitute for health insurance. Nevertheless, if you are interested in a discount plan, check whether the doctors you use participate. Call your providers, as well as others on the plan's list, before you enroll or pay any fees. Some dishonest plan promoters may tell you that particular local doctors participate when they do not, or they might send you outdated lists. Check out every claim, and get the details of the discount plan in writing before you sign up.

Do Not Sign Up on the Spot

Legitimate plans should be willing to point you to written information and give you the chance to check out their claims before you enroll. The pressure to sign up quickly or miss out on a "special deal" is your cue to say, "no thanks."

Some Pitches Are after Your Information

Unfortunately, identity thieves also use pitches for medical discount plans and insurance to get your personal information. Do not give out your financial information to someone who calls you out of the blue, or whose reputation you have not checked out. You can do that with your state insurance department, your state attorney general, your local Better Business Bureau (BBB), and even by entering the company's name and the word complaints or scam in an online search engine to see what others have to say.

CHECKING OUT PLANS

The idea behind medical discount plans—also known as "discount healthcare programs"—is that you will save money on products and services your insurance may not cover, such as dental, vision, hearing, or chiropractic services. Some people automatically get discount programs through their health insurance company.

Many states require medical discount programs to be licensed or registered. Your state insurance commissioner's office can tell you whether a medical discount program—or a health insurance plan—is licensed in your state, and may be able to alert you to a scam. Find your contact at naic.org or consumeraction.gov.

REPORT SCAMS

If you have been targeted by a medical discount scam, report it to the FTC at ftc.gov/complaint.

TIPS TO SAVE YOURSELF FROM SCAMS

Medical discount plans are different from health insurance, but scam artists often try to blur the lines.

- **Medical discount plans do not pay your healthcare costs.** They are not insurance. They offer discounts from certain providers.
- **Some discount plans do not make good on their promises.** Dishonest marketers may make it sound as if the discounts are bigger than they are, or as if they are offering affordable health insurance. You learn the truth when you get a bill.
- **Some plans do not include local providers—or give current lists.** Before you enroll or pay any money, call local providers on the list and check whether they offer the advertised discounts.
- **Some offers are just plain scams.** The plan you get could be worthless or a ploy to steel your information—and then your identity. Check out the company with your state Attorney General or state insurance department.

Chapter 73 | Low-Cost or Free Health Insurance for Children

If your children need health coverage, they may be eligible for the Children's Health Insurance Program (CHIP).

The CHIP provides low-cost health coverage to children in families that earn too much money to qualify for Medicaid. In some states, the CHIP covers pregnant women. Each state offers CHIP coverage and works closely with its state Medicaid program.

SEE IF YOUR CHILDREN QUALIFY AND APPLY FOR THE CHILDREN'S HEALTH INSURANCE PROGRAM

Each state program has its own rules about who qualifies for the CHIP. You can apply right now, any time of year, and find out if you qualify. If you apply for Medicaid coverage to your state agency, you will also find out if your children qualify for CHIP. If they qualify, you will not have to buy an insurance plan to cover them.

There are two ways to apply for the CHIP:

- Call 800-318-2596 (Toll-free TTY: 855-889-4325).
- Fill out an application through the Health Insurance Marketplace. If it looks like anyone in your household qualifies for Medicaid or CHIP, the Centers for Medicare & Medicaid Services (CMS) will send your information to your state agency. They will contact you about enrollment. When you submit your Marketplace application, you will also find out if you qualify for an individual insurance plan with savings based on your income instead. Create an account or log in to an existing account to get started.

This chapter includes text excerpted from "The Children's Health Insurance Program (CHIP)," Centers for Medicare & Medicaid Services (CMS), September 21, 2011. Reviewed December 2019.

WHAT THE CHILDREN'S HEALTH INSURANCE PROGRAM COVERS

The CHIP benefits are different in each state. But, all states provide comprehensive coverage, including:

- Routine check-ups
- Immunizations
- Doctor visits
- Prescriptions
- Dental and vision care
- Inpatient and outpatient hospital care
- Laboratory and x-ray services
- Emergency services

States may provide more CHIP benefits. Check with your state for information about covered services.

WHAT THE CHILDREN'S HEALTH INSURANCE PROGRAM COSTS

Routine well-child doctor and dental visits are free under the CHIP. But, there may be copayments for other services. Some states charge a monthly premium for the CHIP coverage. The costs are different in each state, but you will not have to pay more than five percent of your family's income for the year.

WHAT IF YOUR CHILDREN ARE ELIGIBLE FOR CHILDREN'S HEALTH INSURANCE PROGRAM, BUT YOU WOULD RATHER BUY A MARKETPLACE INSURANCE PLAN

If your children are eligible for the CHIP, they will not be eligible for any savings on Marketplace insurance. The CHIP coverage will probably be more affordable. Remember, you and other family members may be eligible for savings on the Marketplace insurance coverage.

IF YOUR CHILDREN CAN GET CHILDREN'S HEALTH INSURANCE PROGRAM, BUT YOU DO NOT QUALIFY FOR MEDICAID, HOW CAN YOU GET INSURED

You may be able to get an insurance plan through the Marketplace, with savings based on your income.

Create an account or log in to an existing account to get started. If it looks like anyone in your household qualifies for the Medicaid or the CHIP, CMS will send your information to your state agency. They will contact you about enrollment. When you submit your Marketplace application, you will also find out if you qualify for an individual insurance plan with savings based on your income instead.

Chapter 74 | High-Risk Health Insurance

WHAT ARE HIGH-RISK POOLS?

High-risk pools are programs created by states that focus on individuals who cannot afford insurance because of existing health conditions. They are a system of public programs and private markets designed to fulfill the needs of various types of consumers.

More than 30 states have established high-risk health-insurance pools that offer comprehensive health-insurance for people who cannot get it elsewhere.

WHO IS ELIGIBLE FOR HEALTH INSURANCE THROUGH HIGH-RISK POOLS?

State high-risk pools offer health insurance to people who have one or more eligibility criteria of the following:

Medically Eligible

High-risk pools can provide health benefits for people who are otherwise uninsurable. Individuals who:

- Work part-time, and therefore, receive no health-insurance benefits from their employers
- Work in a firm that does not offer health-insurance benefits
- Are unemployed and eligible for high-risk health insurance

Individuals who do not have employer-sponsored insurance (ESI) and who do not qualify for public programs can enroll for high-risk insurance. High-risk pools provide health coverage for people who might be able to afford insurance, but are in poor health and cannot find health insurers willing to sell them health-insurance policies.

These individuals and their fellow pool members must meet specific eligibility requirements in order to qualify for this program, though.

"High-Risk Health Insurance," © 2020 Omnigraphics. Reviewed December 2019.

Health Insurance Portability and Accountability Act Eligible

The Health Insurance Portability and Accountability Act (HIPAA) assures the right to buy an individual health plan based on the following:

- You must be insured for 18 months of continuous creditable coverage.
- The last day of the coverage must be under a group health plan.
- You must have used up all your Consolidated Omnibus Budget Reconciliation Act (COBRA) coverage.
- You cannot be eligible for Medicaid or Medicare.
- You must have maintained the coverage plan without a gap of more than 63 days.

If you meet the above-mentioned conditions, any insurance company can provide access to health insurance regardless of your preexisting health condition. However, health-insurance companies determine which health plan they will provide for these HIPAA-eligible individuals.

MEDICARE ELIGIBLE

Two-thirds of state high-risk pools offer health insurance for individuals who are in need of supplemental coverage.

If an individual had no previous insurance and is unable to obtain insurance on their own, then it is recommended that they contact their state insurance commissioner to determine if their state has a high-risk health insurance pool program.

WHAT IS THE COST OF HIGH-RISK INSURANCE COVERAGE?

The cost of the high-risk pool is set by state law. Each state law sets premium caps at various levels. Almost all state high-risk pools set premium caps at 150 to 200 percent of market rates. For example, the Oregon pool discounts 95 percent premiums for individuals who have income up to 180 percent of the level of poverty. Most pools offer health-insurance plans with various deductibles.

Differences in benefits among high-risk pools and overall insurance costs are the result of rate regulation and enforcement and market forces, which vary by state.

WHAT ARE THE BENEFITS OF THE HIGH-RISK POOLS?

Even though the health-insurance plans provided by the state high-risk pools vary, these pools reflect the same coverage when compared to the private nongroup market. It is noted that state high-risk pools offer more than one plan for enrollees. Cost-sharing requirements and other deductibles also vary by state. Most state high-risk pools have at least one plan which contains a lifetime maximum clause.

WHAT ARE TYPICAL DEDUCTIBLES?

High-risk pools offer health-insurance policies at different deductibles ranging from a minimum amount of $500 up to $10,000 per year, which means you, as the insured individual, must pay this deductible prior to the policy covering the claim. You may also choose to begin a tax-free Health Savings Account (HAS) for the purpose of saving money for the deductibles and other expenses that are not covered in the high-risk pool.

CAN LOW-INCOME PEOPLE OBTAIN INSURANCE THROUGH HIGH-RISK POOLS?

A few states (Connecticut, Colorado, Montana, Washington, New Mexico, Oregon, and Wisconsin) offer premium plans to lower-income people who want to participate in high-risk pools.

References

1. "Health Insurance: State High Risk Pools," EveryCRSReport.com, January 26, 2011.
2. Pollitz, Karen. "High-Risk Pools for Uninsurable Individuals," Kaiser Family Foundation (KFF), February 22, 2017.
3. Hall, Jean P. "High-Risk Pools for People with Preexisting Conditions: A Refresher Course," The Commonwealth Fund, March 29, 2017.
4. "What Is HIPAA?" GoHealth, November 24, 2008.
5. Bihari, Michael. "Health Insurance: Understanding High Risk Pools," Verywell Health, April 7, 2019.

Chapter 75 | Transitioning from the Marketplace to Medicare Coverage

MEDICARE AND THE MARKETPLACE

The Health Insurance Marketplace is designed for people who do not have health coverage. If you have health coverage through Medicare, the Marketplace does not affect your Medicare choices or benefits. This means that no matter how you get Medicare, whether through Original Medicare or a Medicare health plan, you would not have to make any changes to your current Medicare coverage.

If I Have Medicare, Do I Need to Do Anything with the Marketplace during Medicare's Open Enrollment?

No. Medicare's Open Enrollment is not part of the Marketplace.

During the Medicare's Open Enrollment period (October 15 to December 7), you can review your current Medicare health and prescription drug coverage to see if it still meets your needs. Take a look at any cost, coverage, and benefit changes that will take effect next year. If you want to change your coverage for next year, do so during this time. If you feel your current coverage will continue to meet your needs for next year, you do not need to do anything.

If you have Medicare, make sure that you are reviewing Medicare plans, not Marketplace ones.

This chapter contains text excerpted from the following sources: Text under the heading "Medicare and the Marketplace" is excerpted from "Medicare and the Marketplace," Centers for Medicare & Medicaid Services (CMS), August 17, 2012. Reviewed December 2019; Text beginning with the heading "Turning 65 Soon? How to Transition from the Marketplace to Medicare Coverage" is excerpted from "From Marketplace to Medicare Coverage: Turning 65 Soon? How to Transition from the Marketplace to Medicare Coverage," Centers for Medicare & Medicaid Services (CMS), July 31, 2015. Reviewed December 2019.

What If I Already Have Medicare, and Someone Tries to Sell Me a Marketplace Plan?

It is against the law for someone who knows that you have Medicare to sell you a Marketplace plan. During Medicare's Open Enrollment, there is a higher risk for fraudulent activities.

TURNING 65 SOON? HOW TO TRANSITION FROM THE MARKETPLACE TO MEDICARE COVERAGE

If you have a health plan through the Health Insurance Marketplace and will soon have Medicare eligibility, it is not too soon to start planning for your coverage to switch.

If you have a Marketplace plan now, you can keep it until your Medicare coverage starts. Then, you can cancel the Marketplace plan without penalty.

WHEN TO APPLY FOR MEDICARE

Once Medicare eligibility begins, you will have a 7-month Initial Enrollment Period to sign up. For most people, this is 3 months before, the month, and 3 months after their 65th birthday.

It is important to sign up for Medicare when you are first eligible because once your Medicare Part A coverage starts, you will have to pay full price for a Marketplace plan. This means you will no longer be eligible to use any premium tax credit or help with costs you might have been getting with your Marketplace plan. Also, if you enroll in Medicare after your Initial Enrollment Period, you may have to pay a late enrollment penalty. It is important to coordinate the date your Marketplace coverage ends with the effective date of your Medicare enrollment, to make sure you do not have a break in coverage. If you have limited income or resources, you may qualify for help paying costs.

HOW TO CANCEL YOUR MARKETPLACE COVERAGE

If you are the only person on your Marketplace application, you can cancel the whole application.

If you and your spouse (or other household members) are enrolled on the same Marketplace plan, but you are the only one eligible for Medicare, you will cancel Marketplace coverage for just yourself. This way any others on the Marketplace application can keep Marketplace coverage.

Chapter 76 | **Filing a Claim for Your Health or Disability Benefits**

If you participate in a health plan or a plan that provides disability benefits, you will want to know how to file a claim for your benefits. The steps outlined below describe some of your plan's obligations and briefly explain the procedures and timelines for filing a health or disability benefits claim.

Before you file, however, be aware of the Employee Retirement Income Security Act (ERISA), of 1974, a federal law that protects your health and disability benefits and sets standards for those who administer your plan. Among other things, the law and rules issued by the U.S. Department of Labor (DOL) include requirements for the processing of benefit claims, the timeline for a decision when you file a claim, and your rights when a claim is denied.

The Affordable Care Act (ACA) (also called "Obamacare") includes additional requirements for claims processing for group health plans that are nongrandfathered. A nongrandfathered health plan is a plan that was established, or that has made certain significant changes, after March 23, 2010.

You should know that ERISA does not cover some employee benefit plans (such as those sponsored by government entities and most churches). If, however, you are one of the millions of participants and beneficiaries who depend on health or disability benefits from a private-sector employment-based plan.

REVIEWING INFORMATION FROM YOUR PLAN

A key document related to your plan is the Summary Plan Description (SPD). The SPD is the brochure you receive when you first are covered by your employer's plan. It provides a detailed overview of the plan—how it works, what benefits it provides, and how to file a claim for benefits. It also describes

This chapter includes text excerpted from "Filing a Claim for Your Health or Disability Benefits," U.S. Department of Labor (DOL), September 2015. Reviewed December 2019.

your rights as well as your responsibilities under ERISA and your plan. You also can find answers to many of your questions in the Summary of Benefits and Coverage (SBC), a short, easy-to-understand summary of the benefits available under your plan and detailed information on the out-of-pocket costs for coverage. For some single-employer collectively bargained plans, you should also check the collective bargaining agreement's (CBA) claim filing, grievance, and appeal procedures as they may apply to claims for health and disability benefits.

Before you apply for health or disability benefits, review the SPD to make sure you meet the plan's requirements and understand the procedures for filing a claim. Sometimes claims procedures are contained in a separate booklet that is handed out with your SPD. If you do not have a copy of your plan's SPD or claims procedures, make a written request for one or both to your plan's administrator. Your plan administrator is required to provide you with a copy.

FILING A CLAIM

An important first step is to check your SPD and the SBC to make sure you meet your plan's requirements to receive benefits. Your plan might say, for example, that a waiting period must pass before you can enroll and receive benefits or that a dependent is not covered after a certain age. Also, be aware of what your plan requires to file a claim. The SPD or claims procedure booklet must include information on where to file, what to file, and whom to contact if you have questions about your plan, such as the process for providing a required preapproval for health benefits. Plans generally cannot charge any filing fees or costs for filing claims and appeals.

If, for any reason, that information is not in the SPD or claims procedure booklet, write your plan administrator, your employer's human resource department (or the office that normally handles claims), or your employer to notify them that you have a claim. Keep a copy of the letter for your records. You may also want to send the letter by certified mail, return receipt requested, so you will have a record that the letter was received and by whom.

If it is not you, but an authorized representative who is filing the claim, that person should refer to the SPD and follow your plan's claims procedure. Your plan may require you to complete a form to name the representative. If it is an emergency situation, the treating physician can automatically become your authorized representative without you having to complete a form.

When a claim is filed, be sure to keep a copy for your records.

TYPES OF CLAIMS

All health and disability benefit claims must be decided within a specific time limit, depending on the type of claim filed.

Filing a Claim for Your Health or Disability Benefits

- **Group health claims** are divided into three types: urgent care, preservice, and postservice claims, with the type of claim determining how quickly a decision must be made. The plan must decide what type of claim it is except when a physician determines that the urgent care is needed.
  - **Urgent-care claims** are a special kind of preservice claim that requires a quicker decision because your health would be threatened if the plan took the normal time permitted to decide a preservice claim. If a physician with knowledge of your medical condition tells the plan that a preservice claim is urgent, the plan must treat it as an urgent care claim.
  - **Preservice claims** are requests for approval that the plan requires you to obtain before you get medical care, such as preauthorization or a decision on whether a treatment or procedure is medically necessary.
  - **Postservice claims** are all other claims for benefits under your group health plan, including claims after medical services have been provided, such as requests for reimbursement or payment of the costs of the services provided. Most claims for group health benefits are postservice claims.
- **Disability claims** are requests for benefits where the plan must make a determination of disability to decide the claim.

WAITING FOR A DECISION ON YOUR CLAIM

As noted, ERISA sets specific periods of time for plans to evaluate your claim and inform you of the decision. The time limits are counted in calendar days, so weekends and holidays are included. These limits do not govern when the benefits must be paid or provided. If you are entitled to benefits, check your SPD for how and when benefits are paid. Plans are required to pay or provide benefits within a reasonable time after a claim is approved.

- **Urgent-care claims** must be decided as soon as possible, taking into account the medical needs of the patient, but no later than 72 hours after the plan receives the claim. The plan must tell you within 24 hours if more information is needed; you will have no less than 48 hours to respond. Then the plan must decide the claim within 48 hours after the missing information is supplied or the time to supply it has elapsed. The plan cannot extend the time to make the initial decision without your consent. The plan must give you notice that your claim has been granted or denied before the end of the time allotted for the decision. The plan can notify you orally of the benefit determination so long as a written notification is furnished to you no later than 3 days after the oral notification.

- **Preservice claims** must be decided within a reasonable period of time appropriate to the medical circumstances, but no later than 15 days after the plan has received the claim. The plan may extend the time period up to an additional 15 days if, for reasons beyond the plan's control, the decision cannot be made within the first 15 days. The plan administrator must notify you prior to the expiration of the first 15-day period, explaining the reason for the delay, requesting any additional information, and advising you when the plan expects to make the decision. If more information is requested, you have at least 45 days to supply it. The plan then must decide the claim no later than 15 days after you supply the additional information or after the period of time allowed to supply it ends, whichever comes first. If the plan wants more time, the plan needs your consent. The plan must give you written notice that your claim has been granted or denied before the end of the time allotted for the decision.

- **Postservice health claims** must be decided within a reasonable period of time, but not later than 30 days after the plan has received the claim. If, because of reasons beyond the plan's control, more time is needed to review your request, the plan may extend the time period up to an additional 15 days. However, the plan administrator has to let you know before the end of the first 30-day period, explaining the reason for the delay, requesting any additional information needed, and advising you when a final decision is expected. If more information is requested, you have at least 45 days to supply it. The claim then must be decided no later than 15 days after you supply the additional information or the period of time given by the plan to do so ends, whichever comes first. The plan needs your consent if it wants more time after its first extension. The plan must give you notice that your claim has been denied in whole or in part (paying less than 100 percent of the claim) before the end of the time allotted for the decision.

- **Disability claims** must be decided within a reasonable period of time, but not later than 45 days after the plan has received the claim. If, because of reasons beyond the plan's control, more time is needed to review your request, the plan can extend the timeframe up to 30 days. The plan must tell you prior to the end of the first 45-day period that additional time is needed, explaining why, any unresolved issues and additional information needed, and when the plan expects to render a final decision. If more information is requested during either extension period, you will have at least 45 days to supply it. The claim then must be decided no later than 30 days after you supply the additional information or the period of time given by the plan to do so ends, whichever comes first. The plan administrator may extend the time period for up to another 30 days as long as it notifies you before the first extension expires. For any additional extensions, the plan needs your consent. The plan must give you notice whether your claim has been denied before the end of the time allotted for the decision.

If your claim is denied, the plan administrator must send you a notice, either in writing or electronically, with a detailed explanation of why your claim was denied and a description of the appeal process. In addition, the plan must include the plan rules, guidelines, or exclusions (such as medical necessity or experimental treatment exclusions) used in the decision or provide you with instructions on how you can request a copy of these documents from the plan. The notice may also include a specific request for you to provide the plan with additional information in case you wish to appeal your denial.

APPEALING A DENIED CLAIM

Claims are denied for various reasons. Perhaps you are not eligible for benefits. Perhaps the services you received are not covered by your plan. Or, perhaps the plan simply needs more information about your claim. Whatever the reason, you have at least 180 days to file an appeal (check your SPD or claims procedure to see if your plan provides a longer period).

Use the information in your claim denial notice in preparing your appeal. You should also be aware that the plan must provide claimants, on request and free of charge, copies of documents, records, and other information relevant to the claim for benefits. The plan also must identify, at your request, any medical or vocational expert whose advice was obtained by the plan. Be sure to include in your appeal all information related to your claim, particularly any additional information or evidence that you want the plan to consider, and get it to the person specified in the denial notice before the end of the 180-day period.

REVIEWING AN APPEAL

On appeal, your claim must be reviewed by someone new who looks at all of the information submitted and consults with qualified medical professionals if a medical judgment is involved. This reviewer cannot be the same person or a subordinate of the person who made the initial decision and the reviewer must give no consideration to that decision.

Plans have specific periods of time within which to review your appeal, depending on the type of claim.

- **Urgent-care claims** must be reviewed as soon as possible, taking into account the medical needs of the patient, but not later than 72 hours after the plan receives your request to review a denied claim.

- **Preservice claims** must be reviewed within a reasonable period of time appropriate to the medical circumstances, but not later than 30 days after the plan receives your request to review a denied claim.
- **Postservice claims** must be reviewed within a reasonable period of time, but not later than 60 days after the plan receives your request to review a denied claim. If a group health plan needs more time, the plan must get your consent. If you do not agree to more time, the plan must complete the review within the permitted time limit.
- **Disability claims** must be reviewed within a reasonable period of time, but not later than 45 days after the plan receives your request to review a denied claim. If the plan determines special circumstances exist and an extension is needed, the plan may take up to an additional 45 days to decide the appeal. However, before taking the extension, the plan must notify you in writing during the first 45-day period explaining the special circumstances, and the date by which the plan expects to make the decision.

There are two exceptions to these time limits. In general, single-employer collectively bargained plans may use a collectively bargained grievance process for their claims appeal procedure if it has provisions on filing, determination, and review of benefit claims. Multi-employer collectively bargained plans are given special timeframes to allow them to schedule reviews on appeal of post-service claims and disability claims for the regular quarterly meetings of their boards of trustees. If you are a participant in one of those plans and you have questions about your plan's procedures, you can consult your plan's SPD and CBA, or contact the DOL Employee Benefits Security Administration (EBSA) at the phone number below.

Plans can require you to go through two levels of review of a denied health or disability claim to finish the plan's claims process. If two levels of review are required, the maximum time for each review generally is half of the time limit permitted for one review. For example, in the case of a group health plan with one appeal level, as noted above, the review of a preservice claim must be completed within a reasonable period of time appropriate to the medical circumstances but no later than 30 days after the plan gets your appeal. If the plan requires two appeals, each review must be completed within 15 days for preservice claims. If your claim on appeal is still denied after the first review, the plan has to allow you a reasonable period of time (but not a full 180 days) to file for the second review.

Once the final decision on your claim is made, the plan must send you a written explanation of the decision. The notice must be in plain language that can be understood by participants in the plan. It must include all the specific reasons for the denial of your claim on appeal, refer you to the plan provisions on which the decision is based, tell you if the plan has any additional voluntary levels of appeal, explain your right to receive documents that are relevant to your benefit claim free of charge, and describe your rights to seek judicial review of the plan's decision.

IF YOUR APPEAL IS DENIED

If the plan's final decision denies your claim, you may want to seek legal advice regarding your rights to bring an action in court to challenge the denial. Normally, you must complete your plan's claim process before filing an action in court to challenge the denial of a claim for benefits. However, if you believe your plan failed to establish or follow a claims procedure consistent with the Department's rules described in this chapter, you may want to seek legal advice regarding your right to ask a court to review your benefit claim without waiting for a decision from the plan. You also may want to contact the nearest EBSA office about your rights if you believe the plan failed to follow any of ERISA's requirements in handling your benefit claim.

If your appeal is denied and you are in a nongrandfathered health plan, you also have the right to external review of the decision, as discussed below. To find out if your plan is not grandfathered, check the documents from your plan describing the plan's benefits. If your plan is grandfathered, it must be disclosed. If there is no disclosure in your plan's documents, your plan likely is not grandfathered.

ADDITIONAL PROTECTIONS IF YOUR PLAN IS NOT GRANDFATHERED UNDER THE AFFORDABLE CARE ACT

Nongrandfathered health plans, or insurers to those plans, must provide additional internal claims and appeal rights and a process for external review of benefit claim denials. Internal claims and appeals are your health claims or appeals of denials reviewed by your plan. These rights also apply to rescissions (retroactive cancellations) of coverage.

The additional internal claims and appeal protections include:

- Providing you with new or additional evidence or rationale, and the opportunity to respond to it, before a final decision is made on the claim
- Ensuring that claims and appeals are adjudicated in an independent and impartial manner
- Providing detail on the claim involved, the reason for denial (including the denial code and meaning), the internal and external appeals processes that are available, and information on consumer assistance, in all claims denial notices
- Providing, on request, diagnosis and treatment codes (and their meanings) for any denied claim

- Providing notices in a culturally and linguistically appropriate manner
- Allowing you to begin the external review process if the plan fails to follow the internal claims requirements (unless the plan's violation is minimal)
- Allowing you to resubmit an internal claim if a request for an immediate external review is rejected

Nongrandfathered plans also must provide a process for an external review of claims denials by an independent party. The external review process used depends on whether the plan is self-funded or provides benefits through an insurance company. The notice of the denial of your claim from your plan will describe the external review process and your rights. To request an external review of your claim denial, follow the steps provided in your denial notice.

FILING A CLAIM—SUMMARY

- Check your plan's benefits and claims procedure before filing a claim. Read your SPD and SBC. Contact your plan administrator if you have questions.
- Once your claim is filed, the maximum allowable waiting period for a decision varies by the type of claim, ranging from 72 hours to 45 days. However, your plan can extend certain time periods but must notify you before doing so. Usually, you will receive a decision within this timeframe.
- If your claim is denied, you must receive a written notice, including specific information about why your claim was denied and how to file an appeal.
- You have at least 180 days to request a full and fair review of your denied claim. Use your plan's appeals procedure and be aware that you may need to gather and submit new evidence or information to help the plan in reviewing the claim.
- Reviewing your appeal can take between 72 hours and 60 days depending on the type of claim. The law and the Department's rules allow a disability plan additional time if the plan's administrator has notified you beforehand of the need for an extension. For an appeal of a health claim, the plan needs your permission for an extension. The plan must send you a written notice telling you whether the appeal was granted or denied.
- If the appeal is denied, the written notice must tell you the reason it was denied, describe any additional appeal levels or voluntary appeal procedures offered by the plan, and contain a statement regarding your rights to seek judicial review of the plan's decision.
- You may decide to seek legal advice if your claim's appeal is denied or if the plan failed to establish or follow reasonable claims procedures. If you

believe the plan failed to follow ERISA's requirements, you also may want to contact the nearest EBSA office concerning your rights under ERISA.

- If the appeal is denied and your plan is not grandfathered, the denial notice will describe your rights to independent external review of the denied claim. To request external review, follow the steps provided in the notice.

Part 8 | **Additional Help and Information**

Chapter 77 | Glossary of Terms Related to Disease Management

accuracy: A measure of agreement between a test result and an accepted reference value. Example: if you have a standardized reference material at a known value (such as 180 mg/dl of cholesterol), accuracy measures how close the result of the test you are using will get to the known value. You may have a test that is very precise yet very inaccurate, which would be the case if your device measures 180 mg/dl of cholesterol reproducibly as 240 mg/dl.

activities of daily living (ADL): The tasks of everyday life. These activities include eating, dressing, getting into or out of a bed or chair, taking a bath or shower, and using the shopping, doing housework, and using a telephone.

advance directive: A legal document that states the treatment or care a person wishes to receive or not receive if she or he becomes unable to make medical decisions (for example, due to being unconscious or in a coma).

Alzheimer disease (AD): A progressive and fatal disease in which nerve cells in the brain degenerate and brain matter shrinks, resulting in impaired thinking, behavior and memory.

analyte: The part of the sample that the test is designed to find or measure. Example: a home pregnancy test measures human chorionic gonadotropin (hCG) in urine. The analyte is hCG.

anesthesia: A combination of medications administered to a patient to block pain and other sensations, at times rendering the patient unconscious, so that medical or surgical procedures can be performed; anesthesia can be general, regional or local

This glossary contains terms excerpted from documents produced by several sources deemed reliable.

anesthesiology: A medical specialty concerned with purposeful depression of nerve function, characterized by loss of feeling or sensation, usually the result of pharmacologic action by anesthetics, and induced to allow performance of surgery or other painful procedures.

antibiotic: A drug used to treat infections caused by bacteria and other microorganisms.

anxiety: Feelings of fear, dread, and uneasiness that may occur as a reaction to stress. A person with anxiety may sweat, feel restless and tense, and have a rapid heartbeat.

appeal: An appeal is a special kind of complaint you make if you disagree with a decision to deny a request for healthcare services, or payment for services you already received. You may also make a complaint if you disagree with a decision to stop services that you are receiving. For example, you may ask for an appeal if medicare does not pay for an item or service you think you should be able to get. There is a specific process that your medicare health plan or the original medicare plan must use when you ask for an appeal.

approved amount: The fee medicare sets for a covered medical service. This is the amount a doctor or supplier is paid by you and medicare for a service or supply. It may be less than the actual amount charged by a doctor or supplier. The approved amount is sometimes called the "approved charge."

assessment: In healthcare, a process used to learn about a patient's condition.

assistive device: A tool that helps a person with a disability to do a certain task. Examples are a cane, wheelchair, scooter, walker, hearing aid, or special bed.

assistive technology: Any device or technology that helps a disabled person. Examples are special grips for holding utensils, computer screen monitors to help a person with low vision read more easily.

blood: A tissue with red blood cells (RBCs), white blood cells (WBCs), platelets, and other substances suspended in fluid called "plasma." Blood takes oxygen and nutrients to the tissues, and carries away wastes.

blood transfusion: The administration of blood or blood products into a blood vessel.

cancer: A term for diseases in which abnormal cells divide without control. Cancer cells can invade nearby tissues and can spread to other parts of the body through the blood and lymph systems.

cardiology: A medical subspecialty concerned with the study of the heart, its physiology, and its functions.

caregiver: Anyone who helps care for an elderly individual or person with a disability who lives at home.

cell: The individual unit that makes up the tissues of the body. All living things are made up of one or more cells.

Glossary of Terms Related to Disease Management

chaplain: A member of the clergy in charge of a chapel or who works with the military or with an institution, such as a hospital.

chemotherapy: Treatment with drugs that kill cancer cells.

clinical trial: A type of research study that tests how well new medical approaches work in people. These studies test new methods of screening, prevention, diagnosis, or treatment of a disease; also called a "clinical study."

COBRA: An abbreviation for the consolidated omnibus budget reconciliation act of 1986, a law that provides for a temporary extension of health plan coverage from a prior group health plan.

counseling: The process by which a professional counselor helps a person cope with mental or emotional distress, and understand and solve personal problems.

cure: To heal or restore health; a treatment to restore health.

depression: A mental condition marked by ongoing feelings of sadness, despair, loss of energy, and difficulty dealing with routine daily life. Other symptoms of depression include feelings of worthlessness and hopelessness, loss of pleasure in activities, changes in eating or sleeping habits, and thoughts of death or suicide.

diagnosis: The process of identifying a disease by the signs and symptoms.

diet: What a person eats and drinks. Any type of eating plan.

drug: Any substance, other than food, that is used to prevent, diagnose, treat, or relieve symptoms of a disease or abnormal condition.

durable power of attorney (DPA): A type of power of attorney. A power of attorney is a legal document that gives one person (such as a relative, lawyer, or friend) the authority to make legal, medical, or financial decisions for another person.

family practice: A medical specialty concerned with the provision of continuing, comprehensive primary healthcare for the entire family.

genome: An organism's complete set of DNA, including all of its genes. Each genome contains all of the information needed to build and maintain that organism.

home health agency: An organization that gives home care services, such as skilled nursing care, physical therapy, occupational therapy, speech therapy, and care by home health aides.

hospice: A program that provides special care for people who are near the end of life and for their families, either at home, in freestanding facilities, or within hospitals.

infection: Invasion and multiplication of germs in the body. Infections can occur in any part of the body and can spread throughout the body. The germs may be bacteria, viruses, yeast, or fungi. They can cause a fever and other problems, depending on where the infection occurs.

insured plan: A plan which provides benefits through an insurance company or HMO. Check your summary plan description (SPD) to see if your plan is insured.

intended use: A description of what the manufacturer intended to measure with a certain test.

living will: A type of legal advance directive in which a person describes specific treatment guidelines that are to be followed by healthcare providers if she or he becomes terminally ill and cannot communicate.

lung: One of a pair of organs in the chest that supplies the body with oxygen and removes carbon dioxide from the body.

Medicaid: A joint federal and state program that helps with medical costs for some people with limited income and resources. Medicaid programs vary from state to state, but most healthcare costs are covered if you qualify for both medicare and medicaid.

Medicare health plan: Generally, a plan offered by a private company that contracts with medicare to provide part a and part b benefits to people with medicare who enroll in the plan. Medicare health plans include all medicare advantage plans, medicare cost plans, and demonstration/pilot programs. Programs of all-inclusive care for the elderly (pace) organizations are special types of medicare health plans. Pace plans can be offered by public or private entities and provide part d and other benefits in addition to part a and part b benefits.

mental health: A person's overall psychological and emotional condition. Good mental health is a state of well-being in which a person is able to cope with everyday events, think clearly, be responsible, meet challenges, and have good relationships with others.

multidisciplinary: Term used to describe a treatment planning approach or team that includes a number of doctors and other healthcare professionals who are experts in different specialties (disciplines).

neurology: A medical specialty concerned with the study of the structures, functions, and diseases of the nervous system.

nuclear medicine: A subspecialty field of radiology concerned with diagnostic, therapeutic, and investigative use of radioactive compounds in pharmaceutical form.

nurse: A health professional trained to care for people who are ill or disabled.

nursing: The profession concerned with the provision of care and services essential to the promotion, maintenance, and restoration of health by attending to a patient's needs.

Glossary of Terms Related to Disease Management

nursing home: A place that gives care to people who have physical or mental disabilities and need help with activities of daily living (such as taking a bath, getting dressed, and going to the bathroom) but do not need to be in the hospital.

nutrition: The clinical practice concerned with nutrients and other substances contained in food and their action, interaction, and balance in relation to health and disease.

obstetrics/gynecology: The medical-surgical specialty concerned with management and care of women during pregnancy, parturition, and puerperium; the physiology and disorders primarily of the female genital tract; and female endocrinology and reproductive physiology.

occupational therapist: A health professional trained to help people who are ill or disabled learn to manage their daily activities.

occupational therapy: Services given to help you return to usual activities (such as bathing, preparing meals, housekeeping) after illness.

oncology: A subspecialty of internal medicine concerned with the study of neoplasms.

outpatient: A patient who visits a healthcare facility for diagnosis or treatment without spending the night, sometimes called a "day patient."

package insert: Information about the test and/or instructions that come inside the box or package.

palliative care: Care given to improve the quality of life (QOL) of patients who have a serious or life-threatening disease. The goal of palliative care is to prevent or treat as early as possible the symptoms of the disease, side effects caused by treatment of the disease, and psychological, social, and spiritual problems related to the disease or its treatment, also called "comfort care," "supportive care," and "symptom management."

pediatrics: A medical specialty concerned with the physical, emotional, and social health of children from birth to young adulthood.

pharmacology: A clinical specialty concerned with the effectiveness and safety of drugs in humans.

physical examination: An exam of the body to check for general signs of disease.

physical medicine and rehabilitation: A medical specialty concerned with the use of physical agents, mechanical apparatuses, and manipulation in rehabilitating patients who are physically diseased, injured, or recovering from elective surgery (e.g., Hip replacement) to the maximum degree possible. Physicians practicing this specialty are physiatrists.

physical therapist: A health professional who teaches exercises and physical activities that help condition muscles and restore strength and movement.

podiatry: A profession concerned with the diagnosis and treatment of disorders, injuries and anatomic defects of the foot.

provider: A doctor, hospital, healthcare professional, or healthcare facility.

psychological: Having to do with how the mind works and how thoughts and feelings affect behavior.

psychologist: A specialist who can talk with patients and their families about emotional and personal matters and can help them make decisions.

psychology: A clinical profession concerned with recognizing and treating behavior disorders.

pump: A device that is used to give a controlled amount of a liquid at a specific rate. For example, pumps are used to give drugs (such as chemotherapy or pain medicine) or nutrients.

quality of life (QOL): The overall enjoyment of life.

radiology: The specialty concerned with the use of x-ray and other forms of radiant energy in the diagnosis and treatment of disease.

rehabilitation: In medicine, a process to restore mental or physical abilities lost to injury or disease, in order to function in a normal or near-normal way.

related services: A term used in the elementary and secondary school context to refer to developmental, corrective, and other supportive services, including psychological, counseling, and medical diagnostic services and transportation.

saturated fat: Fat that consists of triglycerides containing only saturated fatty acid radicals (i.e., they have no double bonds between the carbon atoms of the fatty acid chain and are fully saturated with hydrogen atoms). Dairy products, animal fats, coconut oil, cottonseed oil, palm kernel oil, and chocolate can contain high amounts of saturated fats.

screening: Checking for disease when there are no symptoms.

screening test: An initial or preliminary test. Screening tests do not tell you if you definitely have a disease or condition. Rather, positive results indicate that you may need additional tests or a doctor's evaluation to see if you have a particular disease or condition.

side effect: A problem that occurs when treatment affects healthy tissues or organs. Some common side effects of cancer treatment are fatigue, pain, nausea, vomiting, decreased blood cell counts, hair loss, and mouth sores.

skilled nursing care: A level of care that includes services that can only be performed safely and correctly by a licensed nurse (either a registered nurse or a licensed practical nurse).

Glossary of Terms Related to Disease Management

social service: A community resource that helps people in need. Services may include help getting to and from medical appointments, home delivery of medication and meals, in-home nursing care, help paying medical costs not covered by insurance, loaning medical equipment, and housekeeping help.

social worker: A professional trained to talk with people and their families about emotional or physical needs and to find them support services.

special enrollment: An opportunity for certain individuals to enroll in a group health plan, regardless of the plan's regular enrollment dates.

speech-language pathology: A clinical profession concerned with the study of speech/language and swallowing disorders and their diagnosis. A clinical profession concerned with the study of speech/language and swallowing disorders and their diagnosis.

stage: The extent of a cancer in the body. Staging is usually based on the size of the tumor, whether lymph nodes contain cancer, and whether the cancer has spread from the original site to other parts of the body.

State Health Insurance Assistance Program (SHIP): A state program that gets money from the federal government to give free health insurance counseling and assistance to people with medicare.

summary plan description (SPD): A document outlining your plan, usually provided when you enroll in the plan.

support group: A group of people with similar disease who meet to discuss how better to cope with their disease and treatment.

supportive care: Care given to improve the quality of life of patients who have a serious or life-threatening disease.

surgery: A medical specialty concerned with manual or operative procedures used in the diagnosis and treatment of diseases, injuries, or deformities.

symptom: An indication that a person has a condition or disease. Some examples of symptoms are headache, fever, fatigue, nausea, vomiting, and pain.

tube feeding: A type of enteral nutrition (nutrition that is delivered into the digestive system in a liquid form). For tube feeding, a small tube may be placed through the nose into the stomach or the small intestine.

waiting period: The time that must pass before coverage can become effective under the terms of a group health plan.

x-ray: A type of high-energy radiation. In low doses, x-rays are used to diagnose diseases by making pictures of the inside of the body.

yoga: An ancient system of practices used to balance the mind and body through exercise, meditation (focusing thoughts), and control of breathing and emotions.

Chapter 78 | **Additional Resources for Information about Disease Management**

GOVERNMENT AGENCIES THAT PROVIDE INFORMATION ABOUT DISEASE MANAGEMENT

Administration on Aging (AOA)
U.S. Department of Health and
Human Services (HHS)
Washington, DC 20201
Phone: 202-619-0724
Fax: 202-357-3555
Website: www.acl.gov
E-mail: aoainfo@aoa.gov

Agency for Healthcare Research and Quality (AHRQ)
Office of Communications
5600 Fishers Ln.
Seventh Fl.
Rockville, MD 20847
Phone: 301-427-1104
Website: www.ahrq.gov

Centers for Disease Control and Prevention (CDC)
1600 Clifton Rd.
Atlanta, GA 30329-4027
Toll-Free: 800-CDC-INFO
(800-232-4636)
Phone: 404-639-3311
Toll-Free TTY: 888-232-6348
Website: www.cdc.gov
E-mail: cdcinfo@cdc.gov

Centers for Medicare and Medicaid Services (CMS)
7500 Security Blvd.
Baltimore, MD 21244
Toll-Free: 877-267-2323
Phone: 410-786-3000
Toll-Free TTY: 866-226-1819
Website: www.cms.gov

Resources in this chapter were compiled from several sources deemed reliable; all contact information was verified and updated in December 2019.

Eunice Kennedy Shriver National Institute of Child Health and Human Development (NICHD)
NICHD Information Resource Center (IRC)
P.O. Box 3006
Rockville, MD 20847
Toll-Free: 800-370-2943
Phone: 301-496-5133
Toll-Free Fax: 866-760-5947
Website: www.nichd.nih.gov
E-mail:
NICHDInformationResourceCenter@mail.nih.gov

Federal Trade Commission (FTC)
600 Pennsylvania Ave., N.W.
Washington, DC 20580
Phone: 202-326-2222
Website: www.ftc.gov

Health Resources and Services Administration (HRSA)
Information Center
5600 Fishers Ln.
Rockville, MD 20857
Toll-Free: 877-489-4772
TTY: 877-897-9910
Website: www.hrsa.gov

National Cancer Institute (NCI)
9609 Medical Center Dr.
BG 9609, MSC 9760
Bethesda, MD 20892-9760
Toll-Free: 800-4-CANCER
(800-422-6237)
Website: www.cancer.gov
E-mail: NCIinfo@nih.gov

National Center for Complementary and Integrative Health (NCCIH)
9000 Rockville Pike
Bethesda, MD 20892
Toll-Free: 888-644-6226
Toll-Free TTY: 866-464-3615
Website: nccih.nih.gov
E-mail: info@nccih.nih.gov

National Health Information Center (NHIC)
U.S. Department of Health and Human Services (HHS)
1101 Wootton Pkwy
Ste. LL100
Rockville, MD 20852
Fax: 240-453-8281
Website: www.health.gov/nhic
E-mail: nhic@hhs.gov

National Heart, Lung, and Blood Institute (NHLBI)
31 Center Dr.
Bldg. 31
Bethesda, MD 20892
Website: www.nhlbi.nih.gov

National Human Genome Research Institute (NHGRI)
National Institutes of Health (NIH)
31 Center Dr., MSC 2152, 9000
Rockville Pike
Bldg. 31, Rm. 4B09
Bethesda, MD 20892-2152
Phone: 301-402-0911
Fax: 301-402-2218
Website: www.genome.gov

National Institute of Arthritis and Musculoskeletal and Skin Diseases (NIAMS)

Information Clearinghouse, National Institutes of Health (NIH)
One AMS Cir.
Bethesda, MD 20892-3675
Toll-Free: 877-22-NIAMS
(877-226-4267)
Phone: 301-495-4484
Fax: 301-718-6366
Website: www.niams.nih.gov
E-mail: NIAMSinfo@mail.nih.gov

National Institute of Diabetes and Digestive and Kidney Diseases (NIDDK)

Toll-Free: 800-860-8747
TTY: 866-569-1162
Website: www.niddk.nih.gov/
health-information/diabetes
E-mail: healthinfo@niddk.nih.gov

National Institute of Mental Health (NIMH)

Office of Science Policy, Planning, and Communications (OSPPC)
6001 Executive Blvd.
Rm. 6200 MSC 9663
Bethesda, MD 20892-9663
Toll-Free: 866-615-NIMH
(866-615-6464)
Toll-Free TTY: 866-415-8051
Fax: 301-443-4279
Website: www.nimh.nih.gov
E-mail: nimhinfo@nih.gov

National Institute of Neurological Disorders and Stroke (NINDS)

NIH Neurological Institute
P.O. Box 5801
Bethesda, MD 20824
Toll-Free: 800-352-9424
Website: www.ninds.nih.gov

National Institute on Aging (NIA)

31 Center Dr., MSC 2292
Bldg. 31, Rm. 5C27
Bethesda, MD 20892
Toll-Free: 800-222-2225
Toll-Free TTY: 800-222-4225
Website: www.nia.nih.gov
E-mail: niaic@nia.nih.gov

National Institutes of Health (NIH)

9000 Rockville Pike
Bethesda, MD 20892
Phone: 301-496-4000
TTY: 301-402-9612
Website: www.nih.gov

National Women's Health Information Center (NWHIC)

Office on Women's Health (OWH)
200 Independence Ave. S.W.
Rm. 712E
Washington, DC 20201
Toll-Free: 800-994-9662
Phone: 202-690-7650
Fax: 202-205-2631
Website: www.womenshealth.gov

Office of Minority Health Resource Center (OMHRC)

U.S. Department of Health and
Human Services (HHS)
Tower Oaks Bldg., 1101 Wootton
Pkwy
Ste. 600
Rockville, MD 20852
Toll-Free: 800-444-6472
Fax: 301-251-2160
Website: www.minorityhealth.hhs.
gov
E-mail: info@minorityhealth.hhs.gov

Substance Abuse and Mental Health Services Administration (SAMHSA)

5600 Fishers Ln.
Rockville, MD 20857
Toll-Free: 877-SAMHSA-7
(877-726-4727)
Toll-Free TTY: 800-487-4889
Website: www.samhsa.gov
E-mail: SAMHSAInfo@samhsa.hhs.
gov

U.S. Equal Employment Opportunity Commission (EEOC)

131 M St., NE
Rm. 6NE25J
Washington, D.C. 20507
Phone: 202-663-4191
Fax: 202-663-4912
Website: www.eeoc.gov
E-mail: legis@eeoc.gov

U.S. Food and Drug Administration (FDA)

10903 New Hampshire Ave.
Silver Spring, MD 20993-0002
Toll-Free: 888-INFO-FDA
(888-463-6332)
Website: www.fda.gov

U.S. National Library of Medicine (NLM)

8600 Rockville Pike
Bethesda, MD 20894
Toll-Free: 888-FIND-NLM
(888-346-3656)
Phone: 301-594-5983
Website: www.nlm.nih.gov
E-mail: custserv@nlm.nih.gov

PRIVATE AGENCIES THAT PROVIDE INFORMATION ABOUT DISEASE MANAGEMENT

AbleData

103 W. Broad St.
Ste. 400
Falls Church, VA 22046
Toll-Free: 800-227-0216
TTY: 703-992-8313
Fax: 703-356-8314
Website: abledata.acl.gov
E-mail: abledata@neweditions.net

Alzheimer's Association

225 N. Michigan Ave.
17th Fl.
Chicago, IL 60601
Toll-Free: 800-272-3900
Website: www.alz.org

Additional Resources for Information about Disease Management

American Academy of Family Physicians (AAFP)
11400 Tomahawk Creek Pkwy
Leawood, KS 66211-2680
Toll-Free: 800-274-2237
Phone: 913-906-6000
Fax: 913-906-6075
Website: www.aafp.org
E-mail: aafp@aafp.org

American Cancer Society (ACS)
250 Williams St., N.W.
Atlanta, GA 30303
Toll-Free: 800-ACS-2345
(800-227-2345)
Toll-Free TTY: 866-228-4327
Website: www.cancer.org

American Health Information Management Association (AHIMA)
233 N. Michigan Ave.
21st Fl.
Chicago, IL 60601-5809
Toll-Free: 800-335-5535
Phone: 312-233-1100
Fax: 312-233-1500
Website: www.ahima.org
E-mail: info@ahima.org

American Heart Association (AHA)
National Center
7272 Greenville Ave.
Dallas, TX 75231
Toll-Free: 800-AHA-USA-1
(800-242-8721)
Website: www.heart.org

American Lung Association (ALA)
National Office
55 W. Wacker Dr.
Ste. 1150
Chicago, IL 60601
Toll-Free: 800-LUNGUSA
(800-586-4872)
Website: www.lung.org
E-mail: info@lung.org

American Medical Association (AMA)
AMA Plaza
330 N. Wabash Ave.
Ste. 39300
Chicago, IL 60611-5885
Toll-Free: 800-896-3650
Phone: 312-464-4782
Website: www.ama-assn.org

Caregiver Action Network (CAN)
1150 Connecticut Ave., N.W.
Ste. 501
Washington, DC 20036-3904
Phone: 202-454-3970
Fax: 301-942-2302
Website: www.caregiveraction.org
E-mail: info@caregiveraction.org

Center for Children's Health Media
300 Longwood Ave.
Boston, MA 02115
Phone: 617-355-5420
Fax: 617-730-0004
Website: cmch.tv
E-mail: cmch@childrens.harvard.edu

Cleveland Clinic
9500 Euclid Ave.
Cleveland, OH 44195
Toll-Free: 800-223-2273
Phone: 216-444-2200
Website: my.clevelandclinic.org

National Healthcare Anti-Fraud Association (NHCAA)

1220 L St., N.W.
Ste. 600
Washington, DC 20005
Phone: 202-659-5955
Fax: 202-785-6764
Website: www.nhcaa.org
E-mail: NHCAA@nhcaa.org

National Patient Advocate Foundation (NPAF)

Washington, DC
Phone: 202-347-8009
Website: www.npaf.org
E-mail: action@npaf.org

National Rehabilitation Information Center (NARIC)

8400 Corporate Dr.
Ste. 500
Landover, MD 20785
Toll-Free: 800-346-2742
Phone: 301-459-5900
Fax: 301-459-4263
Website: www.naric.com

The Nemours Foundation

10140 Centurion Pkwy N.
Jacksonville, FL 32256
Phone: 904-697-4100
Website: www.nemours.org

Chapter 79 | **Directory of Health Insurance Information**

GOVERNMENT AGENCIES THAT PROVIDE INFORMATION ABOUT HEALTH INSURANCE

Agency for Healthcare Research and Quality (AHRQ)
Office of Communications
5600 Fishers Ln.
Seventh Fl.
Rockville, MD 20847
Phone: 301-427-1104
Website: www.ahrq.gov

Centers for Medicare & Medicaid Services (CMS)
7500 Security Blvd.
Baltimore, MD 21244
Toll-Free: 877-267-2323
Phone: 410-786-3000
Toll-Free TTY: 866-226-1819
Website: www.cms.gov

Federal Trade Commission (FTC)
600 Pennsylvania Ave., N.W.
Washington, DC 20580
Phone: 202-326-2222
Website: www.ftc.gov

U.S. Department of Labor (DOL)
200 Constitution Ave., N.W.
Washington, DC 20210
Toll-Free: 866-4-USA-DOL
(866-487-2365)
Website: www.dol.gov

U.S. Department of the Treasury
1500 Pennsylvania Ave., N.W.
Washington, DC 20220
Toll-Free: 800-829-1040
Phone: 202- 622-2000
Website: www.treasury.gov

Resources in this chapter were compiled from several sources deemed reliable; all contact information was verified and updated in December 2019.

PRIVATE AGENCIES THAT PROVIDE INFORMATION ABOUT HEALTH INSURANCE

America's Health Insurance Plans (AHIP)

601 Pennsylvania Ave., N.W., S. Bldg.
Ste.500
Washington, DC 20004
Phone: 202-778-3200
Fax: 202-331-7487
Website: www.ahip.org
E-mail: info@ahip.org

Coalition against Insurance Fraud (CAIF)

1012 14th St., N.W.
Ste.200
Washington, DC 20005
Phone: 202-393-7330
Website: www.insurancefraud.org
E-mail: info@insurancefraud.org

Families USA

1225 New York Ave., N.W.
Ste.800
Washington, DC 20005
Phone: 202-628-3030
Fax: 202-347-2417
Website: www.familiesusa.org
E-mail: info@familiesusa.org

Insurance Information Institute (III)

110 William St.
New York, NY 10038
Phone: 212-346-5500
Website: www.iii.org
E-mail: info@iii.org

Kaiser Family Foundation (KFF)

Website: www.kff.org

National Association of Insurance Commissioners (NAIC)

Central Office
1100 Walnut St.
Ste. 1500
Kansas City, MO 64106-2197
Toll-Free: 866-470-NAIC
(866-470-6242)
Phone: 816-842-3600
Fax: 816-783-8175
Website: www.naic.org
E-mail: help@naic.org

Patient Advocate Foundation (PAF)

421 Butler Farm Rd.
Hampton, VA 23666
Toll-Free: 800-532-5274
Fax: 757-873-8999
Website: www.patientadvocate.org
E-mail: help@patientadvocate.org

Chapter 80 | Directory of Organizations That Provide Financial Assistance for Medical Treatments

ASSISTANCE WITH PAYING FOR MEDICAL CARE AND PROCEDURES
Find A Health Center
Health Resources and Services Administration
5600 Fishers Ln.
Rockville, MD 20857
Toll-Free: 877-464-4772
Toll-Free TTY: 877-897-9910
Website: findahealthcenter.hrsa.gov

Insure Kids Now
7500 Security Blvd.
Baltimore, MD 21244
Toll-Free: 877-KIDS-NOW
(877-543-7669)
Website: www.insurekidsnow.gov

U.S. Department of Health and Human Services (HHS)
200 Independence Ave., S.W.
Washington, DC 20201
Toll-Free: 877-696-6775
Website: www.hhs.gov

FINANCIAL AID FOR MEDICAL TREATMENTS
Association of Maternal and Child Health Programs (AMCHP)
1825 K St.
Ste. 250
Washington, DC 20006
Phone: 202-775-0436
Fax: 202-478-5120
Website: www.amchp.org
E-mail: info@amchp.org

Resources in this chapter were compiled from several sources deemed reliable; all contact information was verified and updated in December 2019.

Families USA

1225 New York Ave., N.W.
Ste. 800
Washington, DC 20005
Phone: 202-628-3030
Fax: 202-347-2417
Website: www.familiesusa.org
E-mail: info@familiesusa.org

Family Voices

P.O. Box 37188
Albuquerque, NM 87176
Toll-Free: 888-835-5669
Phone: 505-872-4774
Website: www.familyvoices.org

National Patient Advocate Foundation (NPAF)

Washington, DC
Phone: 202-465-5013
Website: www.npaf.org
E-mail: action@npaf.org

Patient Advocate Foundation (PAF)

421 Butler Farm Rd.
Hampton, VA 23666
Toll-Free: 800-532-5274
Fax: 757-873-8999
Website: www.patientadvocate.org
E-mail: help@patientadvocate.org

Social Security Administration (SSA)

1100 W. High Rise
6401 Security Blvd.
Baltimore, MD 21235
Toll-Free: 800-772-1213
Toll-Free TTY: 800-325-0778
Website: www.ssa.gov

ASSISTANCE WITH PAYING FOR MEDICATIONS
National Organization for Rare Disorders (NORD)

55 Kenosia Ave.
Danbury, CT 06810
Phone: 203-744-0100
Fax: 203-263-9938
Website: www.rarediseases.org

The Partnership for Prescription Assistance (PPA)

American Academy of Family
Physicians
11400 Tomahawk Creek Pkwy
Leawood, KS 66211-2680
Toll-Free: 800-274-2237
Phone: 913-906-6000
Fax: 913-906-6075
Website: www.aafp.org
E-mail: aafp@aafp.org

ASSISTANCE WITH INSURANCE ISSUES
Centers for Medicare & Medicaid Services (CMS)

7500 Security Blvd.
Baltimore, MD 21244
Toll-Free: 877-267-2323
Phone: 410-786-3000
Toll-Free TTY: 866-226-1819
Website: www.cms.gov

Georgetown University Health Policy Institute (GUHPI)

37th and O St., N.W.
Washington, DC 20057
Phone: 202-687-0100
Website: www.georgetown.edu

Health Care Choices (HCC)

6209 16th Ave.
Brooklyn, NY 11204
Phone: 718-234-0073
Website: www. Healthcarechoicesny. org

Medicaid Waivers

Toll-Free: 888-444-3331
Phone: 727-841-8943
Website: www.medicaidwaiver. org

INDEX

INDEX

Index

Index

Index

Index

Index

Index

Index

Index

Index

sigmoidoscopy
   colorectal cancer screenings 478
   healthcare quality issues 115
"6 Things to Know When Selecting a Complementary Health Practitioner" (NCCIH) 85n
"6 Tip-Offs to Rip-Offs: Don't Fall for Health Fraud Scams" (FDA) 207n
skilled nursing care
   defined 538
   Medicare 489
sleeping drugs, medications 223
smoking
   doctor's office 61
   family health history 10
   heart disease 114
   lung cancer 156, 479
   prescription pain relievers 320
   screening tests 41
   surgical site infections 142
   tobacco use 20
Social Security Administration (SSA), contact 550
Social Security number (SSN)
   federal disability programs 499
   health information 201
   prescription drugs 255
social service
   Americans with Disabilities Act (ADA) 451
   chronic health conditions 428
   defined 539
   financial assistance 386
   Medicare 491
social worker
   defined 539
   legal and financial planning 464
   medical specialties 83
   palliative and hospice care 393
   relaxation techniques 354
   seriously ill child 405
   stress 340
SPD *see* summary plan description
special enrollment
   defined 539
   healthcare benefit laws 484

special-needs camps
   chronic health needs 440
   see also camps
specialists
   choosing a hospital 128
   choosing your doctor 25
   doctor's appointment 60
   end-of-life care decisions 390
   health insurance 496
   healthcare professionals 230
   patient rights and responsibilities 185
   rehabilitative technology 371
   seriously ill child 405
   telemedicine 445
   see also medical specialists
speech-language pathology
   defined 539
   Medicare 489
   rehabilitative technologies 371
SSN *see* Social Security number
SSRIs *see* selective serotonin reuptake inhibitors
stage
   assistive devices 372
   clinical study 95
   defined 539
   legal and financial planning 461
   orphan products 289
   pharmacology 223
   preventive care 153
   seriously ill child 404
   transitional care planning 389
   treatments 69
standalone PHRs, described 197
State Health Insurance Assistance Program (SHIP)
   defined 539
   prescription drugs 255
State Pharmaceutical Assistance Program (SPAP), prescription drugs 255
State Survey Agency (SA), Medicare 133
statistics
   chronic diseases 3, 24
   generic medicines 276
   health literacy 162

Index

Index

Index

WITHDRAWN

$76.50